A well-written exposition on a difficult subject.

—Daniel J. Wallace, MD, clinical the University of California, Los Angeles, School of Medicine

In this outstanding book, Clair Davies aptly explains the rational for the trigger point approach based on the teachings of Drs. Janet Travell and David Simons to the treatment of frozen shoulder. He presents his hypothesis well. It is time for the medical profession to accept alternative therapies in treating this condition, which does not often respond to routine medical care.

—Paul B. Brown, MD, Ph.D., rheumatologist and clinical professor of medicine at the University of Washington

Clair Davies has done it again. He has written a wonderful book that provides insight and practical advice for the treatment of a common problem: frozen or stiff shoulder. He shows where the pain is, what the problems are, and how an individual can treat it, sometimes with the help of a partner. His illustrations and directions are clear. His case examples are helpful. This is a very useful book for those who have had rotator cuff injuries or other shoulder problems.

—Robert D. Gerwin, MD, president and medical director of Pain and Rehabilitation Medicine, Baltimore, MD, and the Janet G. Travell, MD, Seminar Series

Mr. Davies has done an outstanding job of tackling and simplifying a difficult topic that challenges even experienced clinicians. His review of the functional anatomy and kinesiology of the shoulder and the central role of the muscles in the control of the shoulder is a welcome review for physicians and therapists. His simple diagrams and descriptions make this topic understandable to those without formal training as well. Most importantly he shows very concrete ways in which a patient or clinician may effectively treat trigger points, which in my view are the primary cause of shoulder pain and stiffness in the majority of cases. I highly recommend this book to patients with shoulder pain and to clinicians involved in the evaluation and treatment of patients with shoulder pain.

—Bryan J. O'Neill, MD, clinical assistant professor in the Department of Rehabilitation Medicine at Thomas Jefferson University, Philadelphia, PA

From a practical point of view, this is a really exceptional *workbook, which could become a best-seller in its field. It is a wonderful overview concerning trigger points, which are the most common cause of frozen shoulder. I can recommend the book to all who are engaged in treating frozen shoulders, including medical doctors, therapists, and patients together with their partners.*

—Dieter Pongratz, MD, professor in the department
of Neurology at the University of Munich Hospital,
Friedrich-Baur-Institute, in Munich, Germany

The Frozen Shoulder Workbook *is truly a remarkable and comprehensive text that will be indispensable for patients with chronic shoulder pain. Written from a layperson's perspective, it is very readable and well illustrated, but still has plenty of background science and anatomy to satisfy clinicians as well. The book outlines a thorough approach to myofascial pain in the shoulder region and provides multiple treatment strategies to address the clinical variations that are seen. I will highly recommend it to my shoulder pain patients.*

—Steven R. Shannon, MD, Pain and Rehabilitation
Medicine, Baltimore, MD

The Frozen Shoulder Workbook

Trigger Point Therapy
for Overcoming Pain &
Regaining Range of Motion

Clair Davies, NCTMB

New Harbinger Publications, Inc.

Publisher's Note

This publication is designed to provide accurate and authoritative information in regard to the subject matter covered. It is sold with the understanding that the publisher is not engaged in rendering psychological, financial, legal, or other professional services. If expert assistance or counseling is needed, the services of a competent professional should be sought.

Distributed in Canada by Raincoast Books

Copyright © 2006 by Clair Davies
New Harbinger Publications, Inc.
5674 Shattuck Avenue
Oakland, CA 94609

Cover design by Amy Shoup
Illustrations by Clair Davies
Text design by Michele Waters-Kermes
Acquired by Jess O'Brien
Edited by Jasmine Star

Figure 2.11 is reprinted from *Myofascial Pain and Dysfunction: The Trigger Point Manual*, Vol. 1, 2nd edition, 1999, by D.G. Simons, J.G. Travell, and L.S. Simons, with permission from David G. Simons and Lippincott Williams & Wilkins.

All Rights Reserved

Printed in the United States of America

Library of Congress Cataloging-in-Publication Data

Davies, Clair.
Frozen shoulder workbook : trigger point therapy for overcoming pain and regaining range of motion / Clair Davies.
p. cm.
ISBN-13: 978-1-57224-447-4
ISBN-10: 1-57224-447-X (pbk.)
1. Shoulder pain—Physical therapy—Treatment—Handbooks, manuals, etc. 2. Myofascial pain syndromes—Physical therapy—Handbooks, manuals, etc. 3. Self-care, Health—Handbooks, manuals, etc. I. Title.
RC939.D38 2006
617.5'72—dc22

2006017701

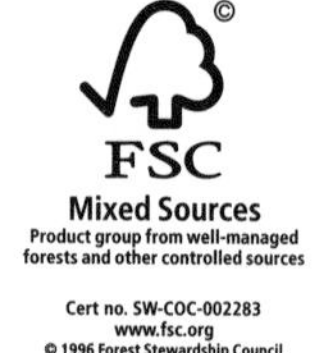

New Harbinger Publications' website address: www.newharbinger.com

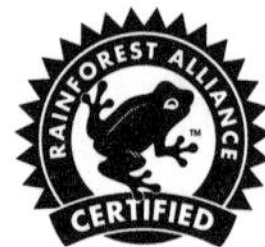

12 11 10

15 14 13 12 11 10 9 8 7

Contents

Foreword

Frozen shoulder is a very common musculoskeletal pain condition that is generally poorly identified and treated because the cause is usually myofascial trigger points that are overlooked in most practitioners' initial education and training. In this book, Clair Davies presents a comprehensive and knowledgeable summary of shoulder problems caused by myofascial trigger points in twenty-four contributing muscles. His unprecedented methods are designed to fit the patient and are much needed.

In his candid introduction, Clair clearly describes the current darkness of inadequate understanding of myofascial trigger points (MFTPs) engulfing many health care professionals. He wisely notes the critical importance of improved attention to MFTPs by schools training those professionals. Fortunately, there is a trend developing to effectively illuminate this darkness. The Philadelphia College of Osteopathic Medicine, the Georgia State University Physical Therapy department, and a number of massage training institutions have effective programs in place.

This book brightly illuminates the shoulder region in this regard in a way that shows patients how to attack the problem for themselves, as Clair did. I hope you read his introduction that so eloquently describes the common plight of so many people suffering from musculoskeletal pain and how he conquered his own shoulder pain. His approach worked and it should be equally helpful to many readers who are afflicted with this problem.

Clair offers a simple manual method that readers can apply to themselves to consistently reduce the pain to fully acceptable levels. This puts you, the patient, in control. You make the decision when to take the time and make the effort to reduce or eliminate the pain. Now the one in charge of your life is *you*, not the pain. Many times, the loss of muscle coordination and strength are as distressing as the pain and are equally important and treatable.

Several points warrant special attention. This book not only presents in working detail the author's massage technique, it also includes a comprehensive review of alternate manual treatments of MFTPs, including the original form of myotherapy introduced by Bonnie Prudden. The essence of Prudden's technique was identified as *ischemic compression* in the first edition of *Myofascial Pain & Dysfunction: The Trigger Point Manual,* which I wrote with Janet Travell. The second edition of our book replaced that term and the method of treatment with a new concept: *Trigger Point Pressure Release*. The essence of this better method is described in Clair's book under Myotherapy (p. 199); in this section he emphasizes the importance of repeated applications of moderate pressure. I would strongly recommend applying this pressure slowly and pausing where the tissue is especially tender. Muscle tissues need time to readjust toward normality—need coaxing, so to speak.

It is now becoming clear, based on yet-to-be-published surface electromyographic research studies, that, although latent (as opposed to active) MFTPs cause no clinical pain complaint, they can be a potent source of dysfunction of the same and associated muscles. These MFTPs commonly cause muscle weakness, incoordination, and substitute functioning by functionally related muscles. These effects can be disastrous in the shoulder and are a major reason for this needed workbook.

A recent research study by Jay Shah and associates at the National Institutes of Health (2005) established unequivocally that there are many highly significant differences in the tissue substances of latent compared to active MFTPs that cause pain and inflammatory reactions. Latent MFTPs affect primarily the motor rather than the sensory nervous system.

The frontier of medicine treads on unexplored and often controversial territory. Under Energy Therapies (p. 202), Clair considers the energy features of acupuncture theory. Possibly related to this is a new treatment modality, *frequency specific microcurrent (FSM)*, that produces unprecedented and remarkably effective results by increasing the energy state of specific tissue components. The many specific frequencies used by FSM energize specific tissues at the molecular level, requiring very low energy because they employ resonant effects. Frequency specific microcurrent has limited application for self-treatment because of the cost of the equipment and the need for some training on how to apply it. Fortunately, there are monthly three-day training programs given around the country that provide the necessary training needed for clinicians to use this novel modality and instrumentation effectively, so some well-trained practitioners are available.

—David G. Simons, MD

Introduction

This book should've been written by a doctor. By rights, a frozen shoulder ought to be in the medical domain. You'd hope that a doctor would know all there is to know about shoulders and could proceed to solve your problem in a knowledgeable and confident manner. But this isn't necessarily true, as you may have already discovered. In general, the medical profession isn't doing too well with shoulders, especially frozen shoulders and common shoulder pain.

If you read the medical literature, you'll repeatedly run into the same disconcerting disclaimer, "We really don't know what causes a frozen shoulder." What remains unsaid, though it's implied, is "We really don't know how to fix a frozen shoulder either." That's a pitiful thing for a doctor to have to admit when the cause of a frozen shoulder and the solution have been available to the medical profession since the 1940s. *Myofascial* (MY-oh-FAH-shul) *trigger points*, or small contraction knots in muscles, are actually the primary cause of a frozen shoulder. In fact, trigger points are the main thing involved in most chronic pain, but you won't find this out from your doctor. If your doctor were able to diagnose and treat myofascial trigger points, you wouldn't have the problem you're having with your shoulder and you wouldn't need this book.

Individual doctors are not really to blame for this. The problem is that doctors have been denied all knowledge about myofascial pain by a system of medical education that's skewed almost exclusively toward surgery and prescription drugs. As a consequence, a legitimate branch of medicine has been disregarded and even maligned in medical education because it doesn't fit into the traditional practice of medicine.

As the author of this book on shoulder trouble, I should have academic credentials validating that I'm an authority on shoulders. But I have no medical education and I'm not a member of the medical establishment. My authority, such as it is, began with a frozen shoulder of my own. Of course, a good many people have had frozen shoulders without gaining any special knowledge whatsoever, except what it's like to suffer unremitting pain with little hope of relief. My frozen shoulder turned out differently than most, however, because I had the good fortune to discover how to overcome it myself with self-applied trigger point massage.

You've probably heard that a frozen shoulder usually takes a year or more to heal, no matter what kind of therapy you undergo, or whether you just live through it without treatment. Curing my own shoulder didn't take a year. It took only about four weeks. I think I was lucky that I didn't learn about shoulders in medical school.

My first efforts at self-treatment fell flat. I tried all the things I'd heard about: I practiced raising my arm with a cane, trying to get my shoulder muscles to stretch. I used a towel to pull my arm up behind my back. I walked my fingers up a wall. I did the Codman exercises, where you try to free up your shoulder by bending over and moving your arm in circles with a can of soup in your hand. But none of those little tricks did a bit of good. They just caused me more pain, and it wasn't long before I could hardly raise my arm at all.

I couldn't reach across to fasten my seat belt. I couldn't pick up my little one-year-old grandson. If I foolishly grabbed at a closing door, I was rewarded with a murderous shot of pain that left me immobile for most of a minute before I could get my breath and go on. The arm was useless for getting anything down from a shelf. If I needed two arms for anything, my good arm had to lift the bad one. I dreaded putting on my coat because of the torture in getting my arm into the sleeve.

The ache in my shoulder got worse when I went to bed. It awakened me repeatedly in the night, and sometimes I couldn't sleep at all. I'd get up and spend an hour rubbing the shoulder with ice. That dulled the pain long enough for me to get back to sleep, but it wasn't a cure. Before morning the pain was back, just as bad as ever. I tried soaking my shoulder in a hot shower to soothe it and try to loosen it up. It felt great, but the effect didn't last. I realized I needed to find someone who knew a little more than I did about what was going on.

Several years earlier, I'd had a good experience with therapeutic massage. A friend had suggested I try it for a back spasm that I'd had for several weeks. Massage seemed a trivial thing and I really didn't hope for much, but the woman fixed my back in just three sessions. It was one of those watershed events, although I didn't recognize it at the time. Up to that time, I'd had no notion that massage actually worked for something serious like pain. The therapist showed me the books she used, a couple of medical books about "trigger points." The books looked interesting, but I was content at the time to just put myself into her hands.

I thought of that therapist again when I ran into a dead end with my shoulder. I was pretty sure she might have the answer. Unfortunately, she had moved away, so I had to find someone else who had similar abilities. I tried a number of massage therapists and inquired about the skills of many others, but their massage was too much of the "feel-good" kind. Nobody really seemed to know how to fix shoulders. I spent a lot of time rubbing my shoulder myself, but I really had no idea what I was doing.

As a last resort, I gave physical therapy a chance, but it didn't go well. The therapist seemed a little patronizing when I told her the stretching exercises were making my pain worse. She insisted that this was the correct therapy and that I just had to keep at it. I found out later that she was hiding the fact that she was suffering from a frozen shoulder at the very time she was treating me! She couldn't fix herself and she couldn't fix me, but it didn't keep her from billing me just the same. In desperation, I renewed my determination to find a way to fix my shoulder myself.

I thought I might possibly find an answer in the books about trigger points I'd been shown by the massage therapist I'd liked so much. She'd been the only person who really seemed to know what she was doing in regard to pain. Absolutely nothing was giving me relief and I was badly in need of some new ideas. I was shocked at the price of medical books, but I swallowed hard and ordered them anyway, the two volumes of *Myofascial Pain and Dysfunction: The Trigger Point Manual*, by Doctors Janet Travell and David Simons

(Simons, Travell, and Simons 1983, 1992). As soon as I began to read, the clouds of mystery around my shoulder problem began to clear away.

The books said that a trigger point was simply a tiny bundle of fibers within a muscle that was staying in a hard contraction, something like what I'd always called a "knot." The little knot could cause ongoing pain, or it could exist silently, causing no pain at all unless pressed on. Usually, however, a trigger point would sneakily send its pain somewhere else. For this reason, the pain from trigger points was called *referred pain.*

I gathered that much of my pain, perhaps all of it, was probably this intriguing displaced pain, this referred pain. I had never been able to figure out why all the rubbing I'd been doing on my shoulder had never done any good, but now I had the reason. The trigger points causing the pain could be several inches away, or even half the body's length away. It was clear that all my trouble lay in the trigger points hiding in various muscles in and around my shoulder, trigger points in twenty-four muscles, as it turned out. I hadn't known what I was doing when I'd tried self-applied massage before, but Travell and Simons offered me the map to the hidden treasure.

Driven by my misery and by my excitement about these new ideas, I studied Travell and Simons literally night and day. I found that my trigger points would soften and go away under the touch of my own hands if I persisted. To my surprise and delight, after only about a month of diligent application of what I was learning, I found I'd succeeded in fixing my own shoulder. I was astounded. The pain was gone. I could sleep through the night. I could raise my arm without being punished. Trigger point massage really worked!

I saw immediately that the world needed to know how well this worked. Somebody should write an accessible and affordable book on the subject! I visualized developing a whole system for dealing with trigger points and thought I could come up with a method for the whole body that anybody could understand and use. Once you knew how to find the trigger points and just exactly how to treat them, it wasn't really all that hard.

Using my own body as a laboratory, I learned something new every day. I found I had trigger points hiding everywhere. Like many people, I always had some kind of pain that I was just living with or trying to outlive. Now I saw that all this pain was actually a blessing, a great opportunity to test my self-treatment methods and make sure they worked. Over a period of three years, with the aid of my daughter Amber, who had also had a tough time with chronic pain, I figured out ways to self-treat trigger points in all 120 pairs of muscles that Travell and Simons dealt with in their books.

By the time I was done, my obsession with trigger points had led me to retire from my lifelong profession as a piano technician and become a professional massage therapist. Eventually I also wrote the book that I thought the world needed, *The Trigger Point Therapy Workbook* (Davies 2001), which was a success almost from the moment it was in print. While I wrote the book, my daughter also became a massage therapist, and later we began giving our trigger point therapy workshops for massage therapists. In our first two years, we taught more than eight hundred therapists from thirty-nine states. Many were seriously afflicted with chronic pain of their own, just like we had been. It was clear that quite a lot of people were ready and eager to learn about trigger points.

Through my daily experience as a massage therapist and from the feedback I got on my book, it became apparent that people everywhere were frustrated by the health care system when it came to pain. I also learned that I wasn't the only one who'd had a bad experience with physical therapy, but physical therapy was where you generally ended up if you went to a doctor with shoulder pain. For pain in joints and muscles, you got a prescription for a painkiller and a referral to physical therapy as a matter of course. Your problem would also be given an official medical label. If you had pain in your shoulder, you had arthritis, tendinitis, or bursitis. If you had a stiff shoulder, you had adhesive capsulitis. Even though these traditional medical explanations for shoulder trouble are contradicted by everything that's known about trigger points, people consistently told me their doctors hadn't said anything about trigger points.

Doctors Travell and Simons believe that the single most important issue regarding shoulder pain is misdiagnosis, and that trigger points are the cause of virtually all shoulder problems. This includes pain, stiffness, and reduced range of motion. But even rotator cuff tears and impingement syndrome are thought to result from the partial disarticulation of the ball-and-socket joint by muscles stiffened by trigger points. Because too few practitioners realize the involvement of myofascial trigger points in these problems, the medical community almost uniformly blames the shoulder joint for shoulder trouble. This is why standard medical treatments so often fail to solve the problem. One of the biggest shortcomings of modern medicine is that the majority of physicians still haven't studied or tried Travell and Simons's trigger point therapy for pain.

After I became a massage therapist, I retained my particular interest in the shoulder. As a consequence, people with shoulder trouble began to seek me out. They told me some very disturbing stories about their experience with the health care system. The more I learned about how doctors were treating shoulders, the angrier I got. A frozen shoulder was obviously one of the worst things you could take into a doctor's office. At best, you got drugs to deaden your pain and a referral for physical therapy. At worst, you got your shoulder wrenched loose under general anesthesia. The bottom line in the medical world was that a frozen shoulder took a year or two to return to normal, whether you got treatment or not. Physicians and physical therapists didn't appear to be making much of a difference in the timeline.

I wrote about frozen shoulder in *The Trigger Point Therapy Workbook* (Davies 2001), and a great number of people have benefited. But since the book had to cover the entire body, I could devote only a couple of dozen pages to the shoulder. Subsequently, my publisher suggested that I write a separate book about the specific problem of frozen shoulder, as there were no books that focused on just that issue and there seemed to be a market for one. I liked the idea because it would allow me to go deeper into what was really my favorite subject. The reality of how people with frozen shoulder were being misdiagnosed and mistreated told me that there was indeed a pressing need for a book that dealt with just this problem in a truly comprehensive way. Maybe I could be of help not only to the public but to health care professionals as well. The success I'd had with my own shoulder and the shoulders of many other people led me to believe I had a great deal more to say.

And now I've said it. Everything I've learned about the shoulder is now in your hands. There's a good chance you can get rid of your own shoulder pain and stiffness just by following the simple instructions you'll find in this book. If for some reason you're physically unable to treat your own trigger points, you'll find alternate techniques that a friend, spouse, partner, or family member can use to help you. In addition, with considerable help again from my daughter, I've also provided a complete set of clinical techniques for physical therapists, occupational therapists, and massage therapists. These hands-on techniques would also be well suited for any physician who's open to trying an efficient method for diagnosing and treating myofascial pain in the shoulder.

You may have already been searching the Internet for solutions to your shoulder difficulty, in which case you know that good information is widely scattered and hard to separate out from the thousands of sales pitches and other nonsense. Even the most authoritative Web sites contain only a rehash of the same antiquated beliefs about what causes frozen shoulder. It's likely that the only therapies you've found are the same parroted dogma about stretching. This book assembles wide-ranging information about shoulder problems in one place and presents an effective, if relatively unknown, concept of therapy to help you make better decisions regarding what steps to take in healing your shoulder. Just as important, you may get a better idea of what things to avoid.

With persistence in applying what you find here, you may never have to make another appointment with anyone for your shoulder, desperately hoping they might actually know how to solve your problem. You can try trigger point massage right now and know within two or three days whether the method will work for you. Most people find that, if done correctly, trigger point massage can begin to relieve pain almost immediately.

If you're not intimidated by the technical side of things, you may want to start with chapter 1 and read straight through the book. If you prefer to get right to the meat of the matter, go to chapter 4 to find out the best way to do trigger point massage. Then go to chapter 5 to begin finding and treating the amazing little knots in your muscles that have been making your life so miserable. The key to an organized approach to self-treatment is the Trigger Point Guide at the beginning of chapter 5 or at the end of the book. You might like to take a look at it now and then decide where to begin.

Chapter 1

Anatomy, Function, and Dysfunction of the Shoulder

Before you can set about healing your frozen or painful shoulder, it's important to understand your shoulder's anatomy. This first chapter will give you a good understanding of how your shoulder works, so you'll have a better idea of why it's not working now. Once you make a commitment to understanding your shoulder, you'll find it's not as hard as you think. Solutions to difficult problems are often surprisingly simple, and that's just the case with the shoulder.

Of course, if you've been living with the full-time agony of a frozen shoulder, you're no doubt feeling worn-out, discouraged, and impatient to find a quick fix. With your energies depleted by months of crisis, just a glance at this chapter may make your head swim. But it won't pay to skim this book looking for an easy answer. You may miss the little tidbit that brings it all together for you. Every page contains something that will increase your understanding of the true cause of your shoulder problem and point the way to its solution. You may feel that you're being asked to sit down and eat an elephant. But you already know how to eat an elephant. Sure, just one bite at a time.

What Is Frozen Shoulder?

Shoulder trouble usually takes a predictable course. When a shoulder muscle is weakened and made dysfunctional by trigger points, associated muscles have to compensate. Under the extra burden, they fall like dominoes, each acquiring trigger points in turn until every muscle in the region has joined the party.

Simple chores become impossible. You can no longer scratch your back, comb your hair, or reach up to get the cereal off the shelf. If you need two hands for something, you have to use your good arm to lift your bad one. You may not even be able to reach across your body to fasten your seat belt. Constant pain disturbs your sleep and makes your job miserable. In its fully developed state, shoulder trouble can persist for months, and sometimes for years (Simons, Travell, and Simons 1999, 604-605; Bonica and Sola 1990, 951).

The term "frozen shoulder" is quite apt as a description of a shoulder condition that is characterized by severely reduced range of motion. But Doctors Travell and Simons make the point that frozen shoulder isn't a true medical diagnosis. This is because, within the medical world, frozen shoulder has neither a well-understood cause, nor a proven method of treatment with a reliable prognosis for recovery (Simons, Travell, and Simons 1999, 604).

In virtually all the medical literature, authors constantly reiterate that frozen shoulder is an enigmatic condition, meaning that its cause is unknown. Travell and Simons, however, assert that the cause of frozen shoulder has been recognized for over sixty years, ever since Janet Travell began writing about it in medical journals. A frozen shoulder can generally be correctly diagnosed if the effects of myofascial trigger points in muscles associated with the shoulder are taken into consideration. What's more, trigger point therapy will usually resolve the problem.

Interestingly, Travell and Simons discovered that trigger points in just a single muscle, the subscapularis, can produce all the symptoms of frozen shoulder. Although there are almost always others muscles involved, the subscapularis on its own can be the cause of reduced range of motion, constant aching deep in the shoulder, sleeplessness, sharp pain on sudden movement, and so on.

The clinical experience of thousands of massage therapists and other health care practitioners has proven that frozen shoulder can be successfully resolved by treating trigger points in the subscapularis and certain other muscles in the shoulder region. And yet, the broader medical community still very rarely considers trigger points in diagnosing or treating frozen shoulder (Simons, Travell, and Simons 1999, 604, 605).

Adhesive Capsulitis

Adhesive capsulitis is just one of many labels that doctors apply to the problem you know as frozen shoulder. Here's a list of some of the other terms applied to this "enigmatic" condition:

- Acromioclavicular arthritis
- Adherent bursitis
- Adherent subacromial bursitis
- Adhesive bursitis
- Arthrofibrosis
- Bursitis calcarea
- Check-rein shoulder
- Degenerative arthritis
- Duplay's syndrome
- Fifties' shoulder
- Glenohumeral synovitis
- Humeral hypomobility syndrome
- Humeroscapular fibrositis
- Idiopathic capsulitis
- Irritative capsulitis
- Joint capsule fibrosis
- Obliterative bursitis
- Periarthritis of the shoulder
- Periarticular arthritis
- Pericapsulitis
- Pitcher's arm
- Scapulohumeral periarthritis
- Scapulothoracic bursitis
- Subacromial bursitis

If you think some of these terms sound a bit contrived, you may be right. They all mean pretty much the same thing, and they mostly represent guesswork, reflecting the fact that most physicians really don't know what causes frozen shoulder.

Among physicians, adhesive capsulitis is the most popular explanation for the symptoms of frozen shoulder. On the surface, this term makes perfect sense. If your shoulder is stuck, there must be sticky stuff in there that's causing the problem. If you can't move your arm, there surely must be adhesions inside the shoulder joint. This is the officially sanctioned rationale taught in medical schools. If you search the Internet, you find this seemingly logical explanation everywhere. The beautifully illustrated pamphlets in your doctor's office promulgate the same notion and set it in stone in the minds of the patients. But the rationale is flawed because adhesive capsulitis isn't the cause of most frozen shoulders. Trigger points are.

Surgery for adhesive capsulitis is becoming more and more the accepted medical treatment for frozen shoulder, in spite of a disturbingly high failure rate. Accepted procedures for treatment of adhesive capsulitis now include manipulation under anesthesia (MUA), pressurized inflation of the joint capsule, severing of the subscapular tendon, removing part of the synovium, removal of the coracohumeral ligament, arthroscopic removal of the adhesions, and open surgical release of the anterior capsule. These procedures are generally not done by physicians who are informed about myofascial trigger points (Simons, Travell, and Simons 1999, 604-605).

The Fundamental Question

The basic issue associated with frozen shoulder is whether it's caused by adhesions or by trigger points. Is the problem in the joint, or is it in the muscles? Does adhesive capsulitis ever actually occur? Are all these shoulder surgeries really necessary?

Medical literature widely recommends that treatment for frozen shoulder begin with three to six months of conservative, nonoperative treatment (Cuomo 1999, 405-407). Conventional physical therapy is the usual choice, in spite of the fact that, for many people, physical therapy either doesn't work or actually makes the problem worse. At least one study shows that no treatment at all may produce better results with shoulder problems than physical therapy, especially intensive, or "aggressive," physical therapy (Diercks and Stevens 2004, 499-502).

Most of the time, a frozen shoulder will resolve on its own, although it can take a full year, or even as long as two and a half years. This means that if you have the courage to tough it out, your shoulder will probably eventually heal itself and return to normal. This alone indicates that frozen shoulder isn't usually due to adhesive capsulitis. The formation of fibrotic tissue (adhesions) tends to be permanent and not so amenable to self-healing.

Travell and Simons say that one frozen shoulder in ten may not heal on its own, in which case surgical relief of adhesions could conceivably be required. But even then they reject resorting to surgery. When adhesions have actually formed, Travell and Simons prefer the use of an antifibrotic medication (Potaba), and this only if restricted range of motion persists after the release of trigger points (Simons, Travell, and Simons 1999, 605).

The reality about adhesive capsulitis is that it's not the norm. Travell and Simons believe that adhesive capsulitis can indeed occur, but only after the muscles afflicted with trigger points have reduced the shoulder's range of motion for an extended period of time, several months or years. It takes time for adhesions to develop. The shoulder has to be already locked in place before adhesions can even to begin to form. In Travell and Simons's view, treatment of trigger points in the muscles of the shoulder complex should be the first line of attack, and the sooner the better, to keep adhesive capsulitis from ever becoming an issue (Simons, Travell, and Simons 1999, 605).

The Shoulder Complex

Think about all the things human beings can do with their hands. The diversity is truly awesome, particularly in sports and the arts. In our world of rapidly proliferating technological devices, human hands and fingers are called on daily to manage subtle, new operations. All of these widely varied actions of the hands depend directly on the strength of the shoulder joints and their ability to move freely. Being deprived of that strength and freedom can leave you seriously handicapped in everything you do.

The structure of the shoulder joint gives it the largest range of motion of any joint in the body. The trouble is that in gaining this extraordinary mobility you lose structural stability. Under normal conditions, stability is rarely at risk if the shoulder muscles remain strong, flexible, and healthy.

Moving the arm into an infinite variety of positions requires extremely fine coordination among all the muscles involved. There are twenty-four muscles that affect the function of each shoulder, including the scalene muscles in each side of the neck. What do the scalene muscles have to do with the function of your shoulders? The answer is that tight scalenes can cause compression of the nerves and blood vessels that supply the shoulders, arms, and hands. Trouble can begin very quickly in these areas when the nerves are hampered and the blood can't circulate freely. So, although the scalenes aren't ordinarily considered to be shoulder muscles, many shoulder problems can be traced ultimately to troubled scalenes.

It's easy to understand the importance of a healthy ball-and-socket joint in positioning the hand and arm for a virtually unlimited variety of actions and operations. Movement of the ball in the socket is the essential action in the shoulder, but movement of the shoulder blade is just as important, if not more so. Think of the shoulder blade as a kind of platform for a crane, the crane being the arm. The shoulder joint is the place where the crane swivels. To maximize the range of motion of the arm, the shoulder blade, lacking the restriction of ligaments, moves freely on the back. To gain this freedom requires an elaborate arrangement of powerful muscles on both the front and the back of the trunk harnessing and controlling the shoulder blade. Of the twenty-four muscles involved with the shoulder, seventeen attach to the shoulder blade.

There are actually three shoulder joints to consider, plus quite a number of ligaments, tendons, and a significant amount of cartilage and connective tissue. You're already familiar with the ball-and-socket joint, technically termed the *glenohumeral joint*. Another, the *acromioclavicular joint*, attaches the shoulder blade to the collarbone. The third, the *sternoclavicular joint*, attaches the collarbone to the breastbone. At each of these joints, strong ligaments keep the bones positioned correctly while still allowing some degree of movement between them. The many tendons of the shoulder complex are the strong fibrous ends of the muscles that anchor them to the bones. The infamous *rotator cuff* is made up of the tendons of the four extraordinarily important muscles that cover the inner and outer surfaces of the shoulder blade.

Amazingly, there's only one conventional bone-to-bone joint attaching the shoulder complex to the rest of the body: the sternoclavicular joint, where the collarbone attaches to the breastbone. Otherwise, the arm is attached to the body only by muscles. Several attach the shoulder blade to the spinal column and the rib cage. Others attach the arm to the shoulder blade or the ribs. One very large muscle on your back, the *latissimus dorsi,* actually connects the upper arm bone, the *humerus,* all the way down to the top of the pelvis! Let's look at some of these parts of the shoulder, starting with the basic framework.

Bones of the Shoulder

As noted earlier, seventeen muscles on each side attach your shoulder blades to your arms and to your body. It's much easier to find these muscles for treatment if you know what the bones of the shoulder look like and can find their bony landmarks (Figures 1.1 and 1.2). The following is the key to both drawings:

A. Superior angle of the shoulder blade (highest point)

B. Medial border of the shoulder blade (inner edge)

C. Lateral border of the shoulder blade (outer edge)

D. Inferior angle of the shoulder blade (lowest point)

E. Acromion (outer tip of the shoulder)

F. Coracoid process (sticking out through the front of the shoulder)

G. Head of the humerus and the glenoid cavity (the ball and socket)

H. Scapular spine (the ridgelike spine of the shoulder blade)

I. Humerus (upper arm bone)

J. Collarbone

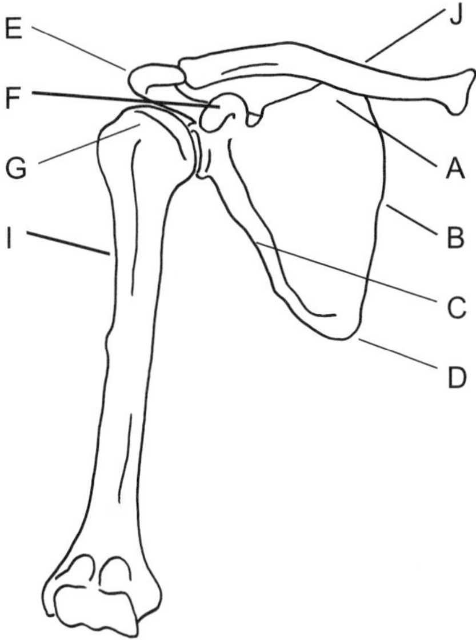

Figure 1.1 Front view of the bones of the right shoulder

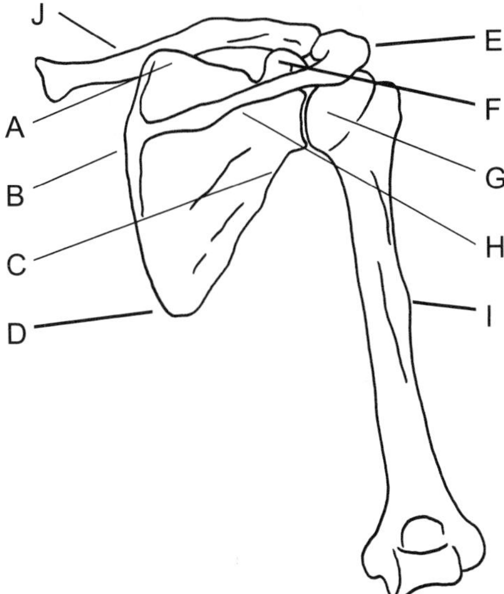

Figure 1.2 Back view of the bones of the right shoulder

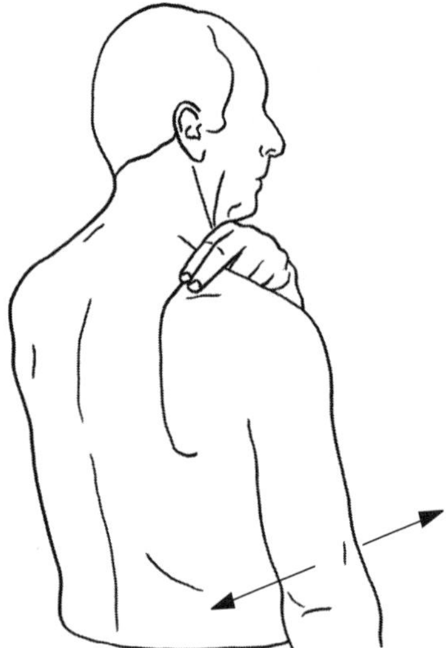

Figure 1.3 Swing the arm to feel the superior angle move under your fingertips.

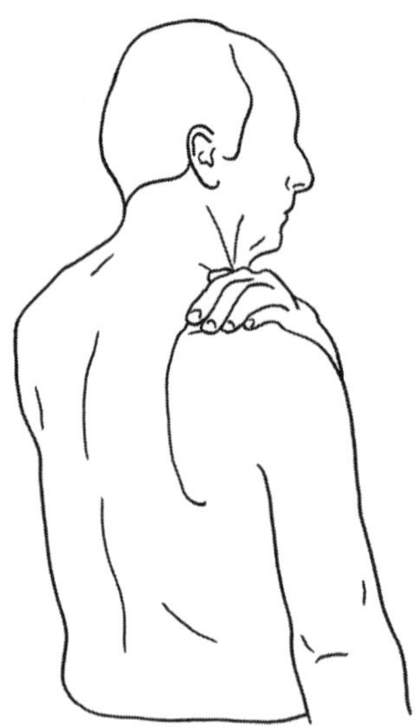

Figure 1.4 Locating the spine of the shoulder blade, one inch down from the superior angle

With the heel of your hand resting on your collarbone, feel for the bony *superior angle* (A) of the shoulder blade just above the scapular spine (Figure 1.3). Swing your arm forward and back to make the superior angle move back and forth under your fingers. This is an important landmark for locating the *supraspinatus*, one of the four rotator cuff muscles.

The most touchable part of the shoulder blade is the *scapular spine* (H). On very slender people, you can see it standing out very clearly beneath the skin (Figure 1.4). See if you can trace it with your fingers. On some people it's nearly horizontal. On others, it angles upward as it goes from the inner edge of the shoulder blade to the outer tip of the shoulder. Even if you're heavy, you should still see an angular bulge behind the shoulder that suggests the presence of this bony ridge beneath the skin.

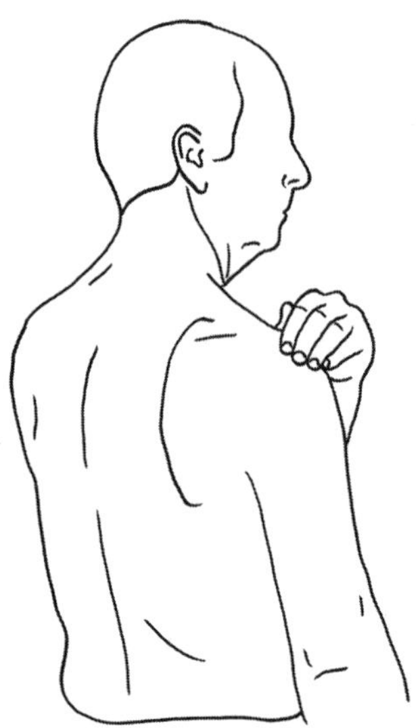

Figure 1.5 The index finger is touching the acromion.

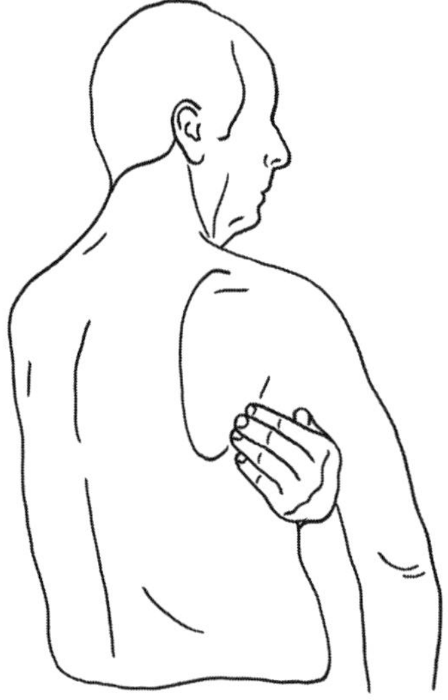

Figure 1.6 Touching the outer border of the shoulder blade

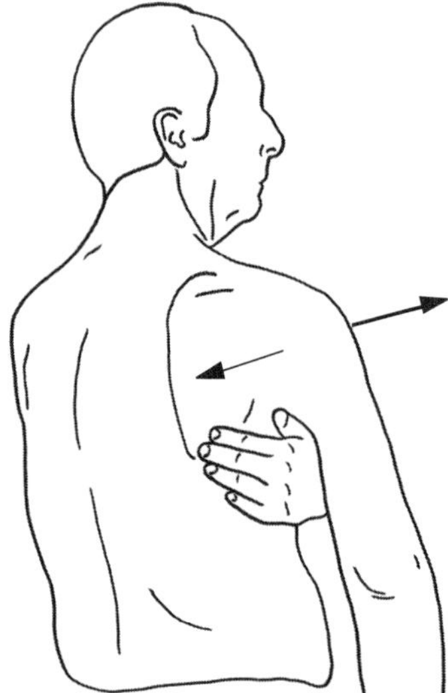

Figure 1.7 Move your shoulder forward and back to feel the inferior angle move.

Now find the *acromion* (E), the flat shelf of bone at the outer tip of the shoulder (Figure 1.5). Feel for a more or less sharp point just behind the shoulder but still on top. In the drawing, the index finger is touching the acromion and the third and fourth fingers are on the head of the humerus. Under your arm at the edge of your back, you should be able to feel the *lateral border* (C) of the shoulder blade (Figure 1.6). This is an important landmark for finding the *subscapularis* muscle, which lines the inner surface of the shoulder blade.

Trace the lateral border down to the lowest point of the shoulder blade, the *inferior angle* (D). To feel it, move your shoulder forward and back to make the inferior angle move back and forth under your fingers (Figure 1.7). If your range of motion isn't hampered by shoulder pain, try reaching all the way across to touch the *medial border* (B), or inner edge, of the shoulder blade (Figure 1.8). Also, try reaching over your shoulder to touch the upper part of the medial border. If you're unsure of the lateral and medial borders, you'll have trouble finding the infraspinatus muscle, which covers the lower two-thirds of the outer surface of the shoulder blade. Infraspinatus trigger points may be the most common cause of shoulder pain.

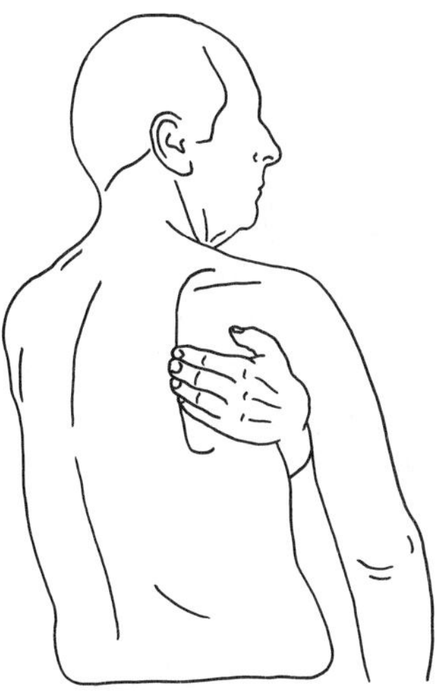

Figure 1.8 Touching the inner border of the shoulder blade

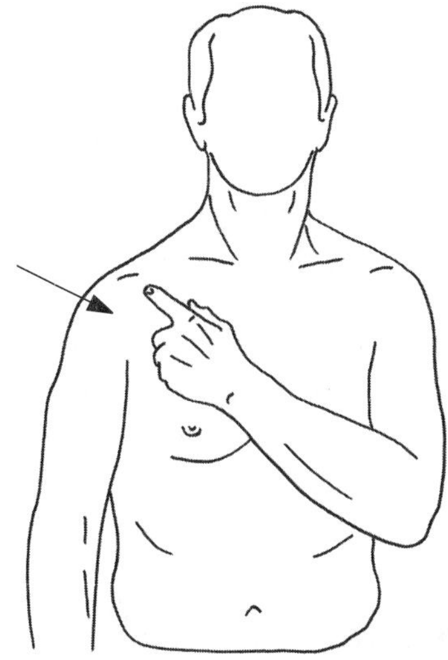

Figure 1.9 Touching the coracoid process; the arrow points to the head of the humerus.

Lastly, search for the *coracoid process* (F). It's part of the shoulder blade but runs all the way through the shoulder and sticks out under the skin in front (Figure 1.9). The coracoid process feels like a marble nestled right under the outer end of the collarbone beside the head of the humerus.

Joints of the Shoulder

Pain and stiffness in the shoulder is too often mistakenly attributed to a problem with the ball-and-socket joint. Among the first words you'll hear are "inflammation," "tendinitis," "bursitis," or "arthritis." Or you may be told that the joint cartilage has deteriorated or that the joint is hampered by tears or adhesions. These conditions do exist, but much less often than you'd think from how often you hear the terms. Usually, the ball-and-socket joint is just fine and it's the muscles that are in trouble. Let's look more closely at the structure of the shoulder joints.

Glenohumeral Joint

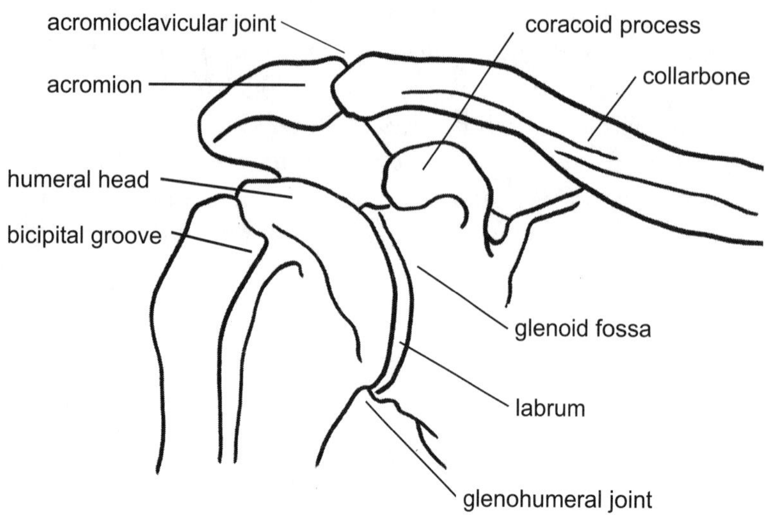

Figure 1.10 Front view of the right shoulder joint

The technical name for the ball-and-socket joint is the *glenohumeral joint* (Figure 1.10). It's also known as a *spheroid joint*. The two parts of the joint are the *head of the humerus* (ball) and the *glenoid fossa* (socket). The word "glenoid" is derived from the Greek word for "cavity."

The glenoid fossa is actually quite shallow, although it's made somewhat deeper by the *glenoid labrum*, a lip or fold of heavy connective tissue around the edge of the cavity. This shallowness, coupled with the flexibility of the labrum, allows maximum freedom of movement of the humeral head. The ball is capable of several kinds of movement in the socket, including inward and outward rotation. It can also rotate upward and downward, slide up and down, and glide forward and back.

Acromioclavicular Joint

The *acromioclavicular joint* links the acromion of the shoulder blade and the outer end of the collarbone (Figure 1.10). Strong ligaments hold this joint together while still allowing it to flex to some extent. This joint permits the two bones to move in the same direction, but also to rotate independently. Your ability to raise your arm all the way overhead depends on freedom in the small movements of the acromioclavicular joint (Smith, Weiss, and Lehmkuhl 1996, 230).

Sternoclavicular Joint

The *sternoclavicular joint* unites the collarbone (*clavicle*) to the breastbone (*sternum*). It's the only joint that actually connects the shoulder to the body (not shown). Because of this firm connection, the sternoclavicular joint restricts movement of the shoulder in all directions, particularly in *protraction*, or movement forward. The posture of the shoulder and entire upper body can be permanently distorted when a broken collarbone heals with overlapping ends or a crooked alignment (Smith, Weiss, and Lehmkuhl 1983, 222).

Scapulothoracic "Joint"

Not a true joint, the association between the shoulder blade and the chest acts like a joint, although an extraordinarily free one. No other articulation of bones in the body is quite like it. While strong muscles couple the shoulder blade to the bony structures of the spine, cranium, and rib cage, there are very few ligaments to keep it from rotating and sliding in a relatively wide range on the rib cage. Without this freedom of movement, the range of motion of the arm would be severely limited.

Connective Tissue of the Shoulder Joints

Connective tissue includes everything that attaches muscle to bone. Muscle is generally too pliant to keep a joint together. Connective tissue, on the other hand, is far more rigid and has much less ability to stretch and lengthen. As a consequence, ligaments, tendons, and other connective tissue are more susceptible to being torn or otherwise damaged than muscle tissue is.

Ligaments

Ligaments are bands or sheets of exceptionally strong, fibrous tissue that serve to hold two or more bones together. Ligaments put limits on the movement between the bones of a joint, which can have both advantages and disadvantages. *Hypermobility* occurs when ligaments are overstretched and become too loose to provide normal support. This can result in a loose joint, which can leave the joint and associated tissues, including the muscles, vulnerable to excessive strain. The injury suffered when a joint is pulled with sufficient force to tear or stretch a ligament is called a *sprain*.

The major shoulder ligaments are shown in Figure 1.11. The *acromioclavicular ligaments* join the acromial process (the tip of the acromion) to the lateral or outer end of the collarbone. In a dislocation of the acromioclavicular joint, or a shoulder separation, these ligaments are usually torn.

The *capsular ligaments* surround the glenohumeral joint, effectively encapsulating or sealing it. Synovial fluid, which lubricates the joint, fills the small space inside the capsule. This sealed capsule helps keep the glenohumeral joint together by creating an internal vacuum when force tends to pull the joint apart (Edgelow 2004, 222). The capsular ligaments are ordinarily quite loose and flexible, however, permitting maximum freedom of movement in the joint.

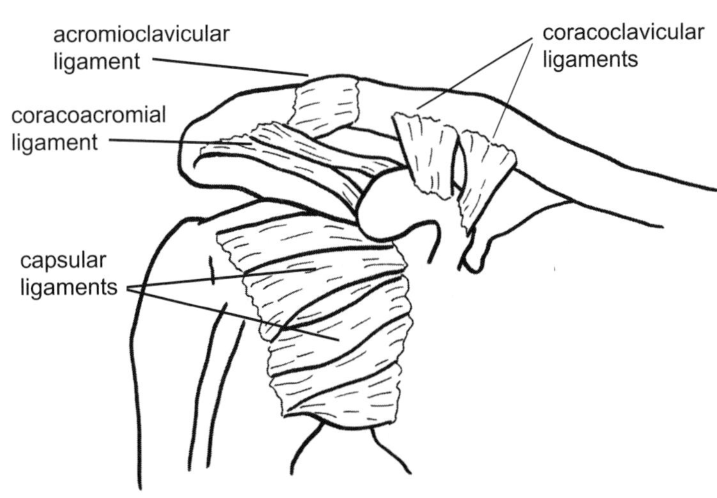

Figure 1.11 Front view of the ligaments of the right shoulder

The *sternoclavicular ligaments* join the medial, or inner, end of the collarbone to the top of the sternum, or breastbone (not shown). They're very important in keeping the shoulder complex attached to the body while allowing some amount of movement between the collarbone and breastbone. Without free movement at this place, you'd have difficulty moving your shoulder or reaching overhead.

The *coracoacromial ligaments* join the coracoid process and the acromion, both somewhat vulnerable projections of the shoulder blade. Their ligamentous attachment allows them to give added support to one another and, together with the acromion, create a kind of roof over the glenohumeral joint.

The *coracoclavicular ligaments* connect the outer end of the collarbone to the coracoid process. They give the shoulder blade a stronger link to the collarbone and ultimately to the body itself through the sternum.

The *coracohumeral ligament* attaches the coracoid process to the *greater tubercle* of the humerus (not shown). The greater tubercle is the larger of the two bulges on either side of the bicipital groove on the upper surface of the head of the humerus. The coracohumeral ligament, like the capsular ligaments, is rather loose and allows maximum movement of the head of the humerus while still giving it strong support at the limits of its movement.

Tendons

Tendons are cords or bands of extremely tough white connective tissue that serve to attach muscle to bone. Tendons are so strong that they are seldom torn. The rotator cuff, sometimes called the *musculotendinous cuff*, is one of the most familiar of the structures of the shoulder, often wrongly getting the blame for shoulder pain. The cuff forms a ring around the upper two-thirds of the humeral head (Figure 1.12) and is made up of the tendons of the teres minor, infraspinatus, supraspinatus, and subscapularis muscles. These are the rotator cuff muscles.

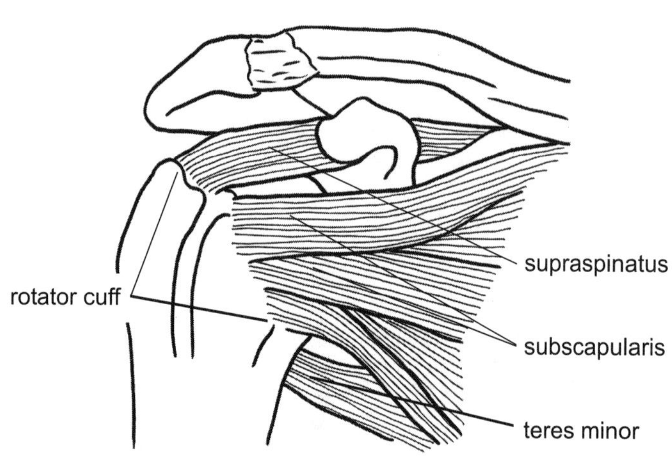

Figure 1.12 The tendons of the rotator cuff muscles. The infraspinatus attaches to the back of the humeral head and is hidden in this view.

Other very important tendons associated with the shoulder are the two *biceps tendons* and one of the *triceps tendons*. The tendon for the long head of the biceps rides in the bicipital groove and attaches to the top of the glenoid fossa (Figure 1.13). The tendon for the short head of the biceps attaches to the coracoid process. The tendon for the long head of the triceps attaches to the underside of the glenoid fossa (Figure 1.14). The biceps and triceps, through their tendons, are extremely important for keeping the ball-and-socket joint together when heavy weight or strong forces threaten to pull it apart.

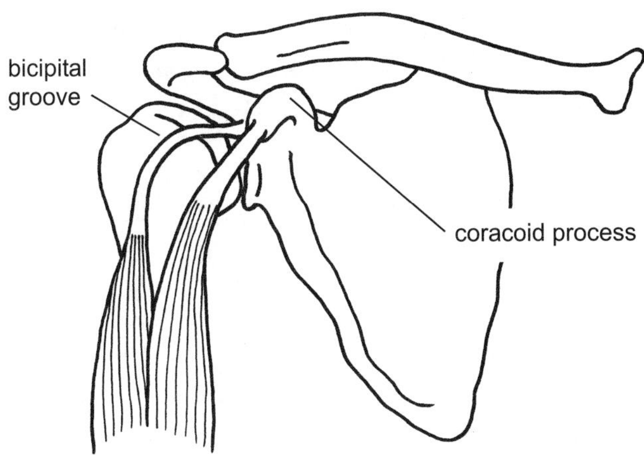

Figure 1.13 Biceps tendon attachments to the shoulder blade—the long head to the top of the glenoid fossa and the short head to the coracoid process

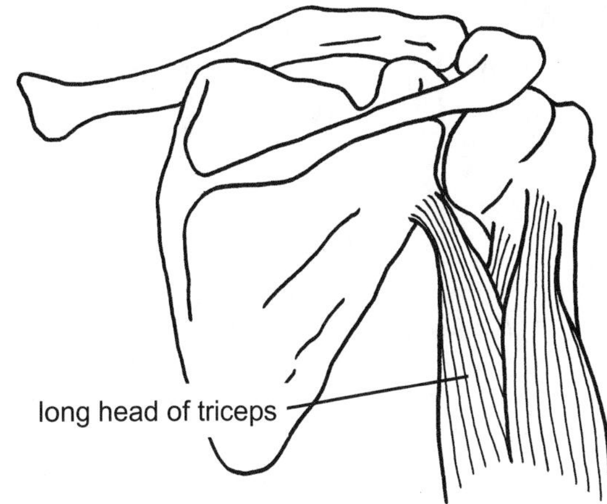

Figure 1.14 Rear view of the right shoulder. The tendon of the long head triceps attaches to the underside of the glenoid fossa; the lateral and medial heads attach to the back of the humerus.

Pain in the front of the shoulder is often wrongly attributed to tendinitis of the long biceps tendon. This supposed bicipital tendinitis is usually simple referred pain from trigger points in the infraspinatus muscles behind the shoulder. This is a classic instance of how misleading myofascial pain can be and an outstanding example of how mistaken a diagnosis can be when it is assumed that the problem is at the place that hurts.

Bursas

The *subacromial bursa,* also called the *subdeltoid bursa,* is a sac filled with thick synovial fluid that insulates the acromion from the supraspinatus tendon at its attachment to the head of the humerus (Figure 1.15). This allows the humeral head to move freely under the acromion without being damaged by direct contact with it. Pain in the top of the shoulder is frequently wrongly diagnosed as bursitis, or inflammation of this bursa, when in reality the pain is coming from trigger points in the supraspinatus muscle a few inches away. True bursitis may occasionally occur, but not as often as commonly believed. Trigger point therapy can quickly clear up any question about the actual cause.

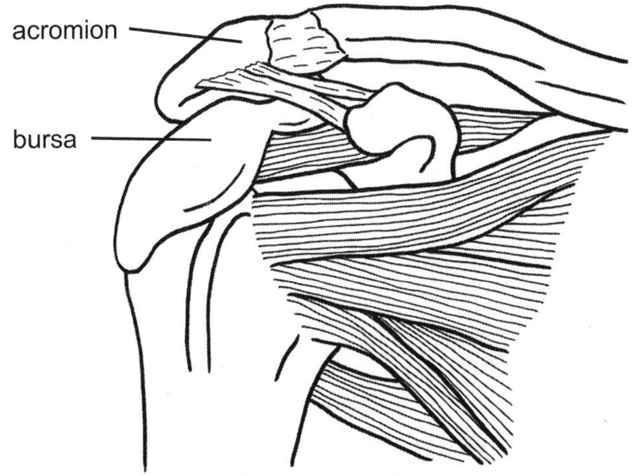

Figure 1.15 Front view of the right shoulder, showing the subacromial bursa

Another bursa, the *subscapular bursa,* lies between the subscapularis tendons and the underlying capsular ligaments (not shown). The subscapularis attaches to the front of the head of the humerus. Pain in the front of the shoulder is sometimes mistakenly blamed on subscapular bursitis, when the practitioner is unfamiliar with the effects of myofascial trigger points.

Capsule of the Shoulder Joint

The shoulder joint *capsule* is a fibrous bag made up of the capsular ligaments and *fascia*. Fascia (FAH-shuh) is an extremely thin, translucent membrane that envelops and separates muscles, groups of muscles, and other bodily structures. Capable of expanding and contracting, fascia's basic purpose is to provide support for tissue that lacks a rigid framework. Lack of activity can cause fascia to shrink and bind the structures it encloses, leading to stiffness and reduced range of motion. Various stretching techniques, however, can restore fascia to its normal resiliency. The word "fascia" is derived from the Latin for "band."

Cartilage

Cartilage is a semi-elastic fibrous material that covers the articular surfaces of all the bones in the shoulder complex. Most important is the cartilage that lines both the humeral head (the ball) and the glenoid cavity (the socket) where they're likely to come in contact. It is thickest on the center of the humeral head and on the periphery of the glenoid fossa. The slickness of cartilage facilitates movement of the joint.

Sometimes practitioners who are unfamiliar with the effects of myofascial trigger points blame thinning of cartilage for shoulder pain, and X-rays or an MRI may seem to substantiate this diagnosis. Nevertheless, trigger points that cause shoulder pain should always be deactivated before drawing conclusions about any possible deterioration of the cartilage. Supposed thinning of cartilage is sometimes used as a justification for surgery that may not be needed.

Glenoid Labrum

The *glenoid labrum* encircles the glenoid fossa but actually provides very little support for the ball-and-socket joint. It is considered by some anatomists to be a redundant or essentially purposeless fold of the joint capsule, although it may contribute in a minor way to preventing disarticulation of the joint. The muscles and ligaments surrounding the joint are what provide its main support and keep it properly articulated (Donatelli 2004, 16).

Practitioners unfamiliar with the effects of myofascial trigger points may credit a supposedly torn or defective glenoid labrum for your shoulder pain and dysfunction. The glenoid labrum is unlikely to have suffered damage unless you've been involved in a violent fall, collision, or sports injury that dislocated your shoulder.

The Twenty-four Muscles Associated with the Shoulder

Muscles involved in the function of the shoulder can be divided into four groups: shoulder blade suspension muscles, rotator cuff muscles, upper arm muscles, and the scalene muscles of the front and sides of the neck.

The shoulder blade suspension muscles are the rhomboids, levator scapulae, subclavius, serratus anterior, and trapezius. These five muscles all attach the shoulder blade to the rib cage and the spinal column. Their function is to help move the shoulder blade into position for all actions of the arm and hand.

The four rotator cuff muscles are the supraspinatus, infraspinatus, teres minor, and subscapularis. They attach the shoulder blade to the top of the humerus, allowing them to rotate the arm and play a primary role in keeping the shoulder joint together.

Ten muscles attach to the upper arm below the humeral head: the pectoralis major, pectoralis minor, teres major, latissimus dorsi, coracobrachialis, biceps, and triceps, and the three deltoids. Only the coracobrachialis, biceps, and triceps are actually part of the arm.

The scalenes, serratus posterior superior, iliocostalis thoracis, brachialis, and diaphragm are not actually involved in controlling the shoulder or arm, but they're included here because their trigger points produce pain in the shoulder and may create satellite trigger points in other muscles of the shoulder complex. You may notice that an additional muscle —the sternocleidomastoid—is covered in chapter 5, Shoulder Treatment, Part A. It isn't included here because it doesn't directly affect shoulder function. Problems in the sternocleidomastoid can have an effect on the scalenes, however, and treating sternocleidomastoid trigger points may be necessary for complete resolution of your shoulder trouble.

The following descriptions of the twenty-four muscles associated with the shoulder will tell you where each muscle attaches and will explain the specific action each muscle contributes to the function of the shoulder and arm.

Trapezius

The *trapezius* (truh-PEE-zee-us) is a superficial muscle covering most of the upper half of the back and extending upward to cover the central part of the back of the neck (Figure 1.16). The word "trapezius" comes from the Greek word for a small table, a reflection of the muscle's relative flatness and four-cornered shape. The muscle attaches to the base of the skull, all of the cervical and thoracic vertebrae, the collarbone, and the acromion and spine of the shoulder blade. The trapezius supports the weight of the shoulder and arm and holds the shoulder blade solidly in place as a base for the finer operations of the

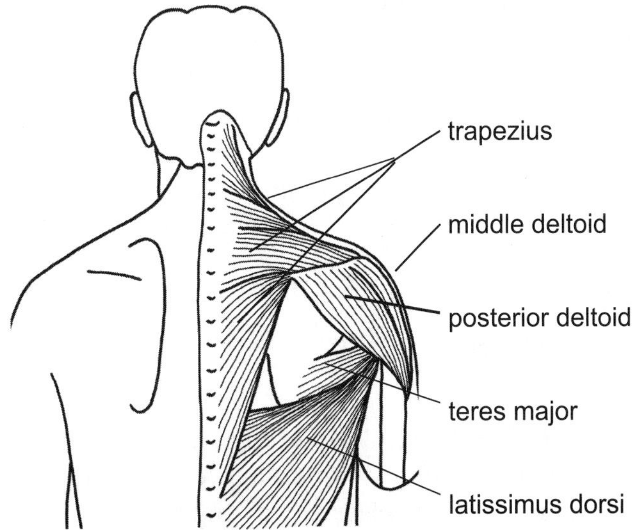

Figure 1.16 Superficial posterior muscles of the shoulder

arm and hand. It must contract strongly to rotate the shoulder blade upward every time you raise your arm.

There are three distinct parts of the trapezius muscle, the upper, middle, and lower. Figure 1.16 shows that the muscle fibers in the three sections are oriented at different angles. This indicates the general direction of pull when that part of the muscle contracts. Each section can work independently of the others, and all can work together.

Posterior Deltoid

The *deltoid* muscle, if flattened out on a table, would resemble the Greek letter delta, which has the shape of a triangle. On the body, the deltoid muscle completely surrounds the shoulder like a cap and covers parts of several other muscles (Figure 1.16). Although the deltoid is technically a single muscle, it has three fairly distinct parts, the anterior, posterior, and middle deltoid, on the front, back, and outer side of the shoulder, respectively. Because of this, the deltoid muscle is often spoken of as "the deltoids."

The deltoids attach to the collarbone, scapular spine, and acromion, the bony point of the shoulder. Their lower attachment is to the *deltoid tuberosity*, a slight lump about halfway down the outer side of the humerus. The function of the deltoids, in conjunction with the supraspinatus muscle, is to raise the arm in any direction—to the front, back, and side. The posterior deltoid is a strong *extensor* of the arm, in that it raises the arm to the rear.

Middle Deltoid

Also called the *lateral deltoid*, the *middle deltoid* is the largest and most powerful of the deltoid heads (Figure 1.16). Its main action is in working with the supraspinatus muscle to raise the arm to the side and bring it up overhead.

Teres Major

The *teres* (TEH-reez) *major* comes together with the latissimus dorsi (luh-TISS-uh-mus DOR-sye) at the back of the armpit and then goes around to attach to the front of the upper arm bone near its top (Figure 1.16). The action of both muscles is to bring the arm down and in toward the chest. With the help of the posterior deltoid, they also extend the arm backward. "Teres major" means "big round muscle." Its attachment to the outer border of the shoulder blade makes it an important part of the shoulder complex. It is often quite a large muscle and forms most of the thick web of muscle at the back of the armpit.

Latissimus Dorsi

Although the *latissimus dorsi* is a muscle of the lower back, it's included with the shoulder muscles because it moves the upper arm and sometimes attaches partially to the inferior angle of the shoulder blade (Figure 1.16). Along with the teres major, the latissimus dorsi can extend, adduct, or inwardly rotate the arm. *Adduction* moves the arm toward the body, "adding" the arm to the body. The teres major and latissimus dorsi can also *depress* the shoulder complex; that is, bring the entire shoulder downward.

Rhomboids

The *rhomboid* (RAHM-boid) muscles lie under the trapezius and attach to several vertebrae of the upper back and to the inner edge of the shoulder blade (Figure 1.17). There are actually two rhomboid muscles, the major and the minor, with slightly different functions. The rhomboid minor is higher and somewhat separate from the rhomboid major, but the two are indistinguishable by touch. The function of the rhomboids is to move the shoulder blade toward the spine, to help raise the shoulder blade, and to hold the shoulder blade still when needed as a solid support for the operations of the arm and hand.

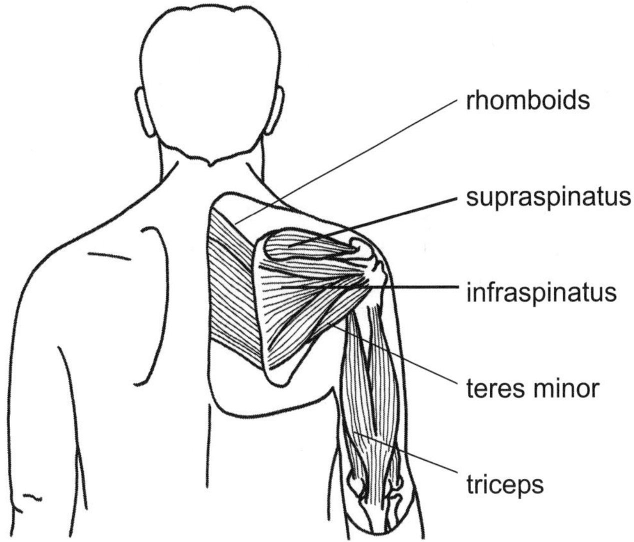

Figure 1.17 Deep posterior muscles of the shoulder

Supraspinatus

The *supraspinatus* (soo-prah-spih-NAH-tus) is one of the four rotator cuff muscles and lies under the upper section of the trapezius. It's buried in a pocket in the top of the shoulder blade above the scapular spine (Figure 1.17). The word "supraspinatus" means "above the spine." At its outer end, the muscle passes under the acromion to attach to the outer side of the top of the head of the humerus. This attachment gives the supraspinatus great leverage for helping raise the arm. It also allows the muscle to help the other rotators hold the joint together.

You'll find the supraspinatus muscle at the top of the shoulder blade, immediately behind the thick roll of the trapezius muscle that lies on top of the shoulder. Place your fingers between the superior angle and spine of the shoulder blade. (Figure 1.3 shows how to find the superior angle.) If your hand is in the right place, your fingertips will be contacting the top edge of the spine of the shoulder blade and the heel of your hand will be resting on your collarbone. To verify by isolated contraction that you're touching the supraspinatus, begin to raise your arm forward and a little to the side. Just as your arm starts to move, you should feel the muscle contract and bulge up under your fingers.

Infraspinatus

The *infraspinatus* (in-frah-spih-NAH-tus) covers almost all of the shoulder blade below the spine of the shoulder blade (Figure 1.17). The word "infraspinatus" means "below the spine." At its outer end, the infraspinatus attaches to the back of the head of the humerus, giving it the ability to rotate the arm outward, as when you pull your arm back to throw a ball or prepare to make a forehand stroke with a tennis racket. Without outward rotation, the arm can't be raised above the level of the shoulder. The infraspinatus is also a strong participant in keeping the head of the humerus in its socket. You can confirm its location by feeling it contract and bulge as you put the arm into outward rotation. The infraspinatus tendon forms part of the rotator cuff.

Teres Minor

The *teres* (TEH-reez) *minor* muscle lies right below the outer end of the infraspinatus on the shoulder blade and has a similar attachment to the back of the head of the humerus (Figure 1.17). The teres minor helps the infraspinatus rotate the arm outward.

Triceps

The *triceps* is a long, broad muscle with three branches, or heads (Figure 1.17). The muscle's attachment to the *ulna*, one of the two bones of the forearm, gives it great leverage for straightening the elbow. The triceps is chiefly responsible for this function, aided only by the small anconeus muscle in the elbow joint. The attachment of the long head of the triceps to the shoulder blade at the bottom of the glenoid cavity helps keep the arm in its socket.

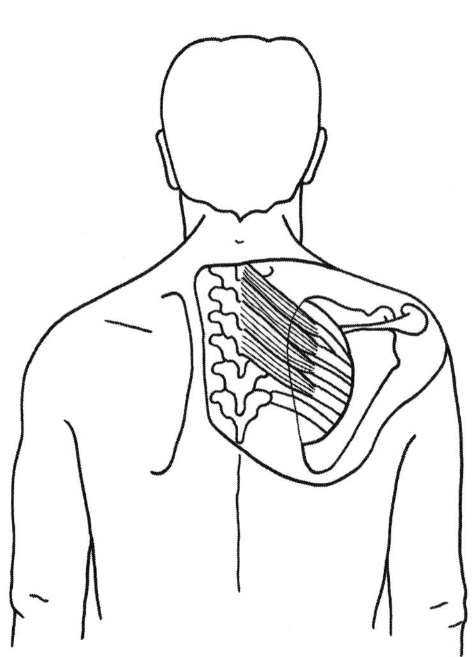

Figure 1.18 Serratus posterior superior

Serratus Posterior Superior

Although the *serratus* (seh-RAY-tus) *posterior superior* muscle attaches to the vertebral column like the rhomboids and runs in the same direction, it doesn't attach to the shoulder blade as the rhomboids do. Instead, it goes underneath the shoulder blade to attach to several upper ribs (Figure 1.18). The function of the serratus posterior superior is to raise the ribs during inhalation to help fill the lungs. The word "serratus," meaning "saw-toothed," relates to its appearance, as it's sequentially attached to several ribs. The word "superior" means that it's the highest on the body of the three serratus muscles. Since the serratus posterior superior doesn't attach to any part of the shoulder complex, it's technically not a shoulder muscle. It's included here because pain from its trigger points occurs deep under the shoulder blade and feels like a shoulder problem.

Iliocostalis Thoracis

The *iliocostalis thoracis* (ILL-ee-oh-kuh-STAHL-iss thor-RA-cis) is a back muscle that runs along and under the inner border of the shoulder blade (not shown). It isn't actually a shoulder muscle, nor is it involved in the shoulder's function, but its trigger points cause pain that feels as though it's in the shoulder.

Levator Scapulae

The lower end of the *levator scapulae* (luh-VAY-ter SCAP-yuh-lee) attaches to the inner edge of the superior angle of the shoulder blade (Figure 1.19). Its upper end attaches to the sides of the top four cervical (neck) vertebrae. This arrangement allows the levator scapulae to help raise the shoulder blade and thereby raise the shoulder. The word "levator" is from the same Latin root as "elevator." *Scapula* is Latin for "shoulder blade." The muscle's name tells its job. In saying the muscle's name in common speech, "scapulae" is usually pronounced like "scapula."

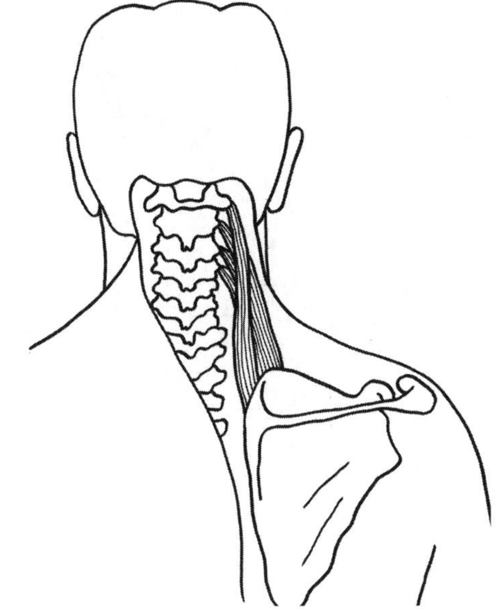

Figure 1.19 Levator scapulae

Pectoralis Major

The *pectoralis* (pek-tur-AH-liss) *major* muscles are the muscular part of the breasts in both men and women (Figure 1.20). The word "pectoralis" comes from *pectus,* Latin for "breast." It's the largest of the four pectoral muscles. The others are the pectoralis minor, subclavius, and sternalis. (Note that the sternalis won't be discussed here, as it has no effect on shoulder sensation or function.)

There are three distinct sections of the pectoralis major. The *clavicular* (upper) section attaches to the collarbone, the *sternal* (middle) section to the breastbone, and the *costal* (lower) section to the ribs and stomach muscles. All come together to attach to the front of the humerus. These attachments allow the pectoralis major to rotate the arm inward and to pull it across the chest (adduction). The upper section also helps raise the arm, and the lower section helps pull the arm and shoulder down. All three sections assist in *protraction* of the shoulder; that is, bringing it forward.

Anterior Deltoid

The main action of the front part of the deltoid, or *anterior deltoid,* is *flexion;* that is, it raises the arm to the front (Figure 1.20). It also assists the posterior and middle deltoid heads in *abducting,* or raising, the arm to the side.

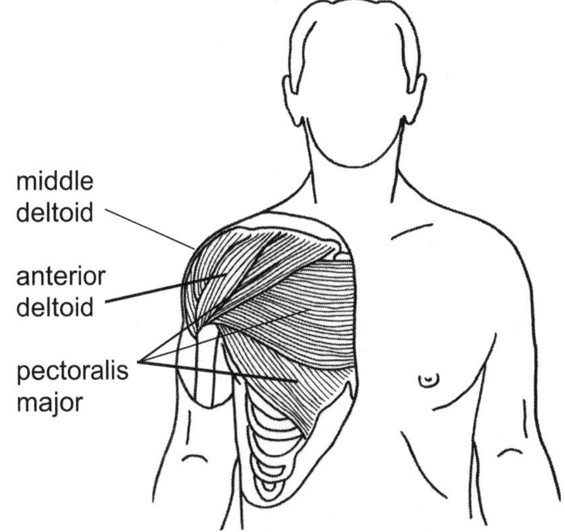

Figure 1.20 Superficial anterior muscles of the shoulder

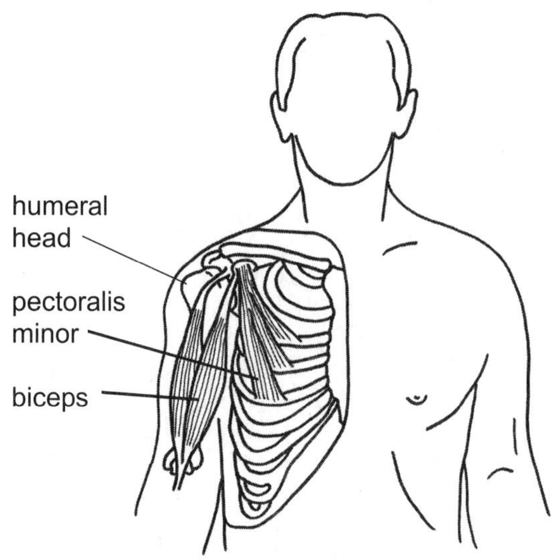

Figure 1.21 Pectoralis minor and biceps

Pectoralis Minor

The *pectoralis* (pek-tur-AH-liss) *minor* muscle lies completely hidden under the pectoralis major and has a different orientation and very different attachments (Figure 1.21). Though generally a smaller muscle, it can still be very strong and thick. The pectoralis minor attaches at its upper end to the coracoid process, an odd little piece of the shoulder blade that sticks through to the front of the shoulder. With your arm at rest in your lap, you can feel the coracoid process as a hard roundness, something like a marble under the skin, just below your collarbone, right next to the head of the humerus.

The lower end of the pectoralis minor muscle divides into three or more sections, which attach to individual ribs in the center of the breast area. The action of the pectoralis minor is to pull down on the coracoid process to fix the shoulder blade in place for various operations of the arm. A secondary function is to pull up on the ribs to assist expansion of the chest during forced breathing, such as in vigorous exercise or sports activity.

You can locate the pectoralis minor by feeling it bulge up when it contracts. To make the pectoralis minor contract without contracting the pectoralis major, put your hand in the small of your back, then push back with your hand against a wall or the back of your chair. If you put your opposite hand on your chest as you would for the Pledge of Allegiance, your fingertips will be in the right position to feel the pectoralis minor contract. The "pledge" hand has to be on the side that you're contracting.

Biceps

The *biceps* has two heads, the short head attaching to the coracoid process alongside the coracobrachialis, the long head attaching to the shoulder blade just above the socket (Figures 1.13 and 1.21). This attachment to the shoulder blade lets the biceps help raise the arm overhead. The leverage of the long tendon of the biceps also prevents it from pressing against the acromion when the deltoids contract strongly. The lower end of the biceps attaches to the bones of the forearm, allowing it to bend the elbow and help turn the hand over, palm side up.

Another extremely important function of the biceps is to participate in keeping the head of the humerus firmly in its socket. Many muscles work to maintain this joint, but without the biceps it would be impossible to carry any weight at all without pulling the joint apart.

Brachialis

The *brachialis* (brah-kee-AH-liss) muscle lies under the biceps on the front of the upper arm (not shown). It has no control over the movement of the shoulder or upper arm, but its trigger points can send pain to the shoulder.

Subscapularis

The *subscapularis* (sub-scap-yu-LEHR-us) is an exceptionally powerful muscle lining the front surface of the shoulder blade (Figure 1.22). It can be as thick as the middle deltoid. Visualize the subscapularis sandwiched between the shoulder blade and the ribs. (In the illustration, the ribs have been removed and you're looking through the body to the back.) The muscle's attachment to the head of the humerus allows it to rotate the arm inward. This attachment also enables the subscapularis to help keep the joint together and center the head of the humerus in its socket.

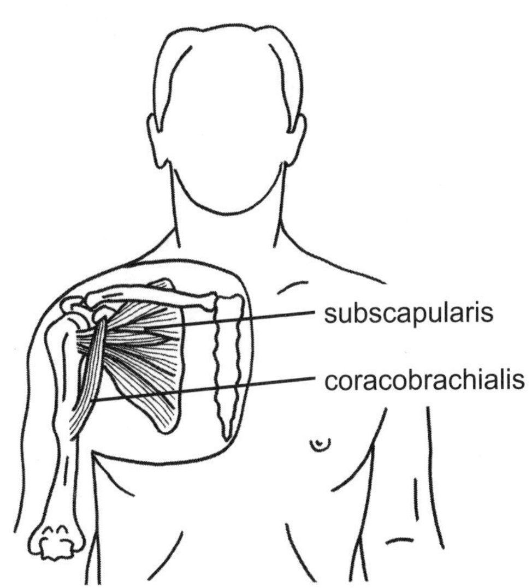

Figure 1.22 Subscapularis and coracobrachialis muscles

You'd think that the subscapularis muscle would be unreachable and untreatable, buried as it is on the front surface of the shoulder blade. Actually, it's surprisingly accessible if you go about it in the right way. This is good news, because the subscapularis is often at the very heart of the problem with frozen shoulder. Trigger points keep the subscapularis from lengthening, which it must do to allow any movement involving outward rotation of the arm, including raising the arm overhead. With a frozen shoulder, knowing how to treat subscapularis trigger points is the key to recovery. Without this knowledge, recovery can be a long time in coming.

Coracobrachialis

The *coracobrachialis* (COR-ah-co-bray-kee-AH-liss) lies between the biceps and the triceps on the inner side of the upper arm (Figure 1.22). The muscle is a little larger than your index finger and about twice as long. At its lower end, it attaches about halfway down the inner surface of the upper arm bone. At its upper end, it attaches to the coracoid process, the little piece of the shoulder blade that sticks through to the front of the shoulder. The action of the coracobrachialis pulls the arm tight against the side.

To locate the coracobrachialis, press your thumb against the inner side of the humerus as high up as you can. You can feel the muscle contract at this location when you clamp your elbow against your side.

Subclavius

The *subclavius* (sub-CLAY-vee-us) muscle lies just under the collarbone (Figure 1.23). It attaches to the middle of the collarbone and to the end of the first rib near where it joins the sternum, or breastbone. Its action is to draw the collarbone down and forward, which assists in depression and protraction of the shoulder.

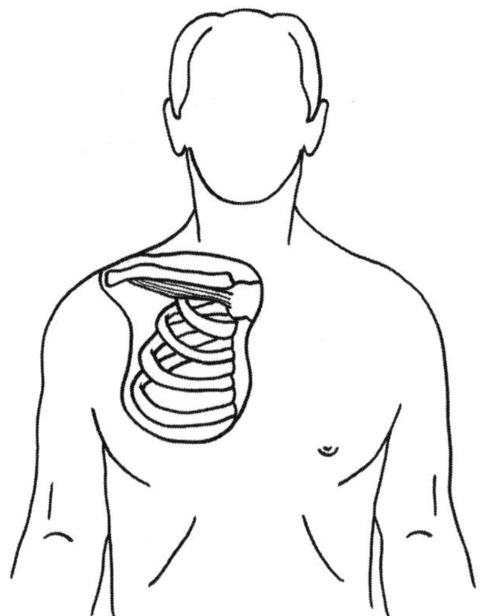

Figure 1.23 Subclavius muscle attaching to the collarbone and sternum

Serratus Anterior

Although the *serratus* (seh-RAY-tus) *anterior* is located under the arm, it's actually a shoulder muscle (Figure 1.24). The muscle's attachments to your ribs and to the inner border of the shoulder blade give it leverage for rotating the shoulder blade so that the socket of the shoulder joint faces more in an upward direction. This allows you to raise your arm all the way overhead. In addition to rotation, the serratus anterior moves the shoulder blade upward and forward on the rib cage. Without this ability to reposition the shoulder blade, you wouldn't be able to raise your arm above the level of your shoulder. The serratus anterior muscles also aid inhalation by assisting expansion of the ribs when you need more air than usual.

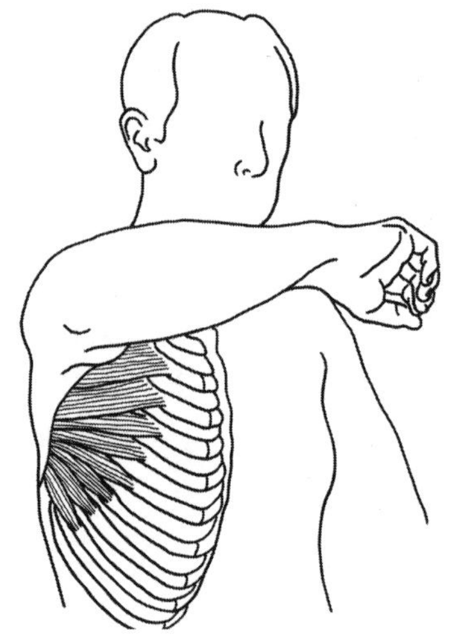

Figure 1.24 Serratus anterior muscle with multiple heads

The Diaphragm

The *diaphragm* is a thin, circular muscle that attaches to the inner surfaces of the lower ribs, separating the chest cavity from the contents of the lower abdomen (not shown). The function of the diaphragm is obviously concerned with breathing and doesn't involve the shoulder. However, diaphragm trigger points are believed to sometimes cause pain in the top of the shoulders, which you may experience as a shoulder problem.

The Scalenes

Although the three *scalenes* (SKAY-leenz) are neck muscles, their trigger points cause a surprising amount of pain in the upper back, shoulder, and upper arm. Scalene trigger points also contribute significantly to pain and other symptoms in the forearm and hand. The scalenes are so important that they should always come first in troubleshooting pain in any of these areas.

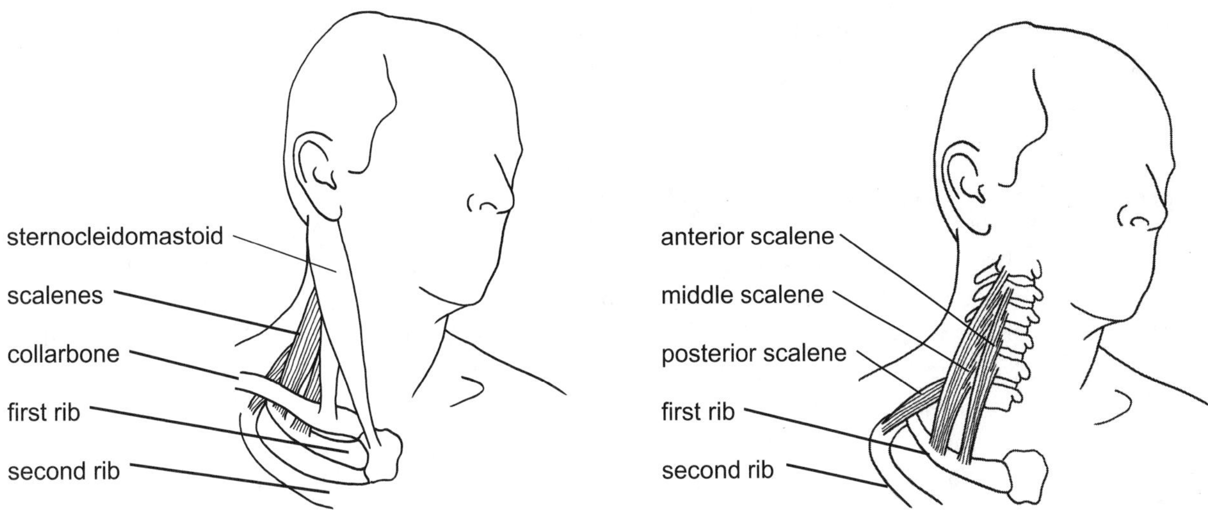

Figure 1.25 Location of the scalenes, behind the sternocleidomastoid

Figure 1.26 Scalene muscles

Success in finding and dealing with the scalenes depends on your understanding of their relationship to the *sternocleidomastoid* (STUR-no-CLY-do-MAS-toid) muscle (Figures 1.25 and 1.26). The *anterior scalene*, the front-most scalene muscle, lies between the sternocleidomastoid muscle and the neck vertebrae and is almost completely hidden. The *middle scalene* is behind the anterior scalene, more on the side of the neck, with its lower half free of the sternocleidomastoid. The *posterior scalene* lies almost horizontally behind and below the middle scalene in the soft triangular depression just above the collarbone and below the front edge of the trapezius. The scalenes cling closely to the neck and feel much firmer than the ordinarily soft, loose, mushy sternocleidomastoids.

The scalene muscles attach to the sides of your neck vertebrae and to your top two ribs. Although the scalenes help stabilize and flex the neck, their main job is to raise the upper two ribs on each side when you inhale. They're active to some degree in every inhalation, and they work extremely hard when your breathing is labored during vigorous activity.

Scalene trigger points cause the muscles to shorten, which pulls the first rib up against the collarbone, entrapping all the nerves and blood vessels that supply the shoulder and arm. Symptoms of pain, numbness, and other abnormal sensations caused by this entrapment are known as *thoracic outlet syndrome*. The complex group of nerves, blood vessels, and lymphatic ducts that pass between the first rib and the collarbone are collectively referred to as a *neurovascular bundle*. It's shown as a heavy black line in Figure 1.27.

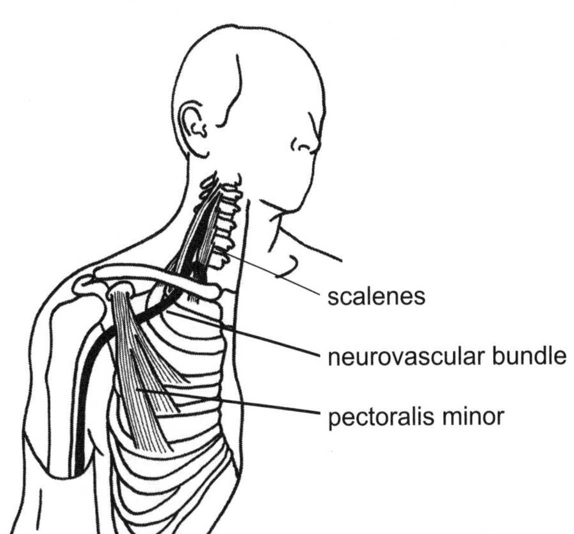

Figure 1.27 Neurovascular bundle (dark line), consisting of the brachial artery, brachial vein, and brachial nerve plexus

Impingement of the nerves and blood vessels that supply the shoulder muscles can be the unsuspected stimulus that initiates the development of myofascial trigger points in the shoulder area. Trouble with the scalenes may sometimes be the mystifyingly distant origin of a frozen shoulder.

Kinesiology of the Shoulder

Kinesiology is the study of movement and the way the muscles cause it to happen. Kinesiology is closely related to anatomy but includes exacting descriptions and measurements of just what the muscles do. The body is treated as a mechanical system, looking at the bones as levers and the muscles as sources of power for moving the bones.

In the fields of physical therapy and occupational therapy, one of the standard textbooks for the study of this complex subject is *Brunnstrom's Clinical Kinesiology* (Smith, Weiss, and Lehmkuhl 1996). For a thorough presentation of the technical aspects of kinesiology, please consult this primary source. Material from this classic text is presented here in a much simplified fashion.

Although primarily a science of normal movement, kinesiology is also concerned with abnormal factors that limit the function of muscles. You'll be better equipped to deal with the muscles causing your shoulder problem when you understand how they're supposed to work. Most problems with the shoulder occur because the muscles that move the shoulder and arm aren't functioning correctly. Trigger points adversely affect the function of muscles. Three effects are especially important:

1. Trigger points shorten muscles and keep them from lengthening.
2. Trigger points cause muscle weakness.
3. Pain from trigger points makes you keep muscles tense. Constant tension in a muscle can make its trigger points worse, leading to an escalating vicious cycle.

It's important to know which muscles control a particular movement so that you'll know which muscles to check when that movement causes pain or is limited. Obviously, certain muscles must contract to make a particular movement. But sometimes it's not so obvious that other muscles must contract at the same time to exert counterforces necessary for fine control and for protection of the vulnerable ball-and-socket joint. It's also important to recognize that there are always muscles that must lengthen to allow the specified movement to occur. Most of the trouble with frozen shoulder comes when particular muscles fail to lengthen when they're supposed to.

Most of the muscles of the shoulder participate in some way in every movement your arm makes. Usually, however, only one or two muscles provide the major force for a given action. Let's look at the fundamental movements in the shoulder's repertoire. Try feeling which muscles are contracting as you make each movement.

Elevation

Elevation is simply the raising of the shoulder. As the shoulder tip rises, the angle of the collarbone can change as much as 60 degrees. The levator scapulae, rhomboids, and upper trapezius elevate the shoulder, with the upper trapezius doing most of the work. Look at Figures 1.16, 1.17, and 1.19 to see how the contraction of these muscles might raise the shoulder. Trigger points in the pectoralis major, pectoralis minor, latissimus dorsi, or lower trapezius tend to limit this movement since they need to lengthen to allow it (Figures 1.16, 1.20, and 1.21).

Depression

From rest position, you can lower your shoulder only 5 to 10 degrees. Starting from maximum elevation of the shoulders, however, *depressing* or lowering the shoulders can be a relatively large, powerful movement. This allows you to lift your body four to six inches with your arms, a necessary action for getting up out of a chair, for example. People confined to wheelchairs depend on this action.

Muscles that depress the shoulder are the pectoralis major, pectoralis minor, latissimus dorsi, and lower trapezius (Figures 1.16, 1.20, and 1.21). The pectoralis major and latissimus dorsi are primary. Since the range of depression from a neutral position is small, it's rarely limited to any extent by *antagonist* muscles, which have an opposing action to the movement in question.

Protraction

Protraction moves the shoulder forward (Figures 1.28 and 1.30). This action requires *abduction* of the shoulder blade, in which the shoulder blade may move away from the vertebral column as much as six inches. This brings the shoulder blade a little way around the side of the body, making part of its front surface accessible for massage. The front surface of the shoulder blade is where the subscapularis muscle resides. Since the subscapularis is usually at the heart of a frozen shoulder problem, learning to access it is vital. Muscles that protract the shoulder are the serratus anterior, pectoralis major, and pectoralis minor, with the pectoralis major having the strongest action (Figures 1.20, 1.21, and 1.24). Trigger points in the rhomboids, middle trapezius, or lower trapezius would limit protraction (Figures 1.16 and 1.17).

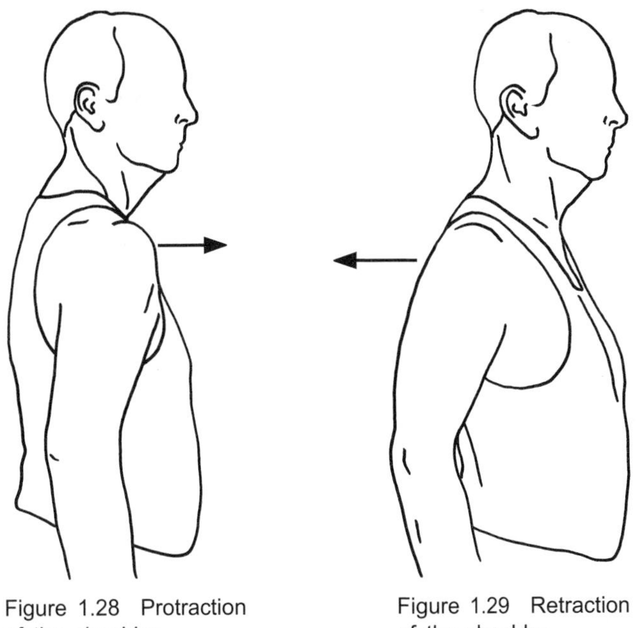

Figure 1.28 Protraction of the shoulder

Figure 1.29 Retraction of the shoulder

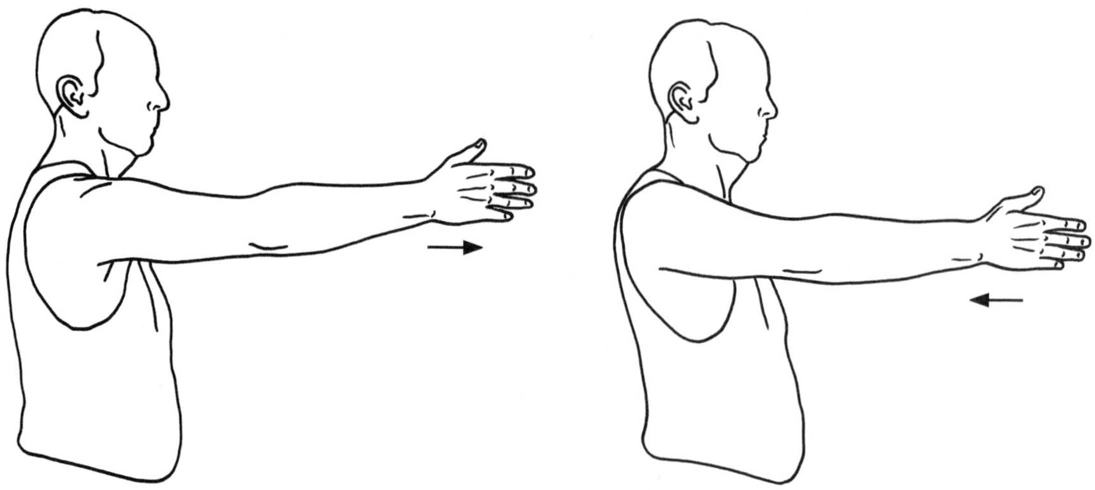

Figure 1.30 Protraction of the shoulder with forward flexion

Figure 1.31 Retraction of the shoulder with forward flexion

Retraction

Shoulder *retraction* is the opposite of protraction and involves pulling the shoulder back (Figures 1.29 and 1.31). This action requires *adduction* of the shoulder blade, which is a movement toward the spinal column. Contraction of the rhomboids and the entire trapezius muscle make the shoulder retract (Figures 1.16 and 1.17). Trigger points in the pectoralis major can limit this action and cause pain in the front of the shoulder (Figure 1.20).

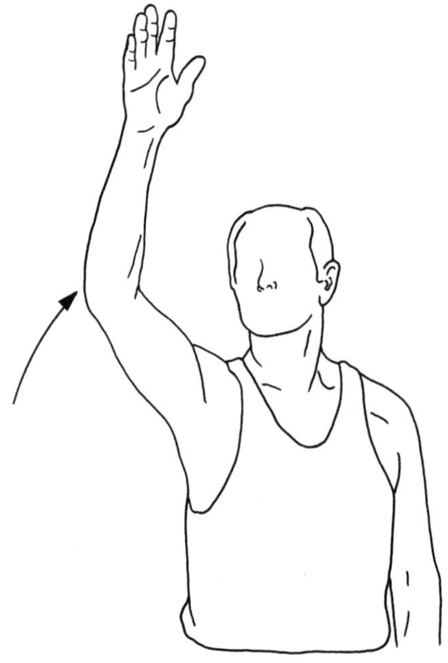

Figure 1.32 Abduction of the arm

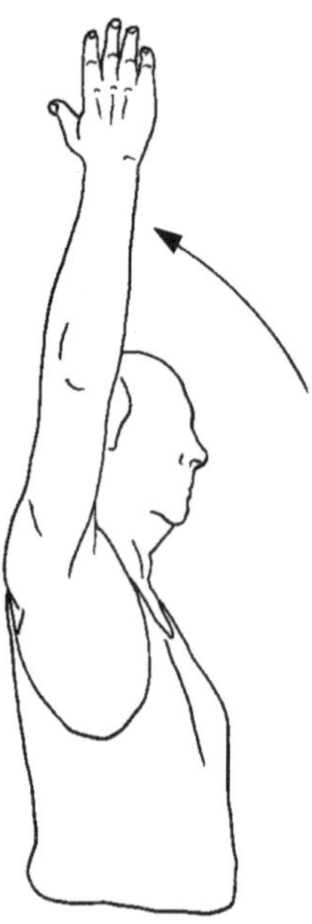

Figure 1.33 Flexion of the arm

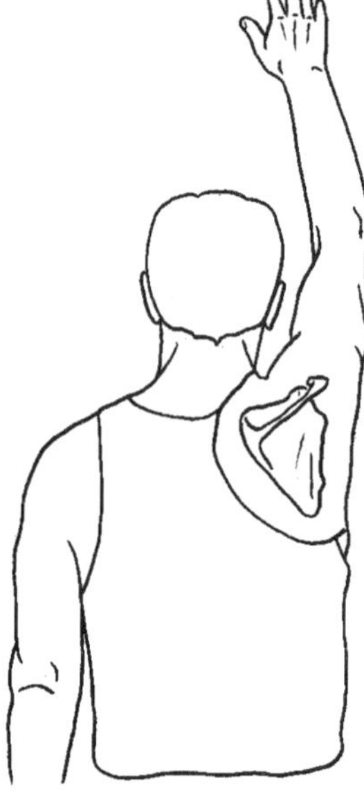

Figure 1.34 Upward rotation of the shoulder blade with abduction and flexion

Abduction

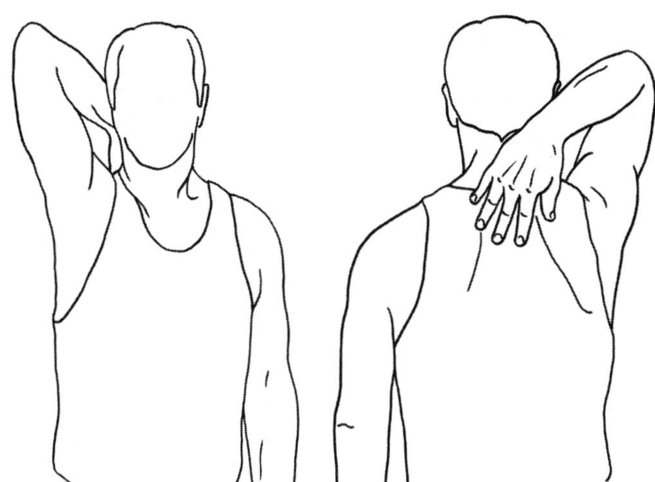

Figure 1.35 Abduction of the arm with flexion of the elbow, showing upward rotation of the shoulder blade

Raising the arm overhead is described as either *abduction* or *flexion*, depending on whether the arm is raised to the side or to the front (Figures 1.32 and 1.33). Figure 1.34 shows how the shoulder blade has to rotate upward for this action to occur. Figure 1.35 shows abduction of the arm along with flexion (bending) of the elbow. Abduction of the arm also requires contraction of the serratus anterior (Figure 1.24) to rotate the shoulder blade upward. The arm itself is moved upward by the deltoids, supraspinatus, and biceps (Figures 1.16, 1.17, 1.20, and 1.21).

To make the entire movement upward, the arm must rotate outward by contraction of the infraspinatus and teres minor (Figure 1.17). Because the subscapularis (Figure 1.22) has to lengthen to permit outward rotation, it's the muscle primarily involved in limiting upward movement of the arm. Subscapularis trigger points tend to prevent outward rotation and cause intense pain to remind you of the problem.

Adduction

Figures 1.36 and 1.37 illustrate *adduction* of the arm; that is, moving it across the body. Muscles that cause adduction are the pectoralis major, teres major, latissimus dorsi, and anterior deltoid, with the pectoralis major making most of the effort (Figures 1.16 and 1.20). Free adduction of the arm can be prevented by trigger points in the posterior deltoid, infraspinatus, teres minor, rhomboids, trapezius, and triceps (Figures 1.16 and 1.17). The infraspinatus would be the main culprit in preventing you from reaching across your body. Note that these antagonist muscles are all on the back of the body.

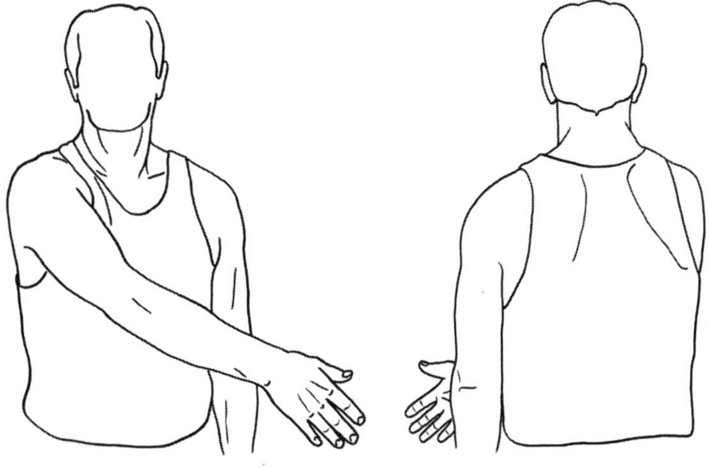

Figure 1.36 Adduction of the arm, the back view showing upward rotation of the shoulder blade

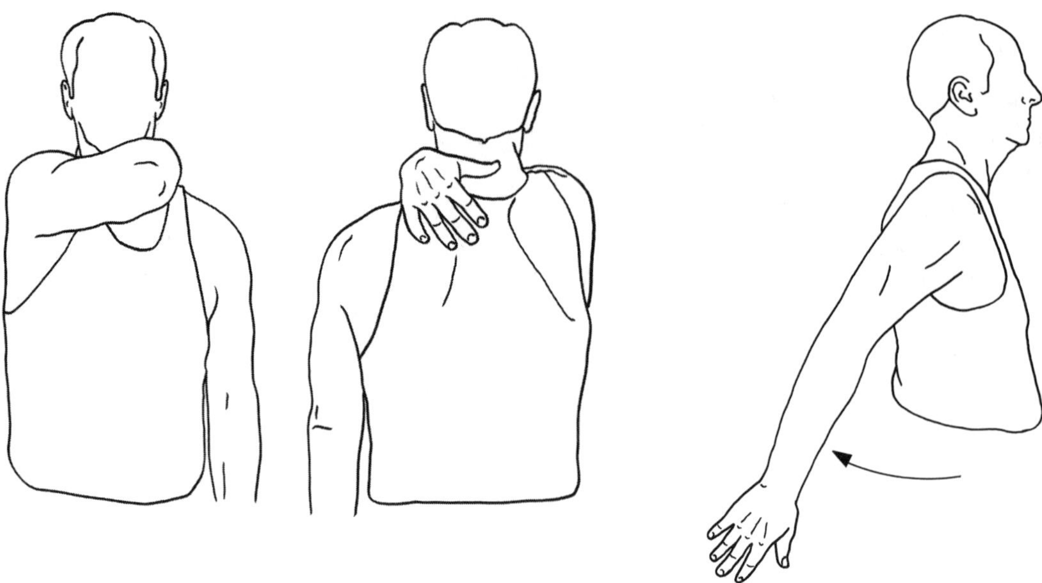

Figure 1.37 Adduction of the arm with flexion of the elbow, the back view showing upward rotation of the shoulder blade

Figure 1.38 Extension of the arm

Extension

Extension is the opposite of flexion. Strictly speaking, the term is *hyperextension* when the arm passes behind the plane of the body (Figure 1.38). The full range of extension can approach 60 degrees and is normally limited only by ligaments in the glenohumeral (ball-and-socket) joint. The muscles that produce extension of the arm are the latissimus dorsi, teres major, triceps, and posterior deltoid (Figures 1.16 and 1.17). Extension can be limited by trigger points in the pectoralis major, anterior deltoid, coracobrachialis, serratus anterior, and biceps (Figures 1.20, 1.21, 1.22, and 1.24).

Inward Rotation

Inward, or *internal, rotation* of the arm is shown in Figure 1.39. Putting your arm behind your back requires a combination of three actions: internal rotation of the arm, extension of the arm, and flexion of the elbow (Figure 1.40).

Rotation of the arm occurs at the ball-and-socket joint and is actuated by the rotator cuff muscles, which attach to the shoulder blade. Several other muscles are involved, depending on whether rotation is inward or outward. The arm's range of motion between maximum inward and outward rotation is a little over 90 degrees, but additional action of forearm muscles increases the hand's range of motion to 270 degrees. To study pure rotation of the arm, the elbow must be bent to take rotation of the forearm out of the picture.

Muscles that rotate the arm inward are the subscapularis, teres major, latissimus dorsi, and pectoralis major, with the subscapularis providing the most force (Figures 1.16, 1.20, and 1.22). Trigger points in the infraspinatus typically place a severe limit on internal rotation of the arm, and trouble in reaching up behind your back is usually traced to the infraspinatus (Figure 1.17).

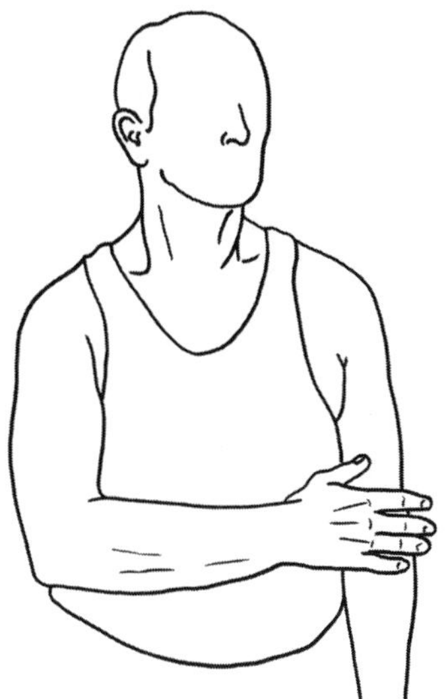

Figure 1.39 Inward rotation of the arm

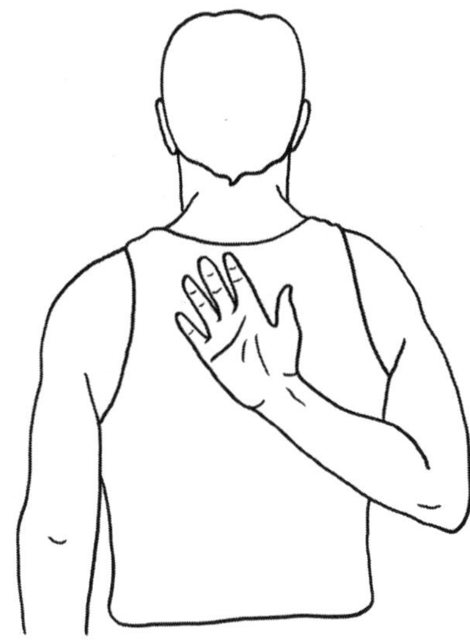

Figure 1.40 Internal rotation behind the back with flexion of the elbow

Outward Rotation

Outward, or *external, rotation* of the arm is pictured in Figure 1.41. Outward rotation calls for adduction of the shoulder blade; that is, moving it toward the spine (Figure 1.42). Muscles that cause external rotation are the infraspinatus, teres minor, and posterior deltoid (Figures 1.16 and 1.17). Working as partners, the infraspinatus and teres minor are the star actors in this scenario. The major villain is the subscapularis, which must lengthen maximally to allow external rotation (Figure 1.22). One of the worst kinds of pain experienced with a frozen shoulder comes when outward rotation is suddenly stopped by a subscapularis stiffened by trigger points.

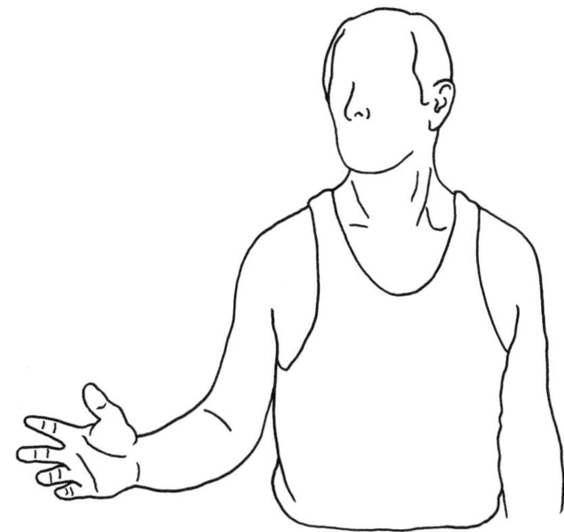

Figure 1.41 Outward rotation of the arm

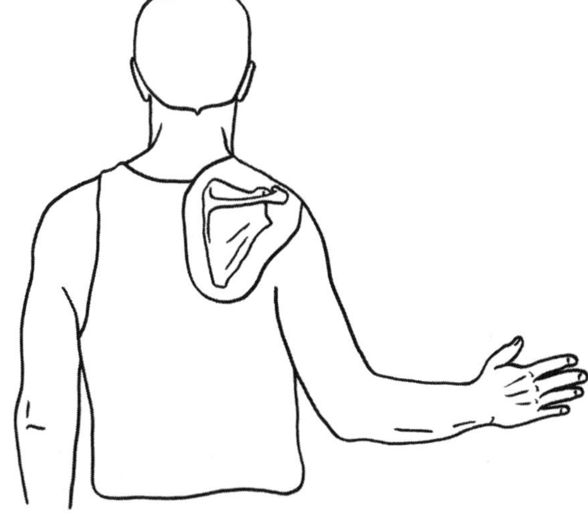

Figure 1.42 Outward rotation of the arm showing adduction of the shoulder blade

Chapter 2

The Science of Myofascial Pain

This chapter explains some of the details of trigger points: what they are, what they aren't, how they work, and the various types of trigger points. But before taking on the science of myofascial pain, you might like to know something about its two foremost proponents, Janet Travell and David Simons. These two extraordinary people dedicated much of their lives to demystifying this complex new science.

Janet G. Travell, MD

Anyone with debilitating shoulder pain will be interested to know that it was Janet Travell's own personal experience with shoulder pain that began her five-decade preoccupation with trigger points and myofascial pain. Dr. Travell tells about her shoulder episode in her autobiography, *Office Hours: Day and Night*, which was published in 1968, after she retired from her position as the first woman White House physician. She described the pain in her shoulder and arm as a steady ache that often kept her from sleeping. She also began having difficulty reaching for things. But it bothered her most that she had to stop playing tennis, her favorite recreation from an early age.

Janet Travell's shoulder trouble started in 1940, when she was thirty-eight years old and had been a practicing physician for over ten years. However, neither her medical education nor her clinical experience gave her any idea of what to do for her shoulder. From the beginning of her career, Dr. Travell loved research every bit as much as the practice of medicine, and she blamed the pain on overuse of her muscles during her many hours spent writing in longhand and doing the demanding laboratory work that she was so interested in writing about. But not being as limber and resilient as she had been at eighteen, an unlucky swing of her tennis racquet could easily have been a contributing factor, if not the actual initial cause (Travell 1968, 250-263).

Physician, Heal Thyself

Dr. Travell was particularly annoyed that she was in more pain than many of her patients but couldn't let on about it. The old adage "Physician, heal thyself" didn't seem to be an option because there really seemed to be no solution to the problem, except to try to outlive it. But Janet Travell wasn't that easily defeated. She was an unusually determined person who was courageous enough to become a physician during a time when women physicians weren't especially welcomed or respected by the men who dominated the field. It made all the difference that her father, Willard Travell, was a successful physician and gave her all his support.

Janet Graeme Travell was born in New York City on December 17, 1901. Influenced by the example set by her father, she and her sister, Virginia, both became doctors, Janet graduating from the Cornell Medical School in 1929. Virginia became a pediatrician. Janet became a cardiologist and pharmacologist.

When Janet Travell's shoulder trouble began, she was sharing her father's practice just above Washington Square in New York. Eager to expand her horizons, she was also engaged as visiting physician at the Sea View Hospital on Staten Island and Beth Israel Hospital in Manhattan. She was very interested in research into heart disease and the effects of cardiac drugs in particular, and both hospitals gave her opportunities to pursue these interests (Travell 1968, 208).

A Curious Coincidence

At the Cardiac Research Clinic at Beth Israel Hospital, Dr. Travell became aware that a number of her heart patients had also developed shoulder pain and stiffness. It appeared to be due to long-term immobility from prolonged bed rest. She was struck by the fact that the patients complained more about their shoulder symptoms than their heart problems.

At Sea View Hospital, which specialized in lung disease, not heart disease, Dr. Travell was intrigued to find that patients were having the same kind of trouble with their shoulders. And just as with her heart patients, the bedridden lung patients were complaining less about their pulmonary problems than about their shoulder pain. The pulmonary physicians assumed that the shoulder pain was somehow a result of disorders of the lungs. Interestingly, the cardiac doctors at Beth Israel had attributed their patients' shoulder pain to heart disease. Dr. Travell surmised that the true cause of shoulder pain in both groups could be related to the shoulder muscles themselves and their enforced immobility (Travell 1968, 252).

Intuition and Exploration

Dr. Travell found herself instinctively massaging her shoulder muscles, seeking any kind of relief from the oppressive, constant aching. She became aware that certain spots in the muscles overlying her shoulder blade were particularly sore. She was greatly astonished to discover that pressing tender spots in the muscles behind her shoulder intensified the pain in the front of her shoulder. When she pressed a spot, she got a shot of pain. She said it was like turning on an electrical switch.

This was Janet Travell's first experience with what she began to call the "trigger area." She knew of no anatomical explanation for the evident pain referral. There were no nerves directly connecting the mysterious tender spots with the places in her shoulder that hurt. She began searching the medical literature for some clue to what was going on.

Almost immediately she found a recently published article that dealt with the very problem she had seen in her bedridden hospital patients, the persistent pain in the shoulder that so often afflicted heart attack patients. The authors of the article told about one of their cardiac patients who found that pressure on the muscles covering his shoulder blade reproduced his shoulder pain—exactly what she had just discovered with her own shoulder (Travell 1968, 252).

Shortly thereafter, Dr. Travell found an article reporting treatment of "tender spots" in back muscles with Novocain injections in an effort to determine whether back pain and sciatica originated in the muscles themselves or in the spine. The authors speculated that if pain persisted in spite of the Novocain-deadened muscles, nerve impingement within the vertebral column must surely be the cause. She was excited to read that in one case the muscle injections had apparently cured the patient's sciatic pain (Travell 1968, 252-253).

A third article seemed to bring it all together. A German physician reported finding that certain tender spots in muscles characteristically referred pain elsewhere. Furthermore, injecting the spots with procaine hydrochloride (a form of Novocain) resulted in "spectacular relief." The author stressed that he got no results when he injected the places that hurt. It was electrifying to read that one of his patients had had the same shoulder pain and the same tender spots that Dr. Travell had found on herself and on her cardiac patients (Travell 1968, 253).

The First Clinical Experiments

In October 1940, Dr. Travell began systematically selecting patients who complained of shoulder pain and injecting their trigger areas with procaine. To her profound delight, the injections achieved long-lasting relief not only of their shoulder pain, but also of the false heart pain caused by tender spots in their chest muscles. She wondered whether she could cure her own shoulder pain with injections. It would be the definitive test.

Her father was extremely interested in her discoveries about pain. He participated in her experiment with enthusiasm. She couldn't reach the trigger areas on her shoulder blade, so he injected them for her. Remarkably, the pain that had oppressed her almost continuously for months melted away in just seconds. She and her father expected the pain might come creeping back as the procaine wore off, but it didn't.

Throughout the 1940s and 1950s, Janet Travell and her father continued sharing a practice in New York City. She never abandoned her interest in cardiology and pharmacology, but she spent more and more of her time researching and writing about pain. As her reputation grew, increasing numbers of her patients were those who suffered from chronic pain. They tended to be people who had sought help from all quarters and had tried everything for their pain. Dr. Travell went on to quietly accumulate twenty years of self-education in a field that few others knew anything about or seemed interested in exploring. She made trigger point therapy her own bailiwick. She became highly skilled and had the satisfaction of seeing her treatments succeed with almost perfect consistency.

The Acquisition of Authority

Among those who now recognize the reality and importance of myofascial pain, Janet Travell is generally recognized as the leading pioneer in its diagnosis and treatment. Many believe that she single-handedly created this branch of medicine. It was not a solo performance, of course. True innovation is seldom the product of a single mind. It's more often a matter of recombining bits and pieces of previous knowledge to solve a new problem.

Dr. Travell read widely, looking for anything she could glean from the work of other people that might address her interests. She discovered that many researchers around the world were beginning to tentatively explore the strange phenomenon of referred pain from trigger areas in muscles. But they all seemed to be working in isolation and largely unaware of one another's thinking. With extraordinary tenacity and persistence, she devoted herself to bringing it all together.

By the time the first volume of her *Myofascial Pain and Dysfunction: The Trigger Point Manual* went to press in 1983, Dr. Travell had been treating trigger points for over forty years and had published more than forty articles in medical journals. Janet Travell's revolutionary concepts about pain have improved the lives of millions of people. Effective techniques used by physicians and physical therapists for the treatment of myofascial pain all over the world wouldn't have existed without Dr. Travell's dedicated energy and intelligence. Trigger point massage, a method used by massage therapists for pain relief, has acquired a scientific foundation based almost entirely on Dr. Travell's insights.

A New Friend and a New Identity

Janet Travell's personal success with one particular patient had a far-reaching effect on history, and it may have been the event that ultimately paved the way for the publication and success of her comprehensive treatise on trigger points and myofascial pain.

Few now remember that Dr. Travell was the White House physician during the Kennedy and Johnson administrations. President Kennedy gave her that position in gratitude for her treatment of the debilitating pain and other ailments that in 1955 had threatened to prematurely end his political career. And in turn, Kennedy's recognition of Dr. Travell's unique knowledge and ability did immeasurable good in advancing trigger point therapy as a bona fide medical procedure. It gave her work validity and recognition that might have been impossible to attain otherwise.

Although in her sixties at the end of her duties at the White House, Dr. Travell had no intention of retiring or even slowing down. She went on developing and teaching her methods with vigor and enthusiasm for the next thirty years. She was past eighty when the first volume of the *Trigger Point Manual* was published and past ninety when the second volume appeared. She always said it was important not to rush into print. She wanted to get it right.

Requiescat In Pace

Doctor Travell spent a long life treating pain. It was part of her identity and a great part of her joy in being a kind and useful person. According to her daughters, Janet and Virginia, their mother was always enthusiastically "on call" at family reunions and holiday get-togethers. Everyone in the family who had a muscle problem would ask her to work on it. The same thing happened with guests at dinner parties. She never failed to respond (Pinci 2005). It's hard to imagine anyone more delightfully in love with their work.

On August 1, 1997, Janet Travell died at the age of ninety-five. She's buried alongside her father, mother, and husband, John Powell, in the Albany Rural Cemetery outside Albany, New York. Her simple gravestone bears her married name, Janet Graeme Powell, with no indication of her professional name, her accomplishments, or her place in history. Perhaps her legacy is more fittingly inscribed in the minds and hearts of those to whom she brought enlightenment and respite from pain.

David G. Simons, MD

Dr. Travell's collaborator, David Simons, shared her inborn single-minded tenacity. It would be hard to imagine anyone more decisive, purposeful, and resolute in the pursuit of their goals. Intent, impatient, and a little short-tempered, Dr. Simons has never let anything stand between him and the scientific truth he seeks. He was the prime mover in getting Janet Travell's immense knowledge and experience into written form and published. Anyone who benefits from trigger point therapy owes as much to David Simons as to Dr. Travell herself.

Man High

David Simons was born on June 7, 1922, in Lancaster, Pennsylvania. His father was a doctor, as Janet Travell's father had been. His father's influence, however, played out differently. David came of age during World War II and was strongly motivated to enlist himself in the battle as so many of his friends were doing. Providentially, the elder Simons took the longer view and insisted that his son go to medical school instead. Ironically, in the end it didn't keep the young man out of the military. David Simons joined the Air Force after medical school with a higher goal than simply being an Air Force doctor. At that time, space flight was just beginning to look like an actual possibility, and he had his eye on becoming an aerospace physician.

Dr. Simons was selected for a program for developing methods of measuring human responses to the stress of weightlessness. As with Janet Travell, David Simons's natural bent toward research found its direction early. Also like his future colleague, his enthusiasm impelled him to employ his own body in his experiments. On a number of occasions, he virtually became the experiment. The literal zenith of his Air Force career was setting the world altitude record for manned balloon flight in August 1957. The project was called Man High, and Dr. Simons actually beat Sputnik to the edge of space by a little over a month. He was featured on the cover of *Life* magazine that year and subsequently wrote *Man High* (1960), a riveting book about his adventure.

In heart-stopping detail, Dr. Simons tells of the real risks to his life and health when he ascended alone to a height of 102,000 feet with only the most primitive equipment to sustain his existence. Although his space capsule with its life-support systems were certainly the best that could be devised, today it looks like nothing more than an oversized tin can. Its primitive technology speaks vividly to Dr. Simon's bravery in the face of the unknown, a more heroic use of his spirit perhaps than carrying a rifle on the front lines would have been a few years earlier. Dr. Simons's flight yielded an enormous amount of information and made the subsequent effort to put humans into orbit much less dangerous than it might have been otherwise.

A Momentous Meeting

David Simons first met Janet Travell while she was still White House physician. She had traveled to the School of Aerospace Medicine at Brooks Air Force Base in San Antonio, Texas, to give a program about trigger points and myofascial pain. Dr. Simons was so intrigued by Dr. Travell's ideas that in 1965 he abandoned the rewards and excitement of his work with the Air Force to begin a long informal apprenticeship in pain medicine under her wing. A remarkable synergy developed between the two during the next two decades, culminating at last in the production of volume 1 of *Myofascial Pain and Dysfunction: The Trigger Point Manual* (1983), a testament to the transcendent power generated when two minds of uncommon intelligence work together.

Dr. Simons's strict attention to detail and adherence to scientific method helped him bring rigorous objectivity to the documentation of myofascial pain. He was the driving force in getting the *Trigger Point Manual* written, doing most of the actual writing himself, with Dr. Travell's vast knowledge and experience as his primary resource.

Unhappily, it must be said that at the present time relatively few physicians have studied this magnificent resource. The vast majority cling to antiquated beliefs regarding the treatment of pain. As a consequence, millions of people with easily treatable myofascial pain continue to suffer needlessly. Hopefully the day is not far away when ordinary people everywhere will know about trigger points and the diagnosis and treatment of myofascial pain will be taught as a standard course in medical schools. The world will then recognize Dr. Simons, along with his mentor, Dr. Janet Travell, as true medical pioneers.

The Trigger Point Manual

Everything of a technical nature in this chapter originated in the second edition of volume 1 of Travell and Simons's *Myofascial Pain and Dysfunction: The Trigger Point Manual* (Simons, Travell, and Simons 1999). Four very lengthy chapters of the *Trigger Point Manual* are devoted to the science of trigger points and myofascial pain and backed up by references to several hundred scientific articles by other researchers. Those first four chapters alone would make up a sizable and very technical book, far too much to impose on the general reader. The object here is to make that valuable material more accessible by condensing it to a single chapter and putting it into words the average reader can understand.

The science of myofascial pain deals only with symptoms that come from trigger points in muscles. Travell and Simons discuss other kinds of pain, such as that caused by disease or physical trauma, only when it's necessary to distinguish them from myofascial pain. In addition, they were mainly concerned with the pain caused by trigger points in individual muscles. Very often, however, a pain problem is a composite of referred pain from several muscles. Pain in the shoulder can be just this kind of composite.

For the purpose of troubleshooting various kinds of pain, Travell and Simons made lists of muscles that send pain to specific areas of the body. The muscles are listed in the order of their probable involvement in the particular pain. As an example, in their section on pain in the upper back, shoulder, and arm, the list for pain in the front of the shoulder includes eleven muscles. This book follows that model, with the addition of the brachialis (Figure 2.1).

Trigger points in the first muscle on the list, the infraspinatus, actually cause most of the pain in the front of the shoulder, but other muscles on the list often contribute part of it. In some cases, the first muscle on the list might play a minor role and another muscle further down would be causing most of the trouble. These lists are the place to start in solving the problem of pain. This book uses similar lists for troubleshooting pain in the shoulder. You can find them in the two-page Trigger Point Guide at the beginning of chapter 5 and at the end of the book.

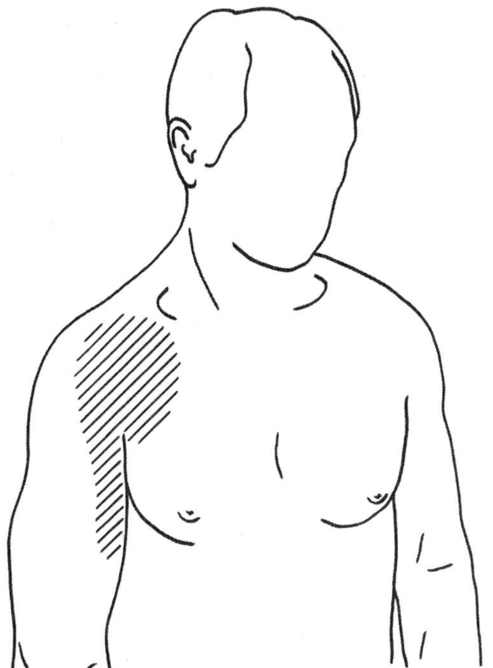

Front-of-Shoulder Pain

1. infraspinatus
2. anterior deltoid
3. scalenes
4. supraspinatus
5. pectoralis major
6. pectoralis minor
7. subscapularis
8. biceps
9. latissimus dorsi
10. coracobrachiallis
11. subclavius
12. brachialis

Figure 2.1 This referred pain pattern is likely to be a composite of pain from trigger points in two or more muscles on the list.

The Scourge of Mankind

Travell and Simons portray trigger points without exaggeration as the "scourge of mankind." Pain from trigger points can be just as harsh as pain caused by a heart attack, kidney stone, or broken bone. Also, pain from a very small muscle can be as bad or worse than pain from a large muscle. Trigger points rarely constitute a risk to life, but the misery they cause can be extremely demoralizing and devastating to quality of life (Simons, Travell, and Simons 1999, 13-14).

Pervasiveness

Trigger points are an extremely common natural phenomenon. It's difficult to imagine anyone escaping them or being in any way immune. In most people, trigger points are present somewhere in their musculature most of the time, at least in a latent state.

Since trigger points are found primarily in muscle tissue, they have a very large territory for creating mischief. You may be surprised to learn that muscle is considered an organ. In fact, muscle is the largest organ in the body, making up an average 50 percent of the body weight. Any of the hundreds of individual muscles in the human body can develop trigger points, and the twenty-four muscles involved in shoulder pain are some of the most common places for trigger points to be found. Pain is the reason given by patients for medical office visits 25 percent of the time. Doctors who specialize in the treatment of myofascial pain have found that trigger points are the main cause of pain 75 percent of the time and that they nearly always contribute to pain problems, even when the pain originates from disease or trauma. The pain inflicted by trigger points may be the biggest cause of disability and loss of time in any workplace or office, in any professional or amateur sport, or simply in day-to-day life (Simons, Travell, and Simons 1999, 12-14).

One of the difficulties in diagnosing and treating trigger points is that their symptoms can mimic many other conditions. Trigger points are known to cause headaches, neck and jaw pain, low back pain, the symptoms of carpal tunnel syndrome, and many kinds of joint pain mistakenly ascribed to arthritis, tendinitis, bursitis, or ligament injury. Trigger points cause problems as diverse as earaches, dizziness, nausea, heartburn, false heart pain, heart arrhythmia, tennis elbow, and genital pain. They can cause sinus pain and congestion, and they may play a part in chronic fatigue and lowered resistance to infection. Even fibromyalgia, which is known to afflict millions of people, is thought in many instances to have its beginning with trigger points (Simons, Travell, and Simons 1999, 12-19; Gerwin 1995, 121; Fishbain et al. 1986, 181-197).

An underestimated trait of trigger points is that they can exist indefinitely in a latent state. Latent trigger points tend to accumulate over a lifetime and appear to be the main cause for the stiff joints and restricted range of motion of old age. The constant muscle tension imposed by latent trigger points tends to overstress muscle attachments even in younger people. Over time, this can do irreversible damage to the joints and may be one of the causes of osteoarthritis.

You may not suspect that you have latent trigger points because they don't cause pain. They're very easy to find, however, because they hurt when you press them. Overactivity can quickly turn latent trigger points into active trigger points that cause spontaneous pain (Simons, Travell, and Simons 1999, 12-21).

Medical Neglect

Despite the importance of muscles as a primary source of common pain, medical students are actually taught very little about them, except as part of the human anatomy. There is no medical specialty devoted to the diagnosis and treatment of muscle disease. In the practice of medicine, attention is directed instead to the joints, bones, bursas, and nerves. This misplaced attention causes a great deal of misdiagnosis and inappropriate treatment (Simons, Travell, and Simons 1999, 13).

The financial cost of the medical community's lack of understanding of trigger points and myofascial pain is enormous, and most of this cost is unnecessary. The tragedy is that physicians continue to be so uninformed, even though the pain-causing knots in muscles have been written about for more than a century (Simons, Travell, and Simons 1999, 14-18).

Early Discoveries

The first research having to do with what we now know as trigger points was published in Germany in 1843 (Froriep 1843). The writer brought attention to tender tight cords or taut strands in muscles that seemed associated with pain. He called them *muskelschwiele* (muscle calluses).

Over the next hundred years in both Germany and England, additional papers were published using new terms such as *muskelhärten* (muscle hardenings) or *myogelosen* (muscle gellings). In their search for understanding, each successive writer, apparently unaware of the writings and terminology of previous authors, contributed to a veritable plague of terms:

muscular indurations, tender nodules, *muskel rheumatismus*, muscle rheumatism, myofascitis, fibrositis, myalgia, and so on.

Interest in muscle pain accelerated during the first half of the twentieth century, although researchers apparently continued to work in isolation, oblivious to one another's labors. In 1919, it was reported in Germany that "muscle gellings" persisted even after death, indicating that they weren't dependent on nervous system activity. It wasn't until 1938 that German and English scientists separately discovered that referred pain was a characteristic of these "muscle hardenings." In 1941, Michael Kelly, an Australian physician, made important systematic links between tender nodules, referred pain, and the chronic pain then widely known as fibrositis and rheumatism.

In 1942, Janet Travell began publishing in the United States. She collated all previous knowledge about referred muscle pain, offered an effective treatment protocol, and introduced the term "trigger point" to describe the critical heart of the matter. The work of the many widely dispersed researchers was extremely important in laying a foundation for the understanding and treatment of myofascial pain, but only Janet Travell's all-encompassing research and carefully perfected clinical applications have withstood the test of time.

What Is a Trigger Point?

Considering the overwhelming importance and pervasiveness of myofascial trigger points, it's incredible that they've remained a mystery as long as they have—and that they're still a mystery to most of the world! The term "trigger point" is still largely unknown to the general public, and you won't find "trigger point" in general dictionaries. Medical dictionaries and other medical references are finally beginning to give trigger points some recognition, but usually no more than a sparse paragraph or two at best.

One thing that has stood in the way of acceptance has been the lack of a clear definition that everybody could understand. It's not easy to say just exactly what a trigger point is. A scientific definition is often easier to produce than something in common language. But sometimes a scientifically precise definition, if you can't understand it, can be very little better than no definition at all.

Defining a Trigger Point

According to Travell and Simons, a trigger point is "a highly irritable localized spot of exquisite tenderness in a nodule in a palpable taut band of muscle tissue." Translated, that just means a trigger point is a knotty place in a muscle that hurts like the devil when you press on it.

The trigger point nodule feels like a small lump in the muscle, usually no bigger than a pea. A trigger point has been described as being like a little piece of partially cooked macaroni or spaghetti. You need a very good sense of touch to feel a trigger point nodule, and not everyone has that ability. Even skilled massage therapists who rely on their sense of touch can have trouble finding trigger points in heavy muscles or those covered with too much fat. In self-treating trigger points, however, you don't have to be able to find the little lumps by feel. You just search around for the spot that feels the most exquisitely tender.

The "palpable taut band" is a tight strand of fibers in the muscle that feels like a cord or small cable (Figure 2.2). A taut band extends from the trigger point in both directions to its

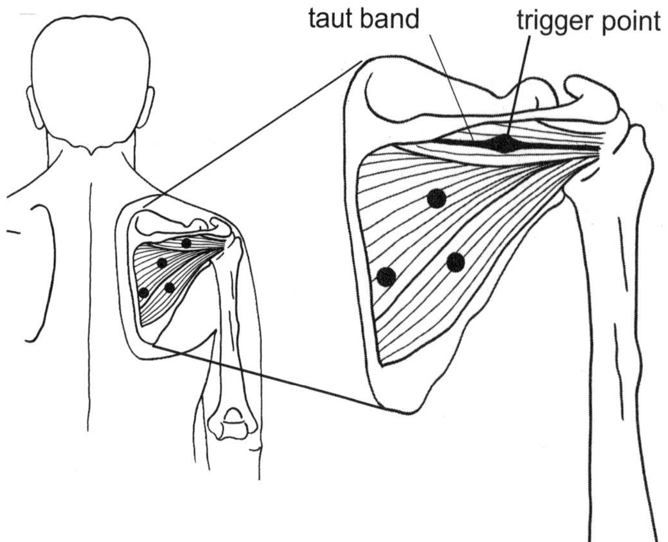

Figure 2.2 Infraspinatus muscle, showing an enlarged view of a trigger point and its associated taut band of muscle fibers. All the black dots are trigger points.

attachments and can easily be mistaken for a tendon. A taut band can be the most troublesome part of the problem because it restricts your range of motion by limiting the muscle's ability to lengthen. Multiple taut bands in your shoulder muscles are, in fact, what make your shoulder stiff, keep you from moving your arm, and ultimately lead to a frozen shoulder.

It's important to grasp that a trigger point is not a muscle spasm, although you will sometimes see them described as such, even in medical literature. A spasm is a sudden, hard contraction of the entire muscle. A trigger point and its associated taut band are a *contracture* of only a small strand within the muscle. A spasm can usually be relaxed in a matter of minutes. Trigger points don't give up that easily.

You shouldn't get too caught up in a search for clearly distinguishable lumps in your muscles. It's better to think in terms of the *sarcomeres*, the smallest units of contraction, that are causing the problem by getting stuck and staying continuously contracted. You can't feel these minuscule sarcomeres individually, but a large number of them in a fairly compact cluster might indeed be felt as a clearly defined nodule (a trigger point or knot).

In actuality, this cluster of sarcomeres is often spread a little more loosely over an area as large as a nickel or a fifty-cent piece. This kind of spot in the muscle could feel somewhat denser, but not necessarily knotlike. In this case, you'd want to think of a trigger point as a trigger "area" and the defining characteristic would be the spot's tenderness, not that you could necessarily feel an actual knot (Simons 2006).

Let's put the scientific definition into everyday words: A trigger point is a very sore spot in a muscle that often feels like a small lump in a tendonlike cord. Even when you can't locate a trigger point by feel, it will always hurt when you press on it.

Facial or Fascial?

When people first hear about myofascial trigger points, they sometimes think they cause pain only in the face, getting "fascial" mixed up with "facial." Trigger points certainly can cause face pain, but myofascial pain can occur anywhere in the body. The prefix "myo" in myofascial refers to muscle. "Fascial" refers to fascia, the thin, translucent membrane that envelops and separates muscles like shrink-wrap. It covers every muscle in your body. (A good place to see fascia is on a chicken leg, after the skin has been removed.) When you have trigger points in a muscle, its fascia typically gets tight and inflexible and becomes part of the problem.

Too Many Points

Janet Travell originally used the term "trigger area" to denote what she later began calling a trigger point. The earlier term did make sense, because the trouble spot was often buried so deeply in the muscle that its boundaries couldn't be clearly defined. When you're trying to find a trigger point, it sometimes does seem more like a small area than a point. Indeed, "trigger point" may not be the best term to use for the phenomenon, but it's so well established now that it would be useless to attempt a change.

Unfortunately, there are other problems with the name. For one thing, the word "trigger" is vastly overused and has a wide variety of connotations. And there are also so many systems of points that people sometimes confuse trigger points with other kinds of points.

Acupressure Points

Many mistakenly believe that trigger points are the same thing as *acupressure points*, or *acupoints*. In reality, they're quite different. The concepts of trigger points and myofascial pain have evolved within the bounds of Western medical research and clinical practice, whereas acupressure points are one of the foundations of the time-honored traditions of Chinese medicine. A similar system of points is used with shiatsu, a Japanese bodywork modality.

An acupressure or acupuncture point is believed to be a kind of blockage somewhere along one of the body's supposed energy pathways, the fourteen meridians. As an example, Figure 2.3 shows the stomach meridian with several of its acupressure points.

It's difficult to prove that the energy meridians and acupressure points exist. They can't be felt or seen, and they aren't aligned with any of the body's systems—circulatory, nervous, skeletal, or muscular. Acupressure points have never been identified by any kind of sensory or physical observation. A trigger point, on the other hand, does have a scientific explanation, and a very credible one at that. A trigger point can also be physically detected and measured in several ways.

A trigger point usually refers pain, whereas an acupressure point does not. You can physically find a trigger point because it's painful to the touch, and sometimes you can feel it in the muscle. You can't find an acupressure point by feel, and it doesn't hurt when pressed unless it happens to coincide with a trigger point. The only material evidence of an acupressure point's existence is a dot and a number printed on a chart.

Despite a lack of objective verification, acupressure enjoys success as pain therapy with a great many people both in the East and in the West. Believers call it "acupressure analgesia." Its effectiveness, however, has been shown to result primarily from the placebo effect and the incidental treatment of trigger points (Simons, Travell, and Simons 1999, 41-42; Melzack, Fox, and Stillwell 1977, 3-23). Perhaps the ancient Chinese who developed the meridian theory were searching for an explanation for the effects of touch on what we now know as myofascial trigger points.

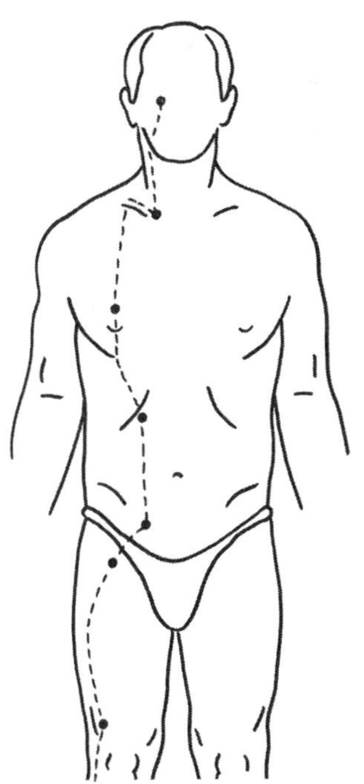

Figure 2.3 Acupressure points on the stomach meridian

Reflex Points

Reflexology is an acupressure-like system wherein pressure or massage is applied to "reflex" points on the feet or hands, purportedly having a healthful effect on specific places in the body. Pressure on the reflex point for the liver, for instance, would stimulate the body's natural healing powers as they affect the liver, increasing circulation and the free flow of energy. There are reflex points on the soles of the feet for each of the major organs and other vulnerable parts of the body, such as the eyes, ears, sinuses, and glands (Figure 2.4). The reflex points are said to be crystalline deposits under the skin created by the sluggish flow of energy in ten vertical zones on the body. Reflex points can be horribly painful spots.

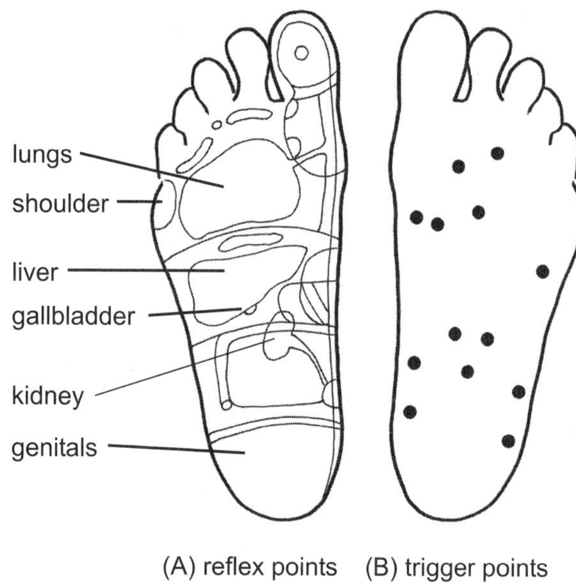

Figure 2.4 (A) Reflex points and (B) trigger points on the bottom of the foot show little relationship.

One of the snags in the reflexology theory is that there are seven muscles on the bottom of each foot that are especially prone to having myofascial trigger points. Although there's little correspondence between the location of reflex points and trigger points, reflexology's rubbing strokes may sometimes incidentally treat trigger points, and this would certainly be therapeutic as far as foot pain is concerned. An enhanced sense of well-being elsewhere in the body could easily be attributed to the relaxing effect of foot pain relief. To be sure, when your feet feel better, you often feel better all over. Practitioners of reflexology, to their credit, usually don't claim that it can cure anything.

Pressure Points

People often say "pressure points" when they can't remember "trigger points." This confusion is understandable because you do press on both. But a *pressure point* or *pulse point* is the place over an artery that you press to stop the flow of blood from a wound. In contrast, the pressure used on a trigger point in the form of massage increases blood flow. Pressure on a pressure point is held continuously until the bleeding stops and the danger is past. The pressure on a trigger point in the form of a repeated massage stroke is relatively brief. There are twelve commonly recognized pressure points. Except for the aorta pulse point, all are present on both sides of the body (Figure 2.5). Pressure points and trigger points can be close to one another, but they are in no way the same thing.

Martial Arts Points

Pressure points are used in the martial arts, too (Figure 2.6). In this case, they're obviously not used for therapy, although after a session of deadly pressure point fighting you may feel the need for treatment of some kind.

Practitioners of martial arts systems such as karate, kung fu, tae kwon do, and jujitsu develop skill in striking their opponent's pressure points for the purpose of self-defense. In

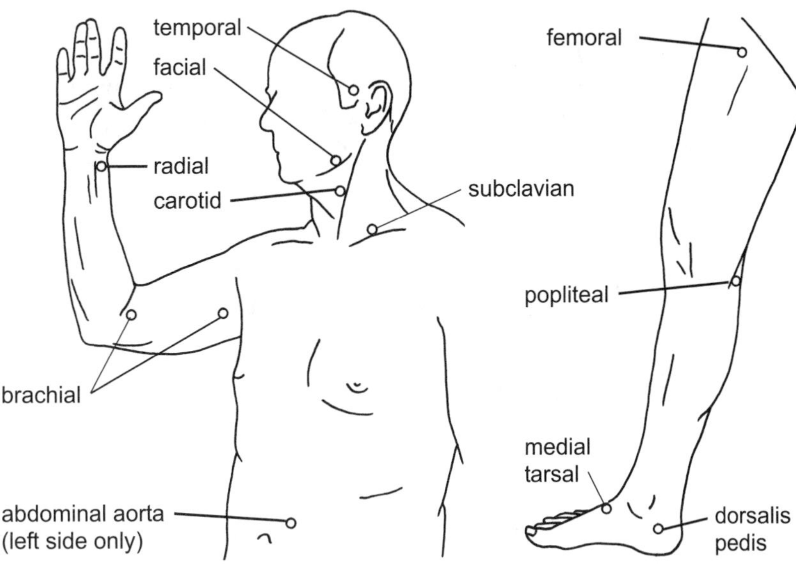

Figure 2.5 The twelve pressure points (pulse points) with the names of the arteries. All pressure points are present on both sides of the body, except the aorta.

pressure point fighting, a blow delivered to an opponent's most vulnerable places can impose several moments of severe immobilizing pain, leaving you free to make a quick escape or disable your opponent further with other techniques.

Sometimes called *vital points, striking points,* or *hit points,* these martial arts defense points are simply vulnerable places on the body. They have no relationship to acupressure points, pressure points for stanching blood flow, or any other system, although many proponents have tried to make such a connection. The deadly reputation of martial arts strike points is largely mythical, having evolved through comic books, movies, and the martial arts industry.

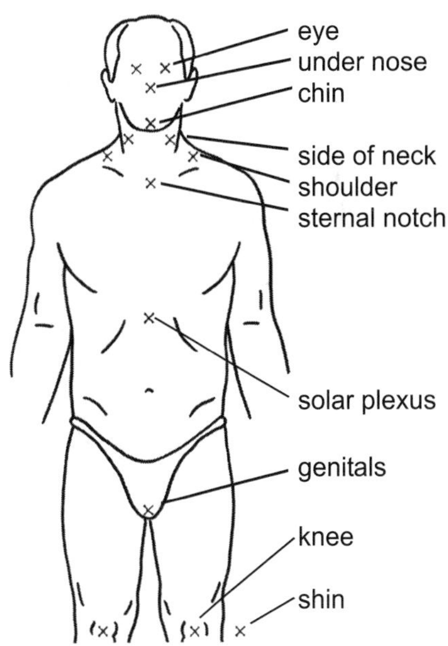

Figure 2.6 The ten strike points of martial arts

Interestingly, two of the striking points in the drawing coincide with places where almost everyone has trigger points: the side of the neck and the top of the shoulder. The extreme tenderness of the trapezius muscle on the top of the shoulder is the origin of the infamous Vulcan death grip from *Star Trek.* You may indeed feel that your life is in imminent danger if someone unexpectedly squeezes you there, but it's extremely unlikely that the Vulcan death grip has actually killed anyone, in this galaxy at least.

Fibromyalgia Tender Points

Trigger points are often mixed up with *tender points,* one of the official criteria for a diagnosis of fibromyalgia. This is a serious mistake when made by a professional, because

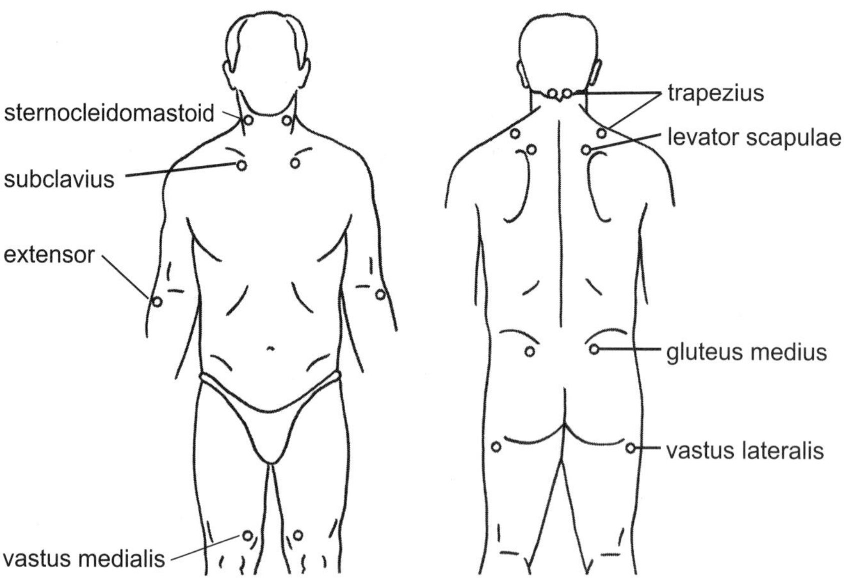

Figure 2.7 Fibromyalgia's eighteen tender points, each coincident with a trigger point in the muscles indicated

fibromyalgia itself has no known cure and tender points can't be treated by any known means. Trigger points, on the other hand, can be treated with good reason to expect relief of symptoms.

There are eighteen officially designated tender points, nine on each side of the body (Figure 2.7). In order to qualify for a diagnosis of fibromyalgia, a person must have had at least eleven of these points for three months and must have tender points in all four quadrants of the body. These standards were established in 1990 by the American College of Rheumatology, and only a medical doctor has the authority to make a fibromyalgia diagnosis. Unfortunately, it's often made in error.

The problem with diagnosing fibromyalgia is that all of the eighteen tender points coincide with the locations of very common myofascial trigger points. There's some question as to whether all of the physicians who are diagnosing fibromyalgia can actually tell the difference between a tender point and a trigger point. You might also question whether the people who established the diagnostic standards knew the difference.

A mistaken diagnosis of fibromyalgia is a gross disservice to someone who suffers from chronic pain. In reality, many people diagnosed with fibromyalgia are afflicted only with widespread myofascial trigger points, which can be treated successfully. Moreover, a great part of the pain experienced in genuine fibromyalgia is often due to trigger points. Massage is widely recognized as the single most effective way to deal with fibromyalgia because it can bring some relief by treating the trigger points that usually accompany this condition.

There are clear guidelines for distinguishing trigger points from tender points. Muscles afflicted with trigger points usually feel firm yet resilient and often seem quite hard and stringy because of multiple taut bands. The muscles of a victim of true fibromyalgia have a soft, doughy quality. A trigger point needs firm pressure to elicit pain, whereas a tender point is typically so painful it can hardly be touched. In addition, tender points cause only local pain. They don't refer pain to another site as trigger points usually do.

People genuinely afflicted with fibromyalgia ordinarily have both types of points concurrently. If they can bear treatment of their trigger points, it often markedly diminishes their pain. The practitioner must have the ability to discriminate between trigger points and tender points, as well as the wisdom to limit treatment to only what the person can tolerate without adverse reactions (Simons, Travell, and Simons 1999, 36-41, 140-142).

The Physiology of a Trigger Point

Physicians who haven't taken the time to study trigger points and myofascial pain tend to doubt they exist. Regarding her resistant peers, Janet Travell often spoke with a twinkle in her eye of her need to "rearrange their prejudices." Her enduring aspiration was to scientifically validate the existence of myofascial trigger points and convert the disbelievers. Although far too many physicians still remain unconvinced, Dr. Travell managed to build a very strong scientific basis for the acceptance of this radical new science among those willing to at least tentatively open their minds and consider the evidence.

The Validation of Trigger Points

One of Dr. Travell's earliest discoveries occurred in 1957 when she found that trigger points generate tiny electrical currents. This allowed the activity of a trigger point to be quantified by measuring these tiny signals with electromyographic instruments. The precise location of a trigger point could also be determined by this same means. A number of other things were revealed by studying these electrical signals.

Muscle tissue is electrically active only when in a state of contraction. It follows that when electrical activity is confined to a very small area, only a small part of the muscle is contracting. Dr. Travell found that pressing on a trigger point increases its electrical activity. Stretching a muscle did the same thing, which may explain why stretching so often makes pain worse, perhaps by irritating the trigger point (Simons, Travell, and Simons 1999, 58-69).

Dr. Travell established that the most convincing practical demonstration of the existence of trigger points was to simply feel for them with the fingers. Active and latent trigger points alike give a distinctively painful response to pressure. If a trigger point is near the surface, sensitive fingers can detect that it's a little warmer than surrounding tissue. This temperature difference, which is due to increased metabolic activity in the trigger point, is measurable (Simons, Travell, and Simons 1999, 29-30).

Being soft tissue, trigger points can't be seen on X-rays. They have been viewed, however, with both electron and light microscopy in fresh human cadavers and in live animal biopsies. In the second edition of volume 1 of the *Trigger Point Manual*, Travell and Simons include a very elucidating microscopic photograph of a trigger point in a dog's leg muscle (Simons, Travell, and Simons, 1999, 69). Dr. Simons permitted use of the photograph in this book and it appears in the next section (Figure 2.11).

Janet Travell's meticulous scientific investigations have great value for the scientifically minded. For practical purposes, however, all the average person really needs to know about trigger points is that they're extremely sore spots in muscles that send pain to other places. With this uncomplicated idea in mind and trigger point charts in hand, a dedicated individual usually has no trouble finding trigger points and successfully treating them.

For those who feel the need to go deeper into the science of myofascial pain, it can be quite a challenge. The physiology of a trigger point is fascinating, but it's complex. Even so, you can simplify the study of trigger points by looking at them in two separate ways: microscopically and electrochemically.

The Microscopic View of a Trigger Point

A muscle fiber actually consists of a bundle of several hundred smaller fibers called *myofibrils*. As seen in Figure 2.8, the muscle fibers themselves make up larger units called *fascicles*. Numerous fascicles, in turn, are bound together by fascia to form a section of muscle. There are approximately one hundred fibers in a fascicle, and each muscle fiber contains between one thousand and two thousand myofibrils. Interestingly, a myofibril is actually a muscle cell, which because of its unusual length contains more than one nucleus.

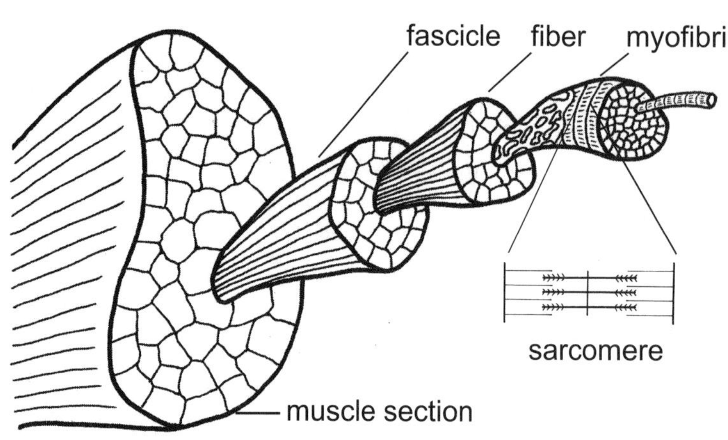

Figure 2.8 Step dissection of muscle tissue, showing a sample muscle section, fascicle, muscle fiber, myofibril, and sarcomere

The smallest unit of muscle contraction that can be seen at the microscopic level is in a tiny part of the myofibril called a *sarcomere* (Figures 2.8 and 2.9). Figure 2.9 shows a sarcomere relaxed (A) and contracted (B). Note that the contracted sarcomere is considerably shorter.

Each myofibril is made up of a chain of sarcomeres connected end to end. An element called a *Z band* separates each sarcomere like a thin wall. Note in Figure 2.9 that the Z bands in the contracted sarcomere have moved closer together. The length of a fully contracted sarcomere can approach half the length of a fully relaxed sarcomere. It's estimated that the average length of an uncontracted human sarcomere is about 1.3 microns, or about 0.00005 inch (Mense and Simons 2001, 252). That's small enough to make a sarcomere seem insignificant, but it's actually where all the action is.

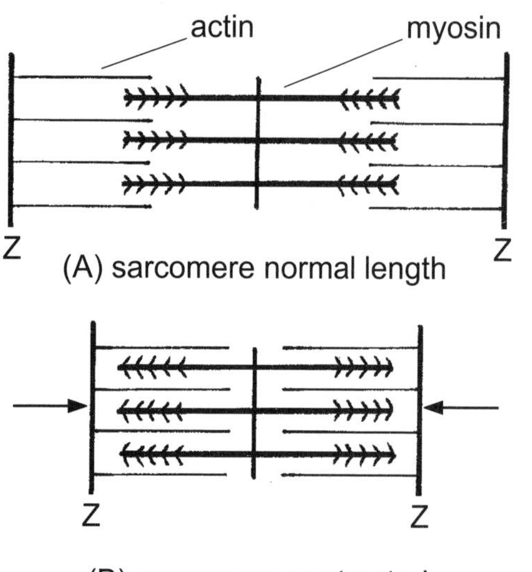

Figure 2.9 The sarcomere, the contractile mechanism of muscle, shown (A) normal length and (B) contracted

The essential parts of each sarcomere are two filament-like protein molecules: *actin* and *myosin*. Contraction occurs in a sarcomere when the actin and myosin molecules are attracted to one another and come together, somewhat like interlocking your fingers to bring your hands together. This action shortens the sarcomere, which in turn shortens its tiny part of the muscle. The shortening of sarcomeres is the heart of muscle contraction. As you can imagine, millions of sarcomeres have to contract in order to make even the smallest movement.

Relaxation of a sarcomere happens when the actin and myosin are repelled from one another and pull apart. They never separate completely. Instead, they stand ready to reunite at the least urging by an impulse from the nervous system. A muscle can be exhausted by any kind of work or play that requires its sarcomeres to contract and relax too often. A trigger point comes into being when exhaustion causes actin and myosin to become stuck in their interlocked state. This locking up of the sarcomeres occurs about midway along the length of the muscle, right where the *motor nerve* enters. The motor nerve is the means for transmitting the signal telling the muscle to contract (Simons, Travell, and Simons 1999, 45-57).

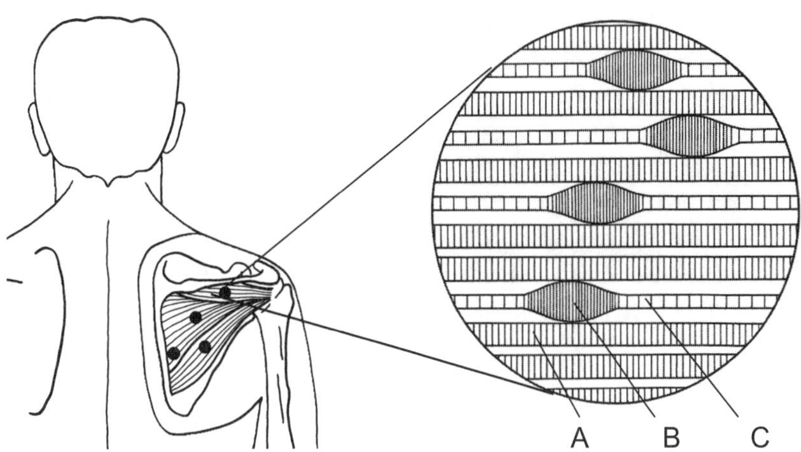

Figure 2.10 Microscopic view of contracted sarcomeres. An actual trigger point may contain several dozen of these tiny knots.

Figure 2.10 depicts several muscle fibers within a trigger point in the infraspinatus muscle of the shoulder. The illustration is a representation of a microscope photograph of an actual sarcomere contracture that makes up a trigger point (Figure 2.11). An examination of Figure 2.10 clarifies what is seen in Figure 2.11.

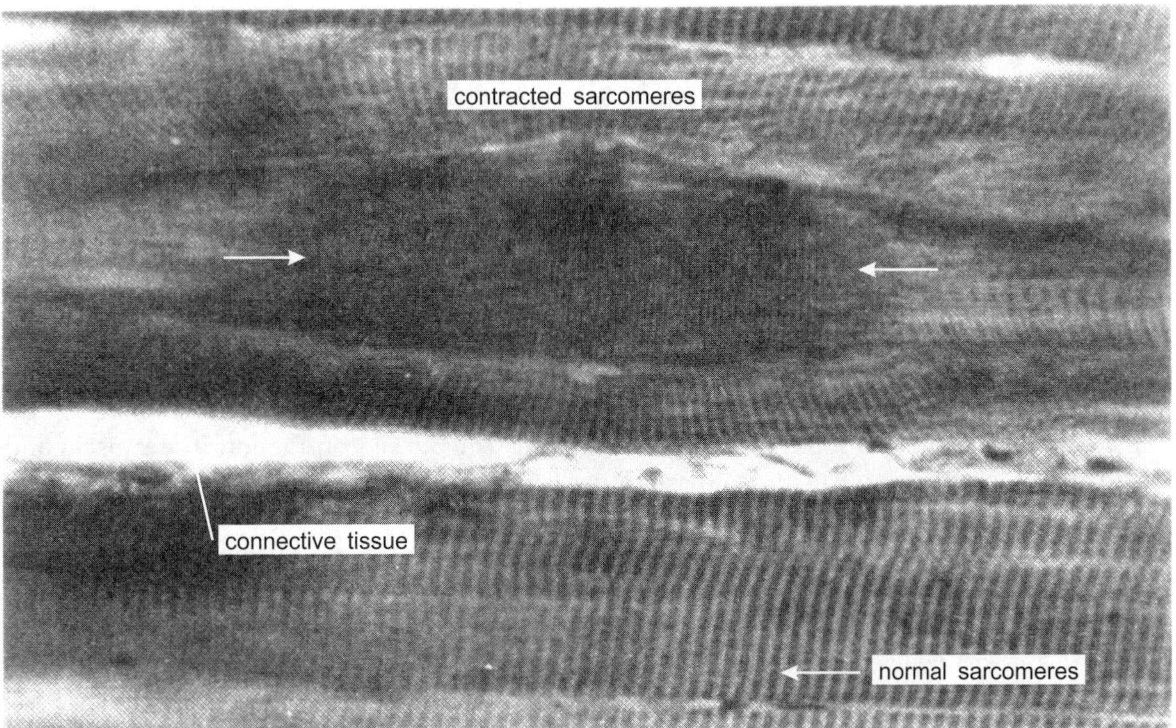

Figure 2.11 A knot of contracted sarcomeres in a myofibril at 240X magnification

Letter A in Figure 2.10 is a muscle myofibril in a normal resting state, neither stretched nor contracted. The tiny vertical Z bands within the fiber mark the ends of individual sarcomeres. The sarcomeres run lengthwise in the fibril.

Letter B is a knot in a myofibril consisting of a mass of sarcomeres in the state of maximum continuous contraction that characterizes a trigger point. The bulbous appearance of the contraction knot indicates how that segment of the myofibril has contracted, with the Z bands of individual sarcomeres now drawn closer together.

Letter C is the part of the myofibril that extends from the contraction knot to the muscle's attachment (to the head of the humerus in this case). Note the greater distance between the vertical Z bands, which shows how the sarcomeres in this part of the myofibril are being stretched by the tension within the contraction knot. These stretched segments are what give tightness and rigidity to the taut band. Therapy should aim at relaxing the knotted sarcomeres, which will allow the stretched sarcomeres along the full length of the fibril to equalize. In this way, the trigger point will release, allowing the taut band to relax.

Normally the action of the sarcomeres, alternately contracting and releasing like tiny pumps, helps the heart circulate blood through the tiny capillaries that supply the sarcomeres' own metabolic needs. When sarcomeres in a trigger point hold their contraction, they squeeze the capillaries shut and blood flow in the area essentially stops. The resulting oxygen starvation and accumulation of the waste products of metabolism causes even more sarcomeres to lock up. When a sufficient number of sarcomeres are disabled, they take on the group identity of a myofascial trigger point, with its characteristic knotlike feel, hypersensitivity, and generation of referred pain (Simons, Travell, and Simons 1999, 57-78).

The Electrochemical View of a Trigger Point

This section will be of interest only if you can handle a little chemistry. Amazingly, high school biology textbooks now deal quite thoroughly with muscle physiology on this level and actually go even deeper into it. But if biology class made your head ache, you can skip this section with little impact on your ability to deal with trigger points.

Muscle Metabolism

The electrochemical processes that occur in the muscles of the body are all part of *muscle metabolism*, which encompasses the basic functions of contracting and relaxing. Two contrasting processes take place in metabolism: *anabolism* and *catabolism*. Anabolism converts nutrients into new body tissue. Catabolism transforms nutrients into energy and heat. The elimination of the waste products of these processes is also part of muscle metabolism, but transforming energy into motion is the primary job. The act of contraction in a muscle and the resultant motion can't occur without muscle metabolism, and metabolism can't occur without an energy source (food).

Metabolism proceeds by transforming the glucose in food into glycogen and fat molecules, which are used for energy storage. When cells need energy, glycogen and fat are converted into the molecule *adenosine triphosphate* (ATP), which then serves as a carrier of energy, transporting it wherever it's needed.

Adenosine triphosphate is a molecule that consists of three main parts: adenine, ribose, and a chain of three phosphates. Although ribose is a form of sugar, the phosphates are the actual power source. Energy contained in the bonds between the phosphates is released when they are broken, which occurs through *hydrolysis*, the addition of a water molecule. When the phosphate bonds are broken, energy is produced and one of the three phosphates is removed, leaving a residual molecule, *adenosine diphosphate* (ADP), with only two phosphates. Interestingly, adenosine diphosphate isn't treated as waste but is processed back into adenosine triphosphate by the addition of phosphate from the diet, thus making very efficient use of the energy source.

Muscle Contraction

Muscle contraction usually begins as an electrical signal from the brain, although reflexive muscle action needs only an impulse from the spinal cord. In both cases, the signal is taken to the muscle by a motor nerve, which is actually a complex sort of cable containing thousands of individual nerve fibers called *axons*. In Figure 2.12, the impulse for contraction is carried from the spinal cord to the infraspinatus muscle by the suprascapular nerve.

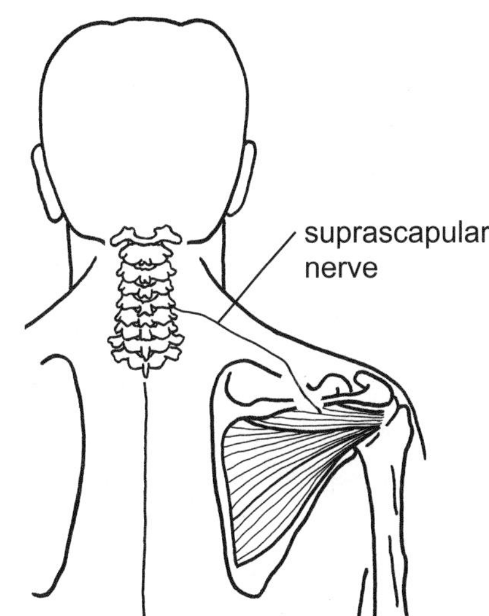

Figure 2.12 Nerve path to the infraspinatus

In a closer view, an axon connects its nerve cell, or *neuron*, to the individual muscle fibers (Figure 2.13). All of the nerve cells that activate muscle contraction reside in the spinal cord. The sensory nerve cells are just outside the spinal cord in the *ganglia*, small bulbous enlargements of the spinal nerves, which exit between the vertebrae. The sensory nerve fibers for the infraspinatus muscle also travel in the suprascapular nerve. The capillaries that supply blood to the area usually parallel the nerve (Figure 2.14). Note that the axon divides into multiple parts and ends just short of the muscle fiber in what is called the *motor endplate zone*. This is about halfway along the muscle fiber's length, midway between its attachments.

The tiny gap between the motor endplate and the muscle fiber is termed the *synaptic cleft*. This is where the electrical signal of the nerve fiber is converted to the chemical messenger *acetylcholine*, which carries the electrical signal to the cell membrane of the muscle fiber. To stimulate contraction, this signal is immediately disseminated throughout the entire muscle fiber.

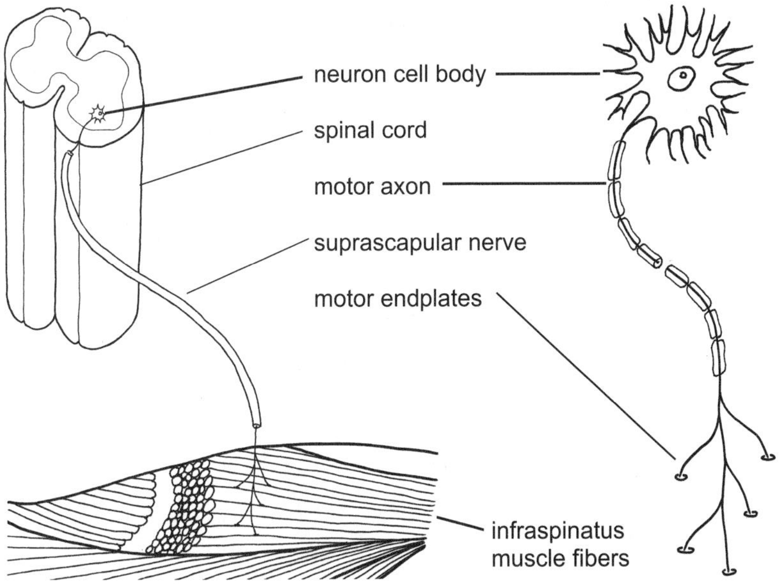

Figure 2.13 A neuron in the spinal cord transmits the neurological signal telling the infraspinatus muscle to contract.

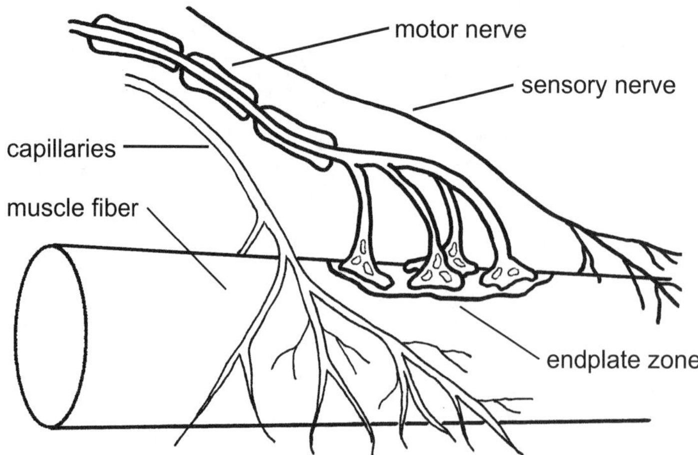

Figure 2.14 The motor endplate zone in a muscle fiber

Figure 2.15 shows an individual neuromuscular junction before the release of acetylcholine, when the sarcomeres are at their full length and relaxed. The *mitochondria* produce the acetylcholine, which is then transported by the acetylcholine vesicles. Figure 2.16 shows how the flow of acetylcholine affects the sarcomeres, causing them to contract and shorten. Acetylcholine is the critical substance in producing contraction of the sarcomeres in the muscles. When the release of acetylcholine gets out of control, muscle contraction also gets out of control. Muscle overload, muscle tension, and sustained rapid movement can all cause excessive release of acetylcholine. This in turn causes sarcomeres to become locked up and unresponsive, beginning what Travell and Simons call an "energy crisis" (Simons, Travell, and Simons 1999, 69-75).

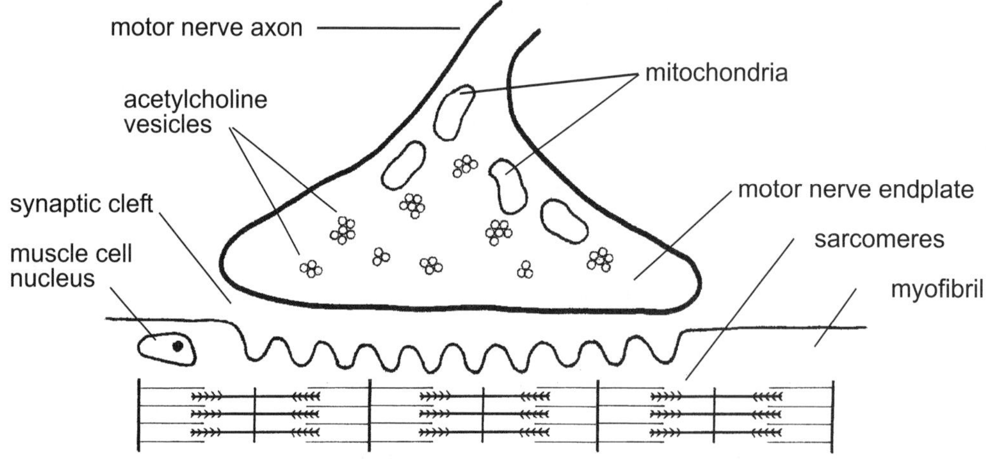

Figure 2.15 Neuromuscular junction with the sarcomeres and the muscle relaxed

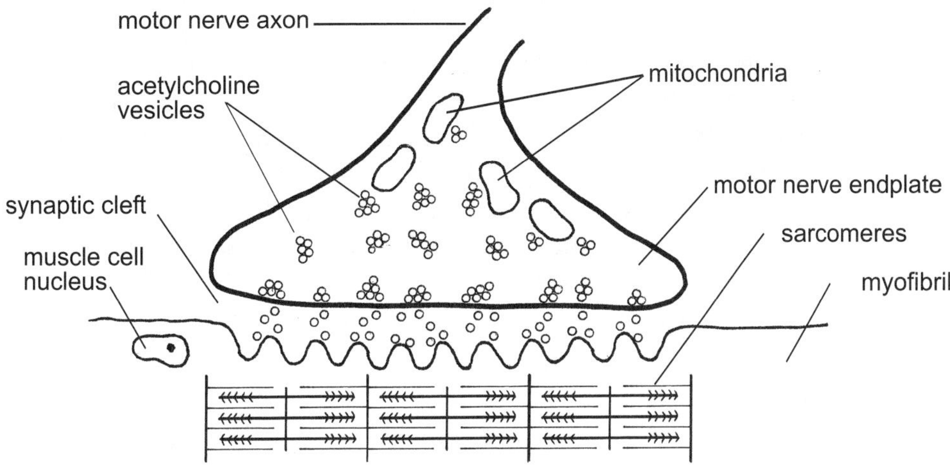

Figure 2.16 Neuromuscular junction with the sarcomeres and the muscle contracted

The Energy Crisis

Travell and Simons's *energy crisis* constitutes a vicious cycle of occurrences at the neuromuscular junction that's believed to be the basis for formation of myofascial trigger points (Figure 2.17). The problem begins with muscle overuse or sustained contraction, which constricts the capillaries that supply the muscle's metabolic needs. Circulation in a muscle fails during a sustained contraction that is more than 30 to 50 percent of maximum effort (Simons, Travell, and Simons 1999, 71). Failed circulation then causes decreased delivery of ATP, the energy molecule. Since energy is needed to detach the myosin filaments from the actin filaments, the absence of ATP leaves the sarcomeres in a shortened and contracted state (Simons, Travell, and Simons 1999, 69-75).

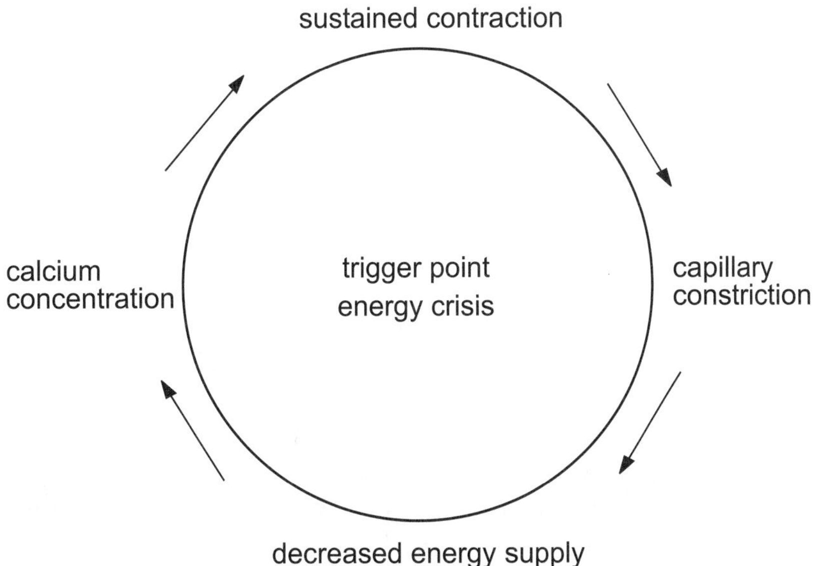

Figure 2.17 The vicious cycle that creates and perpetuates a trigger point

The key process in the energy crisis occurs when reduced ATP stops the reuptake of calcium. This is important because the sarcomeres can't relax and lengthen as long as calcium is present. Calcium ions are the immediate mediators of contraction, being the substance that directly stimulates the actin and myosin elements to link up and shorten. Calcium also acts in the synaptic cleft of the nerve terminal to cause the release of acetylcholine. Because of this, reducing the calcium reuptake leaves an excessive concentration of calcium in the synaptic cleft, promoting an overabundance of acetylcholine, which in turn contributes to maintaining the contraction. This condition at the neuromuscular junction, known as a *dysfunctional endplate,* is the piece that completes the vicious cycle that creates and perpetuates trigger points (Simons, Travell, and Simons 1999, 70-71).

Breaking the Cycle

A trigger point can be deactivated by almost any technique that causes the myosin filaments to release the actin filaments, thereby allowing the sarcomeres to lengthen. However, the muscle can't be forced to relax, nor can it be forced to lengthen without the risk of stimulating further release of acetylcholine. The safest and most effective way to break the vicious cycle that maintains the trigger point is to increase blood circulation, which very quickly increases the supply of oxygen and energy to the muscle tissues.

With the restoration of the energy supply, the reuptake of calcium will begin again, allowing the myosin and actin molecules to part and the sarcomeres to lengthen. Massage of the trigger point is the most direct and risk-free means for establishing renewed circulation through the capillaries in the affected area (Simons, Travell, and Simons 1999, 141-142).

Trigger Point Types

Trigger points can be very different in terms of their importance and their location within the muscle. It's a good idea to be able to recognize the differences before treatment begins because your success may depend on it. It's important to note that all classes of trigger points—central, attachment, primary, satellite, active, and latent—have an important diagnostic characteristic in common: they all hurt when you press on them.

Central Trigger Points

Solving the problem of myofascial pain hinges on locating *central trigger points,* those that occur at the midpoint of the muscle fibers (Figure 2.18). This is usually in the "belly" of the muscle where the motor nerve enters, bringing the tiny electrical impulses that make the muscle contract. This is the same spot where sarcomeres lock up to form a trigger point. Knowing how to find the midpoint of muscle fibers will usually take you right to the central trigger point that's causing your pain (Simons, Travell, and Simons 1999, 47-49).

It can be more complicated to find central trigger points when the fibers don't run from end to end in the muscle. The arrangement of muscle fibers can be very different depending on the job the muscle is designed to do (Figure 2.19). In a muscle made for speed, the fibers are parallel, running straight from attachment to attachment. Its trigger points are easily found at the midpoint of the muscle (A), just as expected.

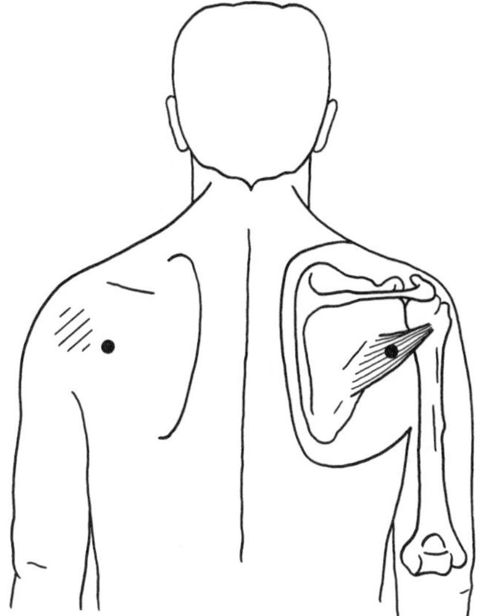

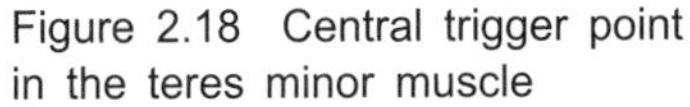

Figure 2.18 Central trigger point in the teres minor muscle

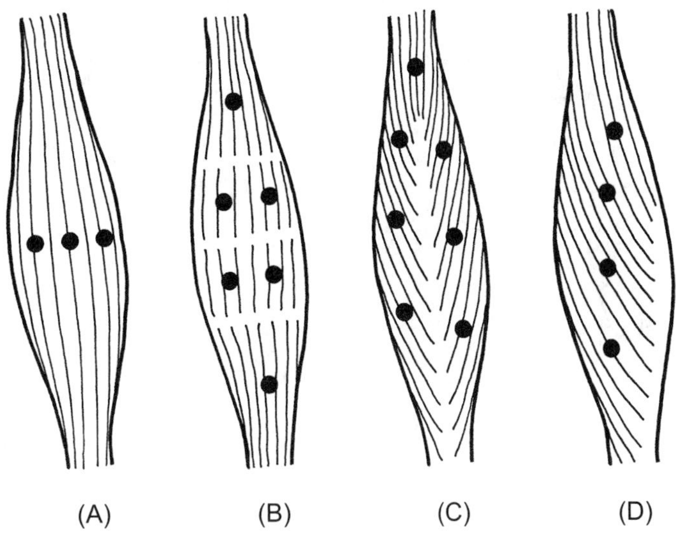

Figure 2.19 Orientation of muscle fibers: (A) Parallel; (B) Parallel with tendinous inscriptions; (C) Bipennate; (D) Unipennate

In a muscle made for power, however, the fibers run at an angle to its length. These fiber arrangements resemble a feather (C) or sometimes half a feather (D). Since trigger points are located at the midpoint of individual fibers, they can be found almost anywhere in muscles with these skewed fibers. (The middle deltoid muscle is constructed this way.) Interestingly, in a muscle with this sort of fiber orientation, all the fibers are the same length (Simons, Travell, and Simons 1999, 49-53).

Another variation is when a muscle is made of several sections, or heads. Often the name of the muscle tells you how many heads it has: the biceps, triceps, and quadriceps, for example, have two, three, and four heads respectively. Each head can have a fiber arrangement quite different from the others. In good anatomical drawings of muscles, the direction of the fibers is usually clearly shown.

Certain other muscles are divided into sections by *tendinous inscriptions*, or cross bands of connective tissue (B). This makes the muscle like a string of sausages, each with its own belly. As a result, trigger points can occur at several sites along the muscle's length. If you're unaware that more than one belly can exist in a muscle, you could easily miss critical trigger points. Examples of this kind of muscle are the rectus abdominis (your stomach muscle), and the gracilis, sartorius, and semitendinosus muscles in the thigh, all of which are long muscles built to exert great power (Simons, Travell, and Simons 1999, 49-53).

Attachment Trigger Points

Exquisitely painful spots are often found where a muscle attaches to bone (Figure 2.20). Travell and Simons believe these *attachment trigger points* are created by central trigger points in the muscle belly. It may be that they're not true trigger points, but rather simply highly sensitized connective tissue that's undergone unusual stress because of continuous muscle tension.

An attachment trigger point is always under the control of the central trigger point, which should be the primary target of treatment. Attachment trigger points generally cease

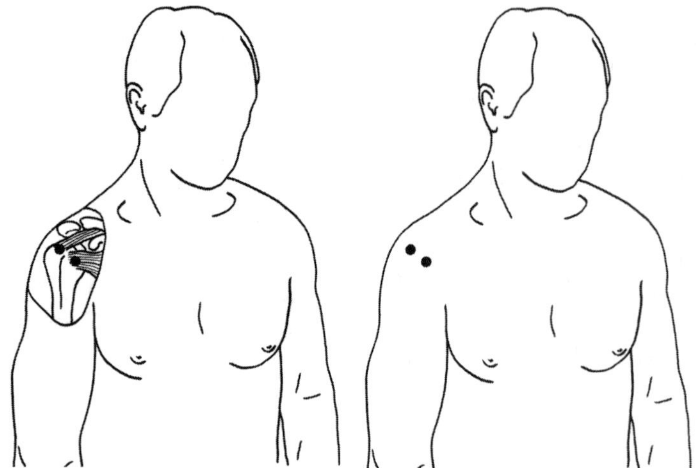

Figure 2.20 Supraspinatus and subscapularis attachment trigger points

to be tender when central trigger points have been deactivated. In chronic conditions where trigger points have been in place for months or years, continuing strain at the site of muscle attachment is believed to cause the degenerative changes that lead to osteoarthritis (Simons, Travell, and Simons 1999, 72, 76, 122; Fassbender and Wegner 1973, 355-374).

Primary and Satellite Trigger Points

A trigger point will very often generate trigger points in other muscles that lie within its pain referral zone (Figure 2.21). These are known as *satellite trigger points* (this term replaces *secondary trigger points*, a term that's no longer recommended). The trigger point sponsoring the satellite is a *primary trigger point* or *key trigger point*. Usually, it's also a central trigger point (Figure 2.18). The distinction between the two is that a central trigger point isn't a primary trigger point unless it has satellites in other muscles.

Long-term chronic pain is often a compound effect from a chain of satellite trigger points, created in a kind of cascade from muscle to muscle, the classic domino effect. It's not unusual for an entire side of the body to be affected. This is how all twenty-four muscles in the shoulder complex can be involved in producing a frozen shoulder.

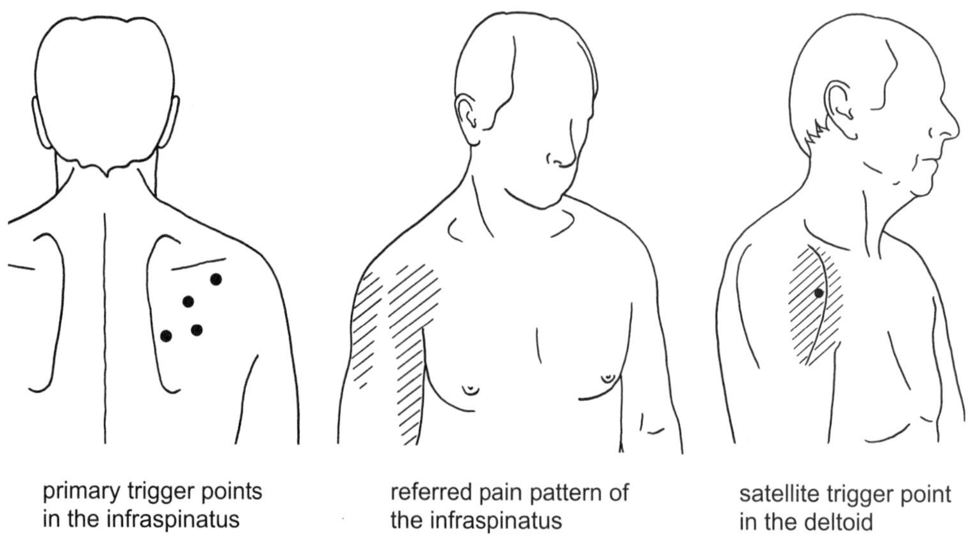

Figure 2.21 Deltoid trigger point created in the referred pain zone of infraspinatus trigger points

Satellite trigger points often resolve without treatment when the primary trigger point is deactivated. By the same token, satellites can be difficult if not impossible to deactivate if the primary trigger point is overlooked. With a frozen shoulder, the critical primary trigger points are usually found in the rotator cuff muscles, particularly the subscapularis and infraspinatus.

Referred pain from diseased internal organs can also promote satellite trigger points, usually in the muscles of the chest, back, and abdomen. This little-known dynamic can lead to trigger points that keep coming back in these areas despite seemingly effective trigger point therapy. In such case, the internal problem would be functioning as a primary trigger, and the recurring trigger points could be viewed as satellites. This circumstance should alert you to a possible internal problem (Simons, Travell, and Simons 1999, 122-123).

Active and Latent Trigger Points

Trigger points are also classified on the basis of their activity or inactivity. *Active trigger points* cause spontaneous pain. Your shoulder (or other part of the body) simply hurts without the provocation of movement or activity of any kind. Not surprisingly, active trigger points are more apt to be a problem during the most active time of life, between the ages of thirty and fifty.

Latent trigger points are inactive and don't cause spontaneous pain. They're distinguished instead by joint stiffness and reduced range of motion. Latent trigger points are far more common than active trigger points, especially in the more sedentary stage of life after age fifty. Travell and Simons believe that accumulated latent trigger points are a primary factor in the characteristic inflexibility and joint stiffness of old age. Latent trigger points are easily converted into active trigger points by stress, strain, or overuse of the muscles involved (Simons, Travell, and Simons 1999, 19).

Chapter 3

Trigger Point Symptoms, Causes, and Perpetuators

Trigger Point Symptoms

The symptoms produced by trigger points are actually quite diverse and aren't limited to pain sensations. Other abnormal sensations can include numbness, tingling, hypersensitivity, and a sense of burning. Physical problems caused by trigger points include weakness, discoordination, stiffness, swelling, and reduced range of motion.

Pain generated by trigger points can range from a vague aching to pain so severe you're completely unable to function. Trigger point pain can also be either acute or chronic. By definition, acute pain is of recent onset, a symptom you've had for just hours or days. In contrast, chronic pain is a condition that has existed for weeks, months, or years. When trigger points have existed long enough to cause chronic pain, they can be much more difficult to get rid of than if they had been treated earlier.

When pain has lasted for as little as three days, the neurological system responds by growing new nerve cells and new synapses between them. (*Synapses* are the electrochemical switches that allow information to pass from one nerve cell to the next.) Chronic pain maintains these new neurological pathways, creating a vicious feedback loop that can make pain essentially self-sustaining. The ideal strategy with trigger points is to treat them before their acute pain becomes chronic pain. When shoulder pain becomes chronic, it has every chance of evolving into a frozen shoulder (Simons, Travell, and Simons 1999, 56).

Referred Pain

Although trigger point symptoms are diverse, their most characteristic effect is referred pain, the displacement of pain from its source to some other part of the body. The concept of referred pain isn't new. Pain sent from internal organs to the musculoskeletal system has been familiar to physicians for many generations.

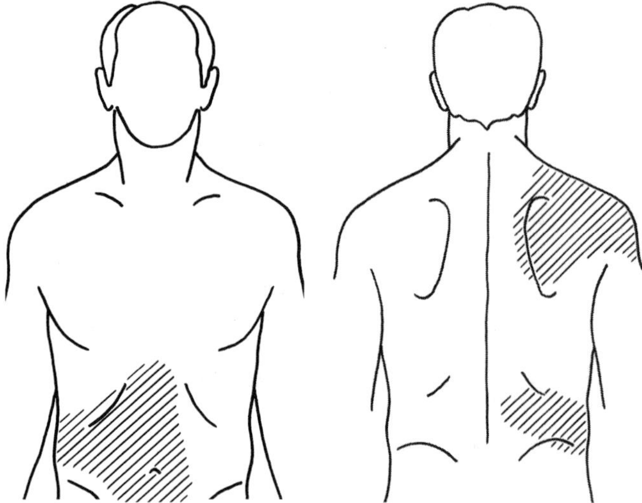

Figure 3.1 Possible sites of pain referral from the gallbladder

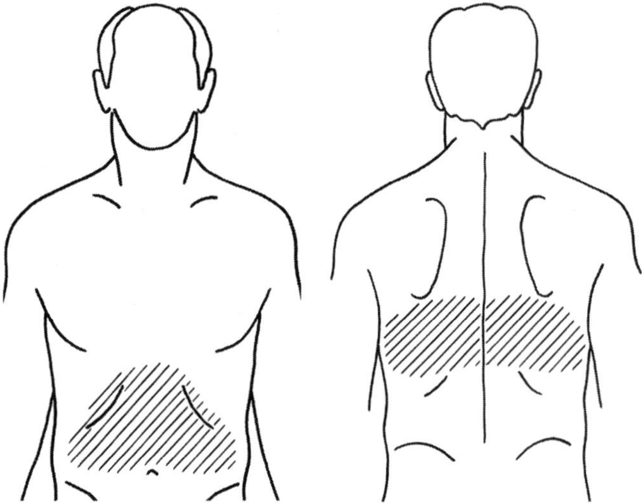

Figure 3.2 Possible sites of pain referral from the pancreas

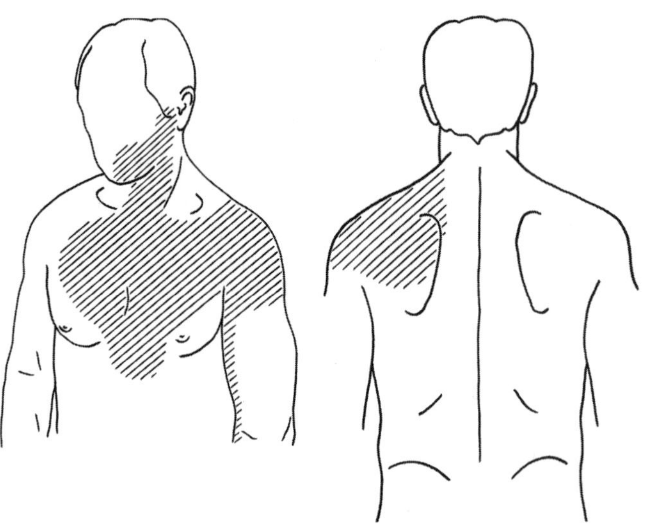

Figure 3.3 Possible sites of pain referral from a heart attack and angina. Pain is sometimes also felt in the right arm and shoulder.

Visceral Referral

The technical term for pain referral from your internal organs is the *viscerosomatic effect*, and it's a very common occurrence (Simons, Travell, and Simons 1999, 959). Symptoms of internal disease are often manifested by some kind of external pain, and the shoulder seems to be a favorite site for visceral pain referral.

An ailing gallbladder, for example, commonly sends pain to the mid back, the upper right quadrant of the abdomen, and the right shoulder blade (Figure 3.1). A diseased pancreas has a similar pattern but without the referral to the shoulder (Figure 3.2). A heart attack or angina can produce pain in the left shoulder, chest, arm, neck, teeth, and jaw (Figure 3.3). It's important to be aware that the referred pain pattern from the heart sometimes includes the right shoulder.

Under certain circumstances, a troubled esophagus, liver, kidney, stomach, or colon can send pain to the shoulder. An aneurysm in the subclavian artery or an arterial blockage in the neck, upper torso, or shoulder area can also refer to the shoulder (Gray 2004, 361-375). Although not a visceral organ, the diaphragm can sometimes be the source of shoulder pain from myofascial trigger points (Simons, Travell, and Simons 1999, 863).

There are five things that should alert you that a visceral problem could be causing part or all of your shoulder pain (Gray 2004, 361):

1. Your shoulder pain is constant and doesn't change with changes in body position or activity.
2. Shoulder pain increases with exertion that doesn't stress the shoulder, such as walking or climbing stairs.
3. Pain increases after eating, during bowel or bladder activity, or while coughing or breathing deeply.
4. Shoulder pain is accompanied by gastrointestinal symptoms like indigestion, nausea, vomiting, diarrhea, constipation, or rectal bleeding.
5. You also have symptoms such as fever, night sweats, pale skin, dizziness, fatigue, or unexplained weight loss. Be aware, however, that trigger points can also cause nausea, dizziness, and fatigue, and that you can have both trigger points and visceral referred pain concurrently.

Pain referral can occur in the opposite direction, sent from your muscles to your internal organs. This is called the *somatovisceral effect*. Visceral pain referred from trigger points in your back or abdominal muscles can make you fear you have an ulcer, gallstones, heart trouble, colitis, or cancer (Simons, Travell, and Simons 1999, 958). Fortunately, trigger points in the shoulder muscles don't usually cause visceral symptoms.

Musculoskeletal Referral

Within your musculoskeletal system, the direction of pain referral from a trigger point is almost always away from the center of the body (Figure 3.4), about 85 percent of the time, in fact. The rest of the time, the pain is shifted more toward the center of the body (Figure 3.5) or occurs locally at the trigger point site (Figure 3.6). Referred pain in all cases is felt as a deep, oppressive ache, although movement can occasionally sharpen it to a lightninglike stab of pain. Referred myofascial pain can be as intense and intolerable as pain from any other cause. It should be noted that the pain level depends more on the degree of trigger point irritability than on the size of the muscle. Trigger points in the tiniest muscle can cripple you with pain (Simons, Travell, and Simons 1999, 96).

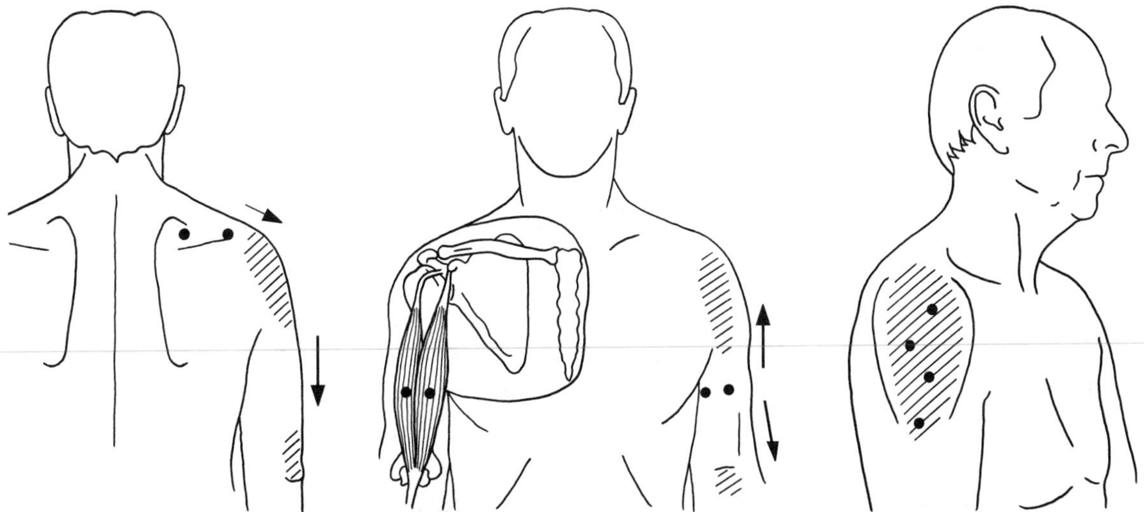

Figure 3.4 Trigger points referring pain away from the center of the body

Figure 3.5 Trigger points referring pain both inwards and outwards relative to the center of the body

Figure 3.6 Trigger points causing only local pain

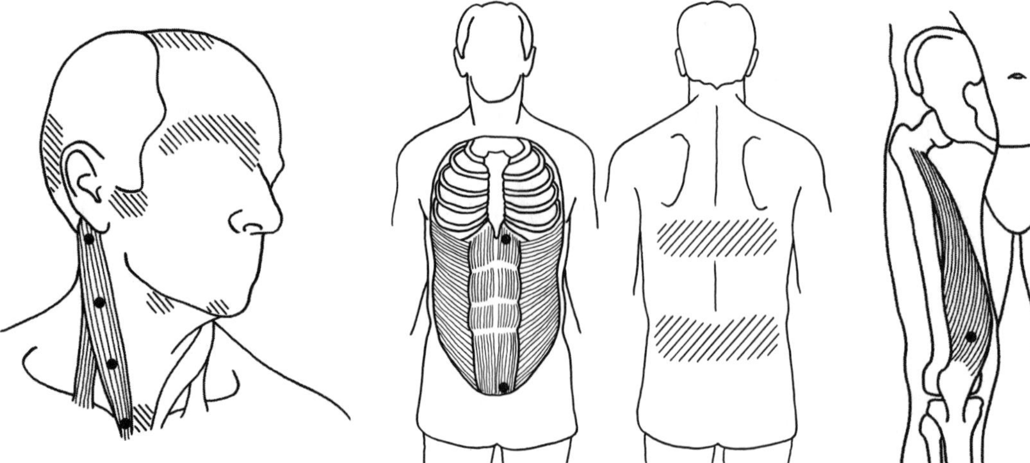

Figure 3.7 Headaches referred from trigger points in the sternocleidomastoid

Figure 3.8 Back pain referred from trigger points in abdominal muscles

Figure 3.9 Quadriceps trigger point that causes knee pain

Common examples of referred myofascial pain include tension headaches caused by trigger points in neck muscles (Figure 3.7), back pain from abdominal trigger points (Figure 3.8), and knee pain referred from trigger points in the quadriceps muscles (Figure 3.9). Sore legs, sore feet, and painful ankles can also be referred pain. Stiffness and pain in a joint should always make you think first, not of arthritis, but of possible trigger points in associated muscles. Pain in such joints as the knuckles, wrists, elbows, shoulders, knees, and hips are classic trigger point symptoms.

A common misconception regarding referred pain is that a painful spot in a muscle isn't a trigger point unless it refers pain when you press on it. Trigger points in certain muscles, such as the infraspinatus and sternocleidomastoid, will frequently respond in this way, but many others don't. You can't depend on it happening as a diagnostic criterion. Very irritable trigger points are more apt to reproduce their pain pattern in response to pressure than those that are less irritable. The only way to reliably verify whether a specific trigger point is causing a specific pain is to deactivate the trigger point and see if the pain remains.

Myofascial pain in the various parts of the shoulder is traceable to trigger points in the same sets of muscles in virtually every case. The patterns of referred pain from trigger points are consistent and predictable, with the same kinds of referral occurring in everyone.

How Referred Pain Works

Perhaps the most common kind of referred pain in the shoulder region originates in the infraspinatus muscle, which covers most of the outer surface of the shoulder blade (Figure 3.10). You'll remember that Janet Travell's interest in referred pain began with her accidental discovery of painful spots in her infraspinatus muscle that seemed to be connected with her own shoulder pain. Pressing the painful spots made the front and side of her shoulder and arm hurt, just as seen in Figure 3.10. There has been an ongoing controversy for several decades about why referred pain should occur, and it hasn't been an easy question to resolve.

Research on referred pain has been difficult because the mechanisms of the nervous system are so unimaginably small. The tiny electrochemical impulses in the nerves can be detected and measured to some extent, but not with accuracy or great discrimination. In addition, there are ethical limits on how far you can go in pain experiments, whether with animals or humans. Nevertheless, scientists have made a number of suppositions about how pain can be displaced from its cause.

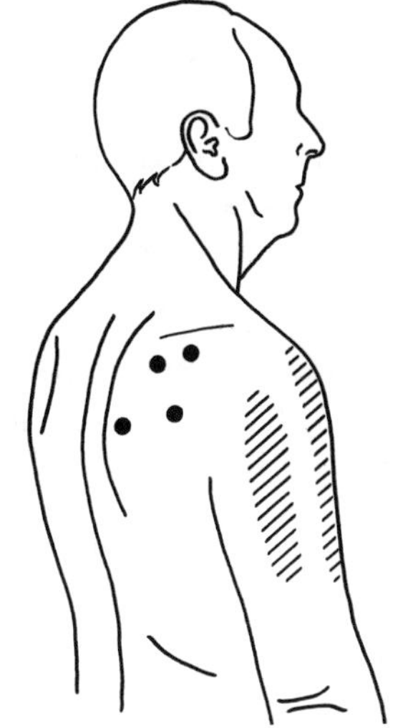

Figure 3.10 Pain referred from infraspinatus trigger points

The easiest theory to accept regarding referred pain is that the signals simply get mixed up and misinterpreted in your neurological wiring (Figure 3.11). This idea was originated by Theodore Ruch and is known by physiologists as the *convergence-projection theory* (Fulton 1947, 397). Dr. Ruch established that single second-order neurons (nerve cells) in the spinal cord actually receive impulses from first-order sensory neurons in several sources: the viscera, the skin, the joints, and the muscles. These electrical signals are integrated and modified at the spinal level before being transmitted to the brain.

Since more than one electrical signal may be processed at the same time in a single cell, it may be possible for one signal to influence another, resulting in mistaken impressions about where the signals are coming from (Simons, Travell, and Simons 1999, 56). The actual neurological processes are undoubtedly far more complex than this. In any case, the pain is clearly not being produced in the area where you feel it, but is in essence an illusion created in the brain from mixed-up or distorted neurological input. Figure 3.11 is a greatly simplified representation of the theory.

Many second-order neurons at the spinal level receive sensory input from two or more muscles. These sensory impulses are then sent up the spinal cord in the spinothalamic tract to the brain, where they synapse with third-order neurons in the thalamus. The impulses are then sent on to the somesthetic area, where they're interpreted (Jacob, Francone, and Lossow 1978, 286).

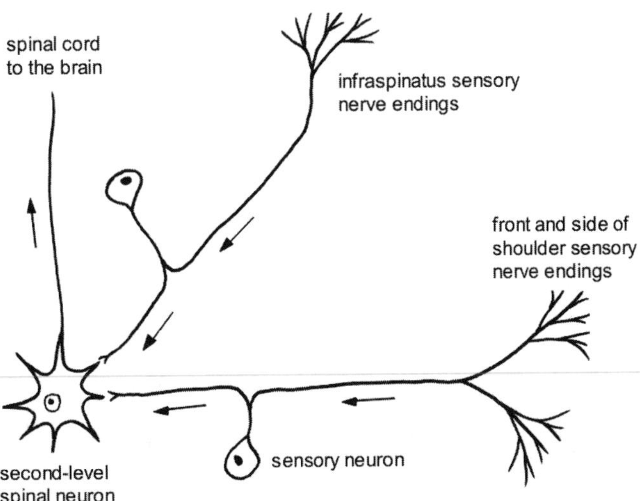

Figure 3.11 Simplified diagram of pain referral from infraspinatus trigger points to the front and side of the shoulder

Luckily, for the practical purpose of treating trigger points, it's not really necessary to understand the neurology of referred pain. You just have to understand that referred pain is real, extremely common, and entirely predictable. As seen in the pain patterns in Figure 3.10, the brain unfailingly concludes that pain signals from the infraspinatus muscle are coming from the anterior deltoid, biceps, and triceps muscles.

Janet Travell's great discovery was that referred pain occurs in very predictable patterns in everyone with only small variations. These patterns seem too consistent to be accidental, and their predictability implies that there may be some functional advantage to the referral of pain. It's notable that referred pain occurs most often in or near a joint, locations where pain is most likely to make you modify the activities or conditions that created the problem (Simons, Travell, and Simons 1999, 96).

Neurological and Vascular Symptoms

Muscles remain under some degree of tension when afflicted with trigger points. This tightness in muscles can cause compression of nerves that pass through the muscles or near them. Nerve compression typically results in abnormal sensations, such as numbness, tingling, burning, hypersensitivity, or an electric kind of pain in the areas served by the nerve. For example, scalene trigger points in the neck that cause shoulder and upper arm pain can also be the source of numbness, tingling, and burning sensations in the forearm, hand, and fingers (Figure 3.12).

Trigger points can also cause a muscle to clamp down on a vein, impeding blood flow in the area served by the vein. When the scalene muscles in the neck tighten, for example, they can cause blood to pool in the hand, which then becomes hot and swollen. Too often medical practitioners are unaware that myofascial trigger points in the neck or shoulders can cause both neurological and vascular symptoms in the hands. Typically, a mistaken diagnosis of carpal tunnel syndrome or nerve disease is then made, which leads to inappropriate and ineffective treatment (Simons, Travell, and Simons 1999, 509-510).

It's also important to understand that compression of a nerve can instigate the formation of trigger points in the areas served by the nerve. For example, a herniated lumbar disk pressing on the motor nerve roots of buttock and leg muscles creates trigger points that are partly responsible for the characteristic buttock and leg pain of sciatica. In the same way, a herniated disk in the cervical spine could foster trigger points in muscles in the shoulder, neck, and upper back and contribute significantly to shoulder pain (Simons, Travell, and Simons 1999, 112).

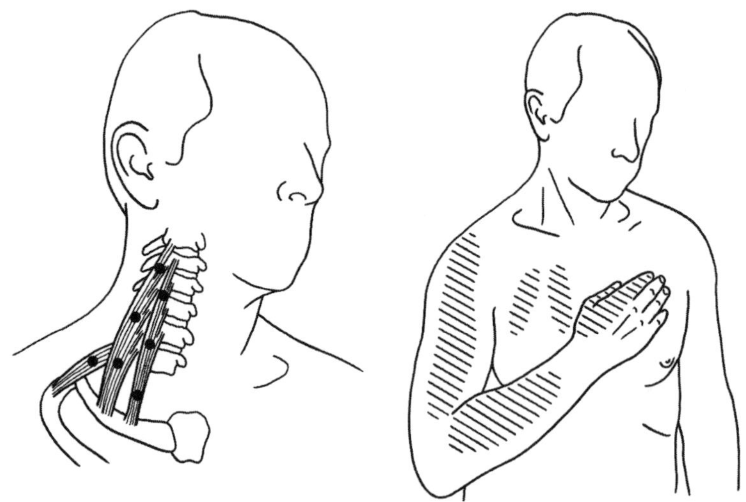

Figure 3.12 Scalene trigger points affecting the shoulder, arm, hand, and fingers with pain, stiffness, tingling, numbness, burning, and weakness

Symptoms of Physical Dysfunction

In addition to pain and other sensory symptoms, trigger points typically disturb the physical functioning of muscles. This can show up as weakness, discoordination, joint stiffness, joint disarticulation, distorted posture, excessive muscle response to load, delayed relaxation, delayed recovery after exertion, and decreased endurance. It's a waste of time to try to fix these things without first attending to the trigger points causing the problem.

Weakness and Discoordination

Trigger points cause a basic weakness in muscles, which can be expressed in a variety of other physical symptoms. For instance, a quadriceps trigger point that sends pain to the knee as shown in Figure 3.9 can also make the knee suddenly give way when you're just innocently walking along. Trigger points in your scalenes, as shown in Figure 3.12, can give you an unreliable grip, causing you to unexpectedly drop your coffee cup and make a mess. Weakening caused by trigger points in the muscles in the front of the lower leg can cause you to trip and stumble unexpectedly, making you seem uncoordinated (Figure 3.13). This kind of muscle weakness doesn't involve true atrophy, so exercise isn't an appropriate therapy. Strength will return quickly when the trigger points causing the problem have been deactivated.

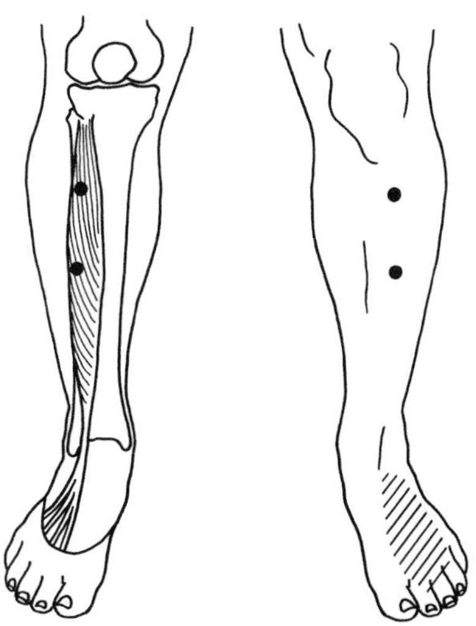

Figure 3.13 Trigger points referring weakness and pain to the foot and toes, a cause of stumbling

Joint Stiffness

Joint stiffness, like pain, is a classic symptom of myofascial trigger points. Stiffness in a joint is seldom due to a problem with the joint but instead is the result of stiffness in the muscles that operate the joint. Trigger points cause stiffness by keeping the muscle from lengthening. Such tightening in muscles associated with a joint is what usually reduces your range of motion. A stiff neck, a back that won't bend, and a frozen shoulder are all examples of joint stiffening caused by myofascial trigger points.

The shoulder's range of motion can be restricted in several ways. A subscapularis muscle shortened by trigger points

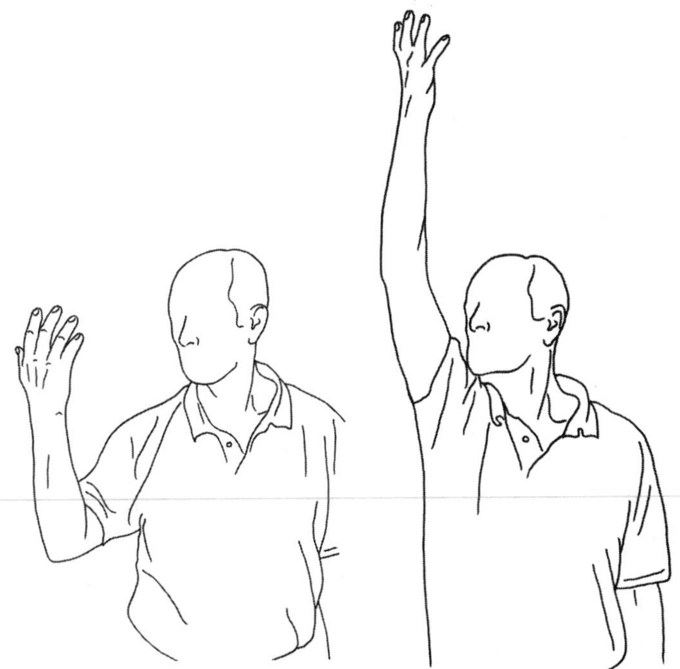

Figure 3.14 Reaching up overhead can be difficult when the arm's outward rotation is restricted by trigger points.

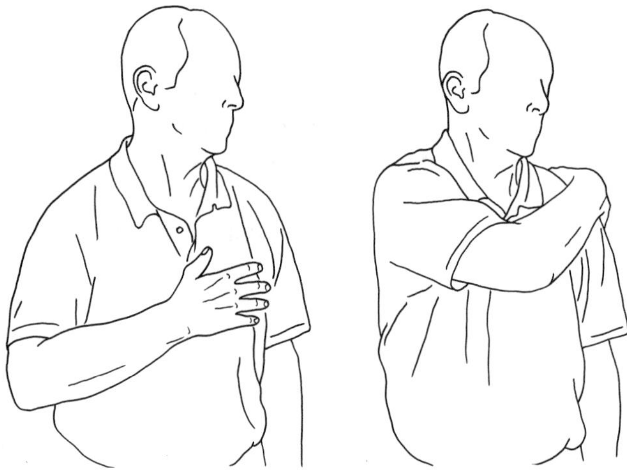

Figure 3.15 Trigger points in the infraspinatus can make it hard to reach across to fasten your seat belt.

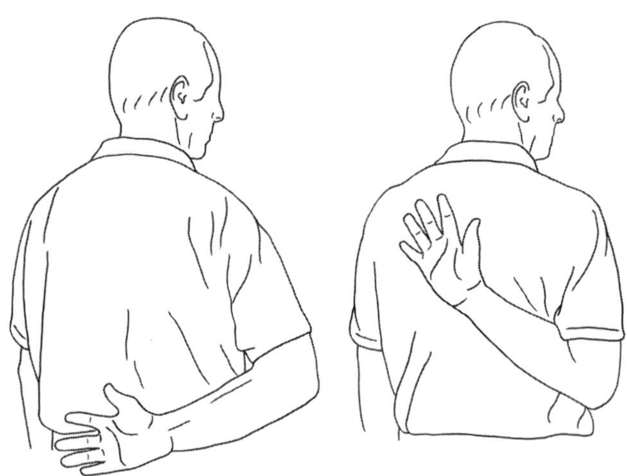

Figure 3.16 Trigger points in the subscapularis and infraspinatus muscles make it difficult to reach up behind your back.

can prevent you from reaching up over your head (Figure 3.14). An infraspinatus muscle shortened by trigger points can keep you from reaching across your body (Figure 3.15). Infraspinatus trigger points can also contribute to an inability to reach up behind your back (Figure 3.16). Other muscles can restrict range of motion in the shoulder, but the subscapularis and infraspinatus are usually the biggest offenders.

Joint Disarticulation

When the muscles controlling a joint have a paradoxical combination of tightness in some of the muscles and weakness in others, it can create an imbalance that results in disarticulation, or partial dislocation. The joint then fails to operate smoothly because the bones catch or rub together abnormally. This is the reason for clicking and popping noises in joints. A thumb joint that catches and won't bend, a clicking in your jaw, an ankle that crackles when you turn your foot, or a popping in your shoulder when you move your arm—are all the result of joint dislocations, often only subtle ones, that may be caused by trigger points.

A noisy shoulder can usually be traced to the effects of trigger points in the rotator cuff muscles. The so-called impingement syndrome affecting the top of the shoulder has the same origin. The ball rides up in the socket and squeezes the supraspinatus tendon against the acromion, all because of trigger points in the rotator muscles.

Distorted Posture

Muscles that stay chronically shortened because of trigger points can be the ultimate source of distorted posture involving the head, neck, upper back, and shoulders. Tight pectoral muscles, for example, can cause your shoulder blades to stick out in back, a condition called "winging." Shortened pectorals are responsible for keeping the shoulders rolled forward and for sponsoring the humped upper back associated with a habitual stoop (Figure 3.17). In older women, shortened pectoral muscles may be as much to blame for the familiar dowager's hump as osteoporosis.

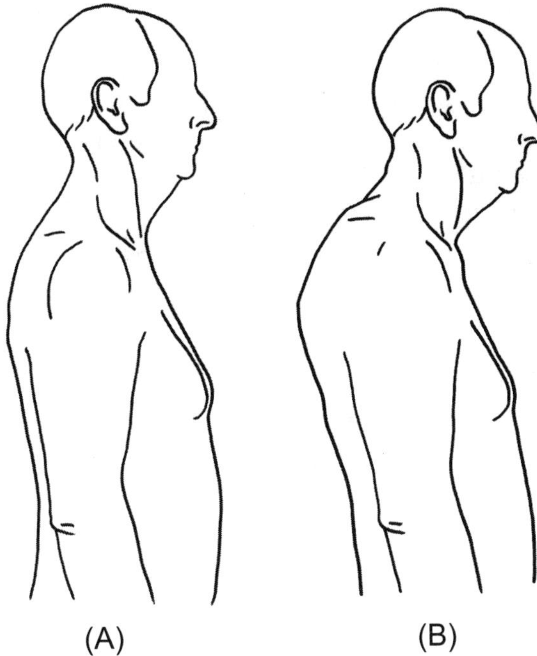

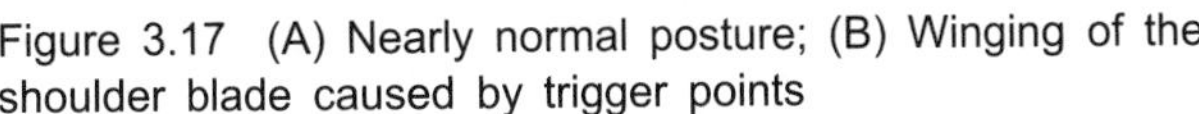

Figure 3.17 (A) Nearly normal posture; (B) Winging of the shoulder blade caused by trigger points

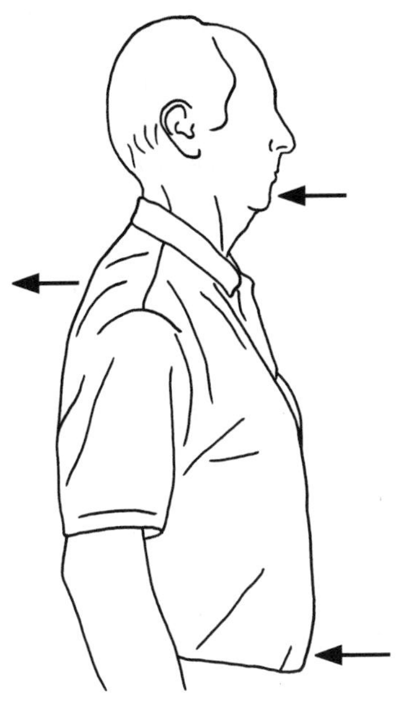

Figure 3.18 Keeping the shoulders back and the chin and stomach pulled in causes tight muscles in the upper back, neck, and stomach.

An artificial, military-style posture with the shoulders back and the chin and stomach pulled in looks really great (Figure 3.18), but in reality it's a wretched way to treat your body because it sponsors unnecessary tension in the upper back, shoulders, and neck. This in turn promotes trigger points in all these places.

You can achieve the most healthful posture by simply raising the crown of your head and letting the muscles in your shoulders, stomach, and the front and back of your neck relax. With the head positioned correctly, everything else falls into a balanced position naturally (Figure 3.19). If you still look and feel saggy, a little exercise to strengthen your body would be a better plan than keeping your muscles tight for sake of appearance. Long-established habits of posture can't be corrected by self-discipline alone. Permanent postural change can, however, be accomplished with the assistance of trigger point therapy, which makes it possible for the tight muscles to lengthen properly (Mense and Simons 2001, 217-219).

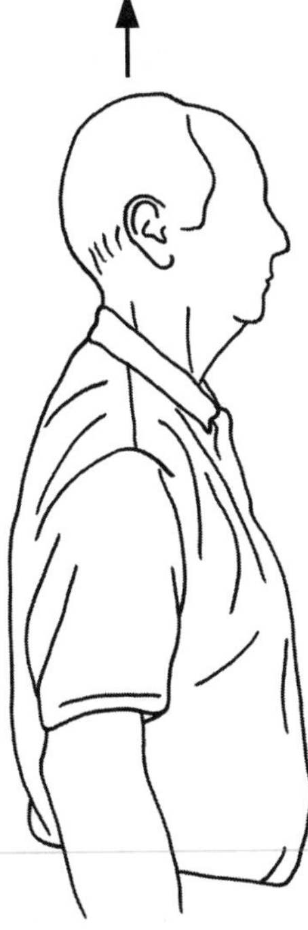

Figure 3.19 Shoulders in neutral position, with the crown of the head raised and muscles relaxed

Excessive Muscle Response

Oddly, muscles work harder than they need to when they're under the influence of trigger points. The self-sustaining neurochemical feedback loop stemming from the energy crisis in the sarcomeres establishes a vicious cycle of tension in muscle tissue that's hard to break. In effect, the tension in the trigger point feeds on itself. Trigger points seem to put muscles into a permanent state of neurotic readiness. They're jumpy. They're too eager. They overrespond to the demands made on them. This brings on a cascade of secondary effects that stem directly from this tendency of muscles to excessive effort.

Delayed Relaxation

In maintaining unnecessary tension in muscles, trigger points make it difficult for the muscles to return to a neutral, relaxed state after contracting. If they relax at all, they're slow to do so. During work and play, muscles tend to remain in that permanent state of readiness. Your shoulders stay hiked up, your brow stays knitted, your mouth and stomach stay tight, or your fists stay clenched. You may feel as though you're always bracing for the worst. If you try to relax, everything tightens up again, as though it were under the control of a big spring.

You may be conscious of a nervous habit of keeping your shoulders up around your ears (Figure 3.20). This posture is not only exhausting for the muscles, it also makes you look older than your years. You can take ten years off just by putting your shoulders down (Figure 3.21). Unfortunately, it's nearly impossible to make a lasting correction of this problem without addressing the trigger points in the upper trapezius, the levator scapulae, and the other muscles that elevate the shoulders.

You could identify the tightness in your muscles as a sign of nervous tension, and you'd be correct to a large degree. Muscle tension is a fundamental expression of nervous tension. But it's important to recognize that trigger points in muscles play a hidden part in sustaining tension.

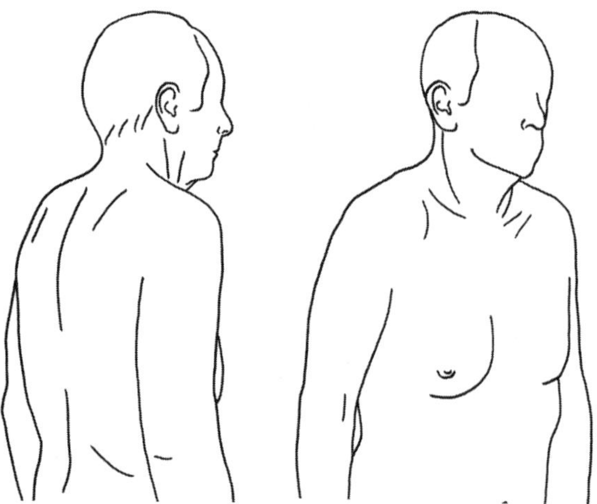

Figure 3.20 Shoulders held high by unnecessary tension in the levator scapulae and upper trapezius muscles

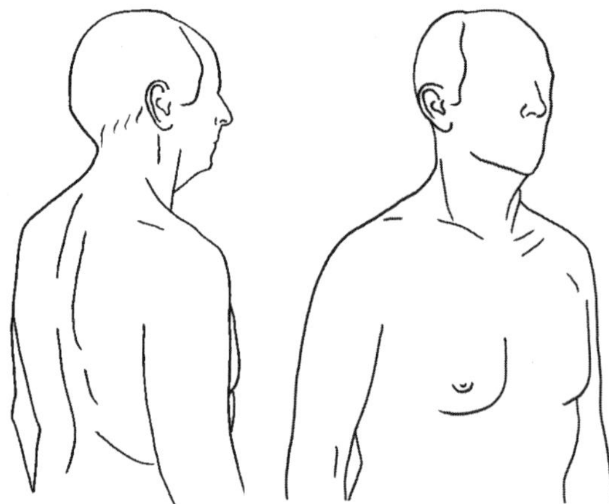

Figure 3.21 Shoulders down, with relaxed levator scapulae and trapezius muscles

Delayed Recovery and Decreased Endurance

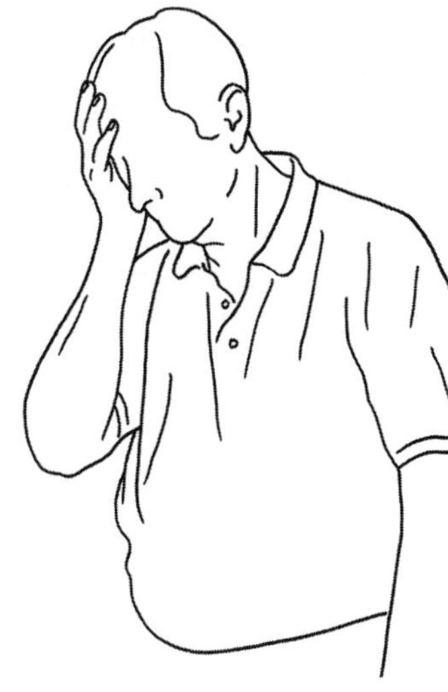

Figure 3.22 Chronic fatigue from widespread trigger points

Trigger points make it difficult for the muscles to recover after exertion. Muscles afflicted with trigger points never really get a chance to rest, which causes them to tire unnecessarily. Until you come to understand just how pervasive the effects of myofascial trigger points can be, you may never recognize the real reason why you become tired so easily, why you've lost your endurance and tolerance for work, or why you seem to have mysteriously acquired what feels like chronic fatigue syndrome (Figure 3.22). Exercise, an improved diet, herbal remedies, and prescription drugs can't be expected to solve your energy problem if myofascial trigger points are handicapping the basic functioning of your muscles. Obviously, quick energy boosters like junk food, chocolate, caffeine, and nicotine can provide only a temporary solution, if that.

When your endurance and stamina are down, you tend to stop using your muscles. You become guarded and conservative in your movements, and you stop reaching up for things if you don't have to. For weeks at a time, you might rarely raise your arms above your head. This kind of routine inactivity lays a solid foundation for the development of a frozen shoulder.

Autonomic Disturbances

Trigger points can be responsible for a number of additional physical symptoms that you wouldn't think they could cause. These symptoms are very different from one another and have little to do with pain, so you may find it hard to believe they're caused by trigger points. Your skepticism may not diminish until you've experienced some of these effects yourself and have gotten relief through trigger point therapy.

These odd symptoms are expressions of unusual activity in the autonomic nervous system, which regulates the glands, the smooth muscles of the digestive system, the blood vessels, the heart, the respiratory system, and activity in the skin. Travell and Simons list some of the known autonomic effects of trigger points as reddening and excessive tearing of the eyes, blurred vision, a droopy eyelid, excessive salivation, and a persistent runny nose (Simons, Travell, and Simons 1999, 308-311). Trigger points in neck muscles can bring about dizziness, poor sense of balance, a chronic cough, sinus congestion, and chronic sinus drainage. Ear stuffiness and a kind of fluttering sensation in the ear can come from trigger points in the masseter muscles of the jaw. These same trigger points cause the exasperating deep ear itch that nothing seems to reach (Figure 3.23). The deep ear itch can be quickly fixed, by the way, with just a little massage to a trigger point in the masseter muscle right in front of the ear lobe.

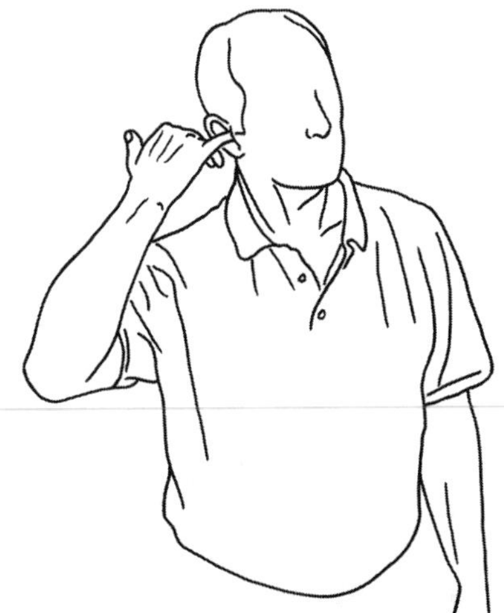

Figure 3.23 Deep ear itch from a masseter muscle trigger point

The autonomic nervous system has influences throughout the body, and the autonomic effects of trigger points are very nearly as widespread. Abdominal trigger points, for instance, can produce nausea, vomiting, and chronic diarrhea. Trigger points in a pectoral muscle can cause an erect, hypersensitive nipple. Amazingly, there's a trigger point on the front of the rib cage that can cause an irregular heartbeat. Certain trigger points can even cause excessive sweating and goose bumps (Simons, Travell, and Simons 1999, 21).

The explanation for all these bizarre phenomena could simply be that muscles afflicted by trigger points are compressing the nerves and blood vessels that serve the areas involved. Watch for possible connections between autonomic symptoms and your shoulder problem. If it turns out that trigger points in your neck muscles are contributing in some way to your shoulder pain, you may find they are also producing some of these autonomic symptoms.

Causes of Trigger Points

Most of the activities and events that create myofascial trigger points are obvious and understandable: accidents, falls, muscle strain, and the infinite varieties of muscle overuse. A one-time episode of overdoing, for example, is notorious for ending in debilitating pain that long outlasts the activity. You've probably lifted too much or carried an unreasonable load on occasion, or ambitiously overexercised when out of condition. Some time or another you've hammered away too long and too hard at some unaccustomed type of work.

Any of these misadventures has the potential to get a shoulder into trouble. Even if you know exactly how your problem started, it's a good idea to look more closely at the question in the interest of heading off a recurrence. This is especially important if your other shoulder hasn't yet been affected. You don't necessarily have to avoid an activity or a sport that has gotten you into trouble with a shoulder. There may simply be an uncommon factor that you've overlooked. The idea is to learn which muscles are at risk in a particular activity and stand ready to treat trigger points in them at the very first twinge of pain. Self-applied trigger point massage is a skill that will give you a wonderful advantage throughout your life. It lets you nip problems in the bud before they deteriorate into an unmanageable condition.

Preventable Muscle Abuse

It's important to remember that the basic function of the shoulder is to make a solid base for the operations of the arm and hand. In almost everything you do, your hands are reaching out in one direction or another while applying some kind of force or lifting some kind of weight. Your shoulder muscles continually have to contract and stay tight to hold your arms and hands in position for whatever they need to do. You have a choice regarding whether your shoulder muscles function safely and efficiently or go at their work in a wasteful manner.

The World of Work

The pain from routine overuse of muscles in work situations is so widespread and universal these days that it has earned a number of imposing labels. If your shoulder problem is associated with your job, you're likely to be diagnosed with overuse syndrome, repetitive motion injury, repetitive strain injury, cumulative trauma disorder, or occupational myalgia.

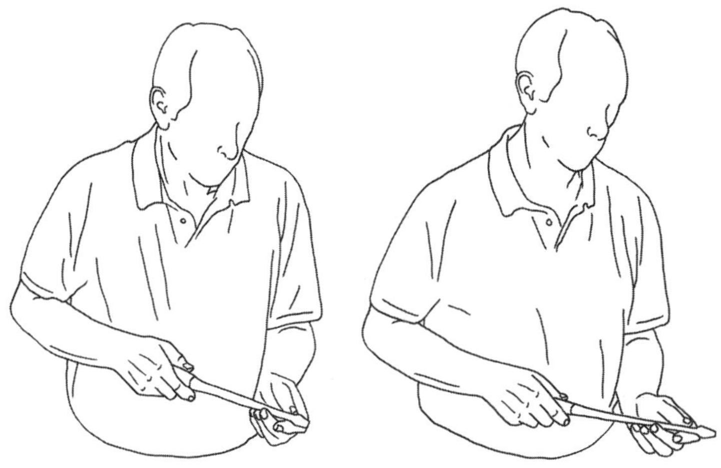

Figure 3.24 The man on the left is working tight, with excess tension in his upper back, shoulders, and neck. The man on the right is giving some attention to keeping those areas relaxed.

These terms look impressive on an insurance claim, but none of them means anything other than that you've unwisely worked a group of muscles beyond their endurance and now they're making you pay for it.

It's important to look critically at a work situation that causes pain. Although trigger points are actually quite easy to deal with when you understand them, they can come back very quickly if you don't change the conditions that bring them on. There are many issues of work style that can be examined, but all of them come down to a question of economy of motion and efficient use of energy. Thoughtless positioning of the body, for instance, is a fundamental cause of the poor body mechanics and inefficient movement that result in muscle strain. Working with your shoulders held high and tight, for example, seems so natural that you may work like that all day without giving it a thought, although it may be a significant cause of your repetitive strain problem (Figure 3.24).

In your own work situation, you can do a great amount of good for yourself no matter what is imposed on you by management and circumstance. Be on the lookout for ways you can use your tools and place your materials and supplies that will reduce unnecessary strain and effort. Mindfulness in this regard can make a tremendous difference in preventing overuse of muscles.

A great example is the computer, which is universally recognized as a major cause of repetitive strain. Ergonomic guidelines for working at a computer are posted and published everywhere, but they're often ignored, especially by those who are annoyed by rules. But chronic shoulder pain is a high price to pay for disdain of these things. Trouble caused by overuse tends to sneak up on you, especially with something like working at a computer keyboard, which can seem harmless at the time you're doing it because it feels so effortless. You may not be aware of the accumulating damage done by holding yourself in a subtly strained position all day, and you probably don't think about the injury that might be caused by the thousands of keystrokes and mouse clicks your fingers perform without rest or relief. Digging ditches could hardly give your muscles more grief.

Use elbow and wrist support to make it easier for your arms, neck, upper back, and shoulders. Position the keyboard so you don't have to hold the weight of your arms out in front of you. Get the monitor up high enough so you can sit up with your head balanced on your neck, not with your neck bent and your head hanging forward (Figures 3.25 and 3.26).

The mouse is an insidious cause of trouble, not only for the fingers and hand, but also, surprisingly, for the shoulder. When the mouse is placed to the far right of the keyboard beyond the number pad, it puts the arm into nearly maximum outward rotation. This requires the infraspinatus muscle to contract every time you use the mouse, adding up to a significant amount of overuse in the course of a day. A troubled infraspinatus muscle refers pain to the front of the shoulder. If you suffer chronic pain in that area, a right-handed

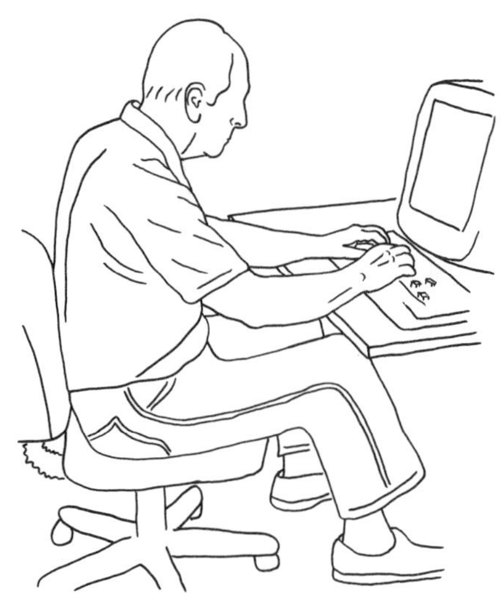

Figure 3.25 Strain at the computer, with tight muscles in the shoulders, neck, upper back, and stomach

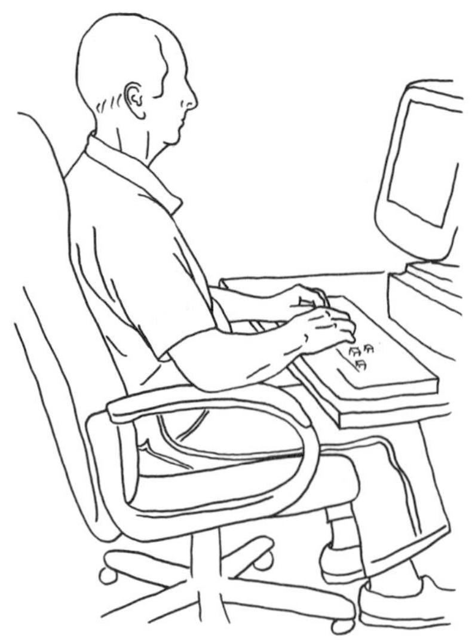

Figure 3.26 Good erect posture at the computer, with the elbows supported and the monitor higher

mouse could be the sole problem. Left-handed people have an advantage in not having to reach so far to the side to use the mouse. It's really not much of a trick for a right-handed person to learn to use the mouse left-handed and give their right shoulder a break.

A touchpad mouse is an even better ergonomic solution, requiring only a light tap on the pad to execute a click instead of contraction of finger and forearm muscles. In many laptop computers, the touch pad is placed in the middle of the keyboard right in front of the keys. This allows you to share the workload by switching hands if you like. If you use a desktop computer with a separate keyboard, consider an ergonomic keyboard with angled keys. They cause much less strain on the wrists and the forearm muscles.

Staying in any position too long, even a comfortable position, is hazardous to muscles. A static position favors the formation of trigger points because it hampers circulation. Muscles need a certain amount of contracting and relaxing to stay healthy. Many jobs are static by nature, particularly anything done sitting at a desk. Unfortunately, sedentary or inactive work gives you the impression that your work is easy, that you're not straining anything. On the contrary, you might well be under a great deal of subtle physical strain and not recognize it.

At the other end of the scale, intensity can be just as much a danger as sedentary work. Intensity is the work style of the type A personality, who sees every job as incredibly important and needing to be done extremely well and as fast as possible. Type A personalities work like they're killing snakes. If you're one of these folks, make a commitment to combating intensity. Train yourself to work loose. Tune in to your muscles while you're working and hone your awareness of unnecessary tension and any part of the job that encourages it. If you apply yourself, you can learn to selectively relax the muscles you aren't actually using for the task at hand.

There's almost always a calmer, slower, and ultimately more efficient way to do something if you just stop and think about it. Lack of commitment to making improvements may be the biggest obstacle of all to reducing repetitive strain and overuse of muscles in the workplace. The changes don't have to be big ones. Small changes can make a huge difference.

Janet Travell had a great tip for housework that could be applied to almost any kind of job. She recommended scrambling housework, not spending too long a time on any one task. Do a little bit of one job, then come back to it after doing a little of something else. This allows you to come back fresh to each task after a kind of mini break, rather than getting locked into a knotted-up position for an unreasonably extended period of time. This little change in work style can be a lifesaver.

Muscle Abuse in Sports

The springing up of sports injury clinics everywhere these days should alert you to the realities of athletic activity. People who engage in sports often know very little about how their muscles actually work. As a consequence, they don't recognize the signs of impending injury in time to prevent it. But if you're aware of trigger points when they first start up, you can treat them, stay in the game, and stay out of the sports injury clinic.

Certain sports tend to cause certain kinds of muscle overuse injuries. Tennis strokes, for example, involve both maximum contraction and maximum lengthening of all the shoulder muscles. You're apt to overstretch your infraspinatus muscle with your backhand stroke or overcontract it in drawing back your arm in preparation for your forehand stroke (Figures 3.27 and 3.28). The serve and the forehand stroke can overwork your subscapularis muscle. The infraspinatus and subscapularis are critical in the development of frozen shoulder and are exposed to risks in all the racquet sports—badminton, lacrosse, table tennis, and even handball—where your hands and arms are used in similar ways.

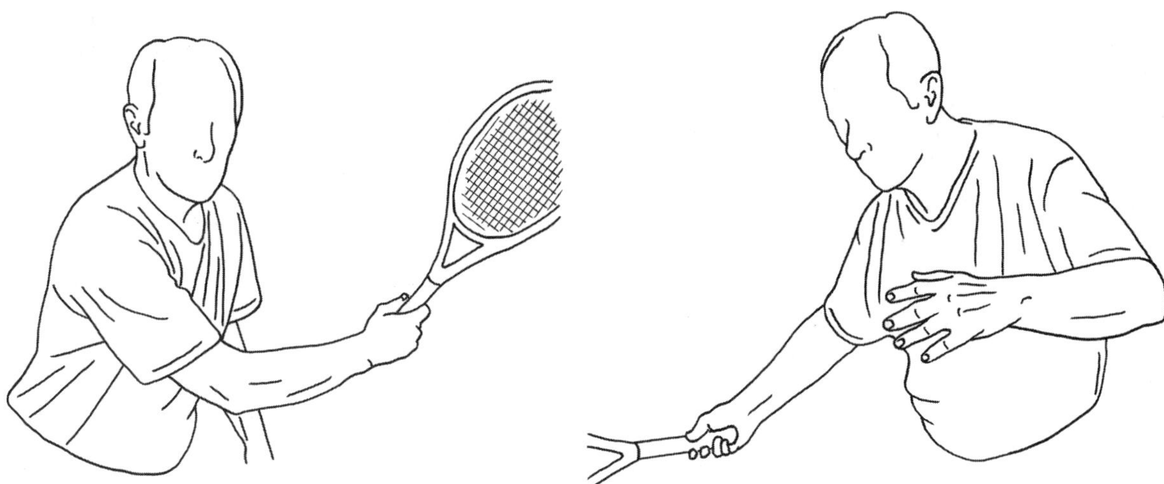

Figure 3.27 The tennis backhand stroke can overstretch the posterior deltoid, infraspinatus, and teres minor.

Figure 3.28 The tennis forehand stroke can both overstretch and overcontract the subscapularis.

Several other muscles are at risk when playing tennis, particularly the supraspinatus, which remains under contraction almost continuously during play because it's a primary muscle for lifting the arm. The extensor muscles in the forearm are also easily overworked simply by the weight of the racquet and the leverage it exerts at the wrist. Trigger points near the elbow in the extensor muscles are the primary cause of the pain known as tennis elbow.

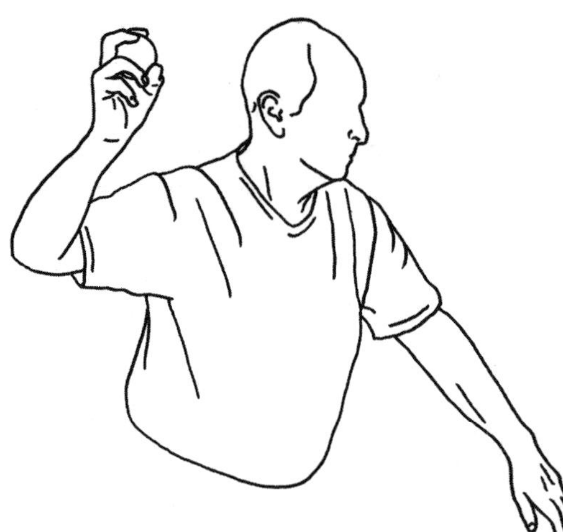

Figure 3.29 Cocking the arm in preparation for throwing a ball can overstretch the subscapularis and pectoralis major.

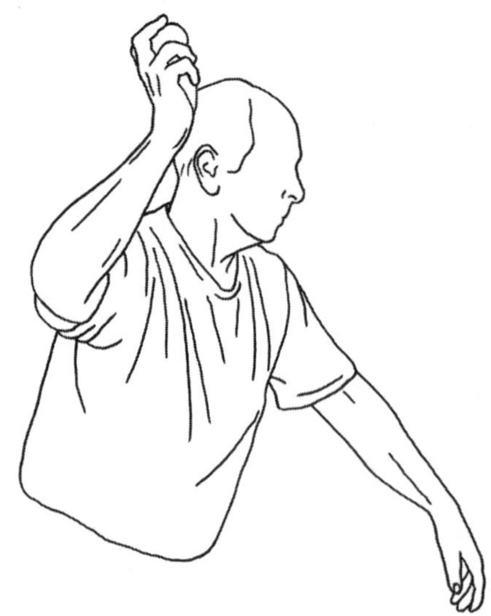

Figure 3.30 Throwing can overcontract the anterior deltoid, pectoralis major, and subscapularis muscles.

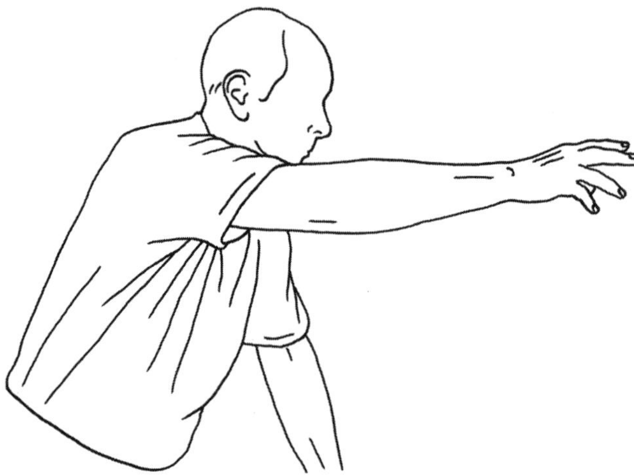

Figure 3.31 As the throw is completed, the anterior deltoid, subscapularis, and pectoralis major are in maximum contraction.

In any sport that requires throwing something—a basketball, baseball, softball, football, shot put, discus or javelin, for instance—the shoulder muscles can easily be worked beyond their strength and endurance. The four rotator cuff muscles are at special risk of overuse and overload. The function of shoulder muscles is basically the same for any kind of overhand throwing (Figures 3.29, 3.30, and 3.31).

Name your sport—golf, bowling, Frisbee, hiking, climbing, skating, hockey, wrestling, or running—all present potential dangers for certain muscle groups. Frisbee, presumably the least strenuous of the forenamed sports, can easily overwork the muscles responsible for outward rotation of the arm (Figures 3.32 and 3.33). Ironically, the flick of your wrist when you let the Frisbee go can overwork the extensor muscles of your forearm and give you tennis elbow.

Golf makes extraordinary demands on the muscles of both shoulders, requiring maximum lengthening and maximum contraction of the pectorals, deltoids, rhomboids, and rotator cuff muscles (Figure 3.34 and 3.35). Trigger points in any of these muscles can profoundly affect coordination. Few golfers, amateur or professional, are aware of how trigger points can undermine their game. Getting good at treating your trigger points can keep you on the greens and might even lower your score.

No matter what your sport, it would be good to figure out which muscles it works the hardest. Special attention should be given to muscles that are required to stretch to their maximum length. Then devote yourself to learning how to monitor them during the sport

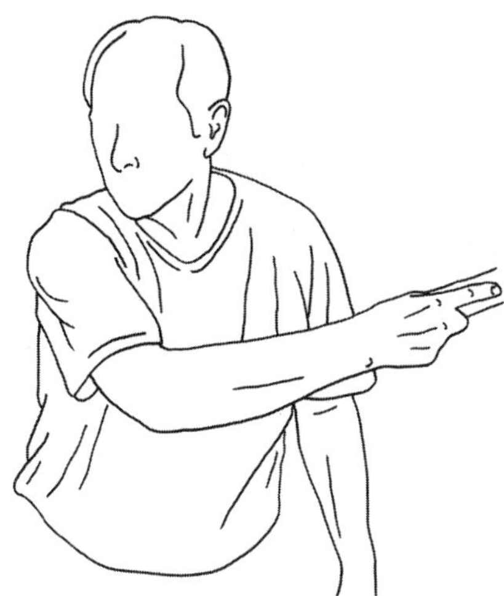

Figure 3.32 Throwing a Frisbee can strain the biceps, pectoralis major, anterior deltoid, supraspinatus, and subscapularis muscles.

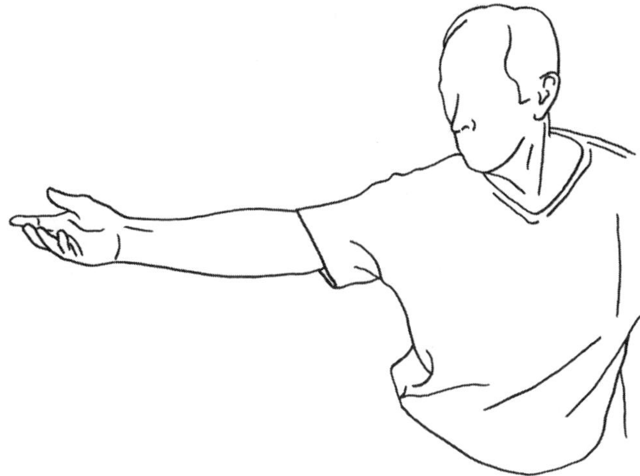

Figure 3.33 A hard throw of a Frisbee can overcontract the infraspinatus, teres minor, posterior deltoid, supraspinatus, trapezius, and rhomboid muscles.

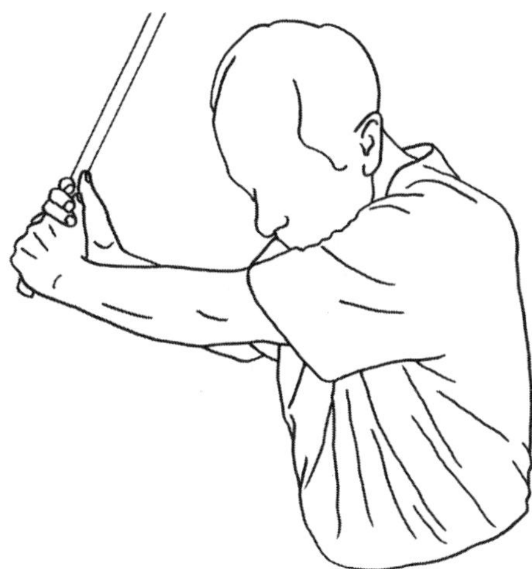

Figure 3.34 The backswing in golf can either overcontract or overstretch almost any of the muscles in both shoulders.

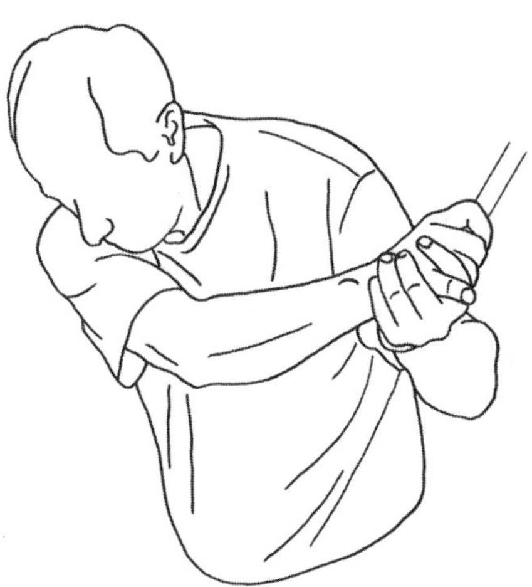

Figure 3.35 The muscles that had to lengthen in the backswing must now contract, and ones that contracted must lengthen.

and how to massage their trigger points when you've worked them too hard. Muscles that are especially vulnerable should be treated before you play, as well as afterward. Trigger point massage is more effective than stretching because it goes directly to the source of the problem.

Swimming is an example of how insidiously harmful a sport can be. You'd think it would be among the safest and most healthful of athletic activities, but it's extraordinarily demanding of the shoulder muscles. In the crawl stroke, for instance, the subscapularis muscles have to work exceptionally hard to pull you forward. The crawl actually puts subscapularis muscles in double jeopardy because they undergo a near-maximum stretch when you reach forward to begin each stroke (Figure 3.36). If you overwork these muscles and fail to treat trigger points as they arise, you may well be setting yourself up for a frozen shoulder.

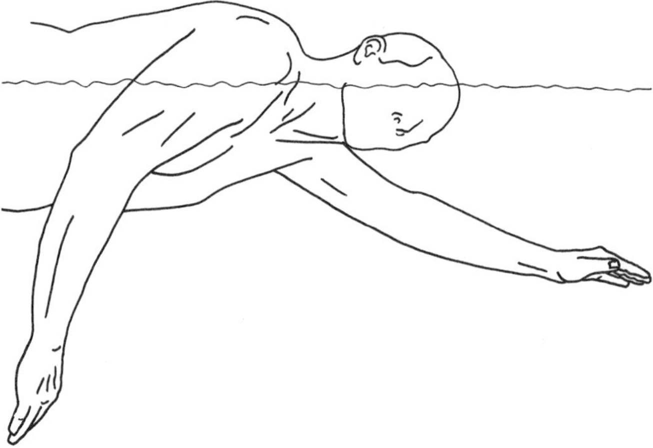

Figure 3.36 Swimming puts many of the shoulder muscles at risk for strain and overuse. You can keep swimming if you treat trigger points before and after going in the water.

Trigger points in the subscapularis give you a deep ache in the back of the shoulder. They also inhibit lengthening of the muscle, making it hard to reach upward or back. When the subscapularis is handicapped by trigger points, almost any movement of your arm aggravates the problem.

Committed athletes do stretching routines faithfully as preventative therapy. Ironically, overly ambitious stretching programs can actually create trigger points. It might be better to implement a regular routine of self-applied trigger point massage for both the treatment and the prevention of myofascial injuries. Remember that muscles with trigger points in them are more vulnerable to pulls and tears because they actively resist stretching. If you believe in stretching, you can make better use of it after you have your trigger points under control.

Exercise is a classic source of myofascial trigger points when overdone or done unwisely. Doing even more exercise in the hope of healing trigger points—working through the pain—is not a good idea. It may be an effective strategy for postexercise soreness, but not for trigger points. To differentiate between trigger point pain and postexercise soreness, search for trigger points. The soreness of a trigger point occurs at a specific spot in the muscle. With postexercise soreness, the entire muscle or entire limb hurts.

Other Avoidable Kinds of Muscle Abuse

Along with mindlessly overdoing it at work and play, there are an unlimited number of other, less obvious, ways to abuse muscles and create trigger points. To begin with, being out of shape and overweight sets you up for the overuse of muscles and the onset of trigger points. If your body is out of shape and your weight out of control, you may feel that the last thing you need is another lecture. But you do need to understand that trigger points can be very difficult to treat effectively when you have to work through layers of excessive fat. Beyond a certain limit, you can't even find them. Excess weight can put a severe limit on your ability to solve your shoulder problem and get rid of your pain.

If you start a conditioning program, however, remember that exercise can be overdone. Even reputedly safe activities like low-impact aerobics and yoga can exacerbate your trigger points and myofascial pain. If you already have shoulder pain, and certainly if you have a frozen shoulder, get a start on your trigger points before getting into extensive exercise.

What other sneaky things promote trigger points? Awkward sleep positions can do it, especially positions that keep a muscle or group of muscles in a shortened state for hours on end. The pain you have when you wake up can give you a clue to which muscle you may be subjecting to this kind of abuse. As an example, pain in the front of the shoulder may indicate that you're spending too much time with your arm in extreme outward rotation, which keeps

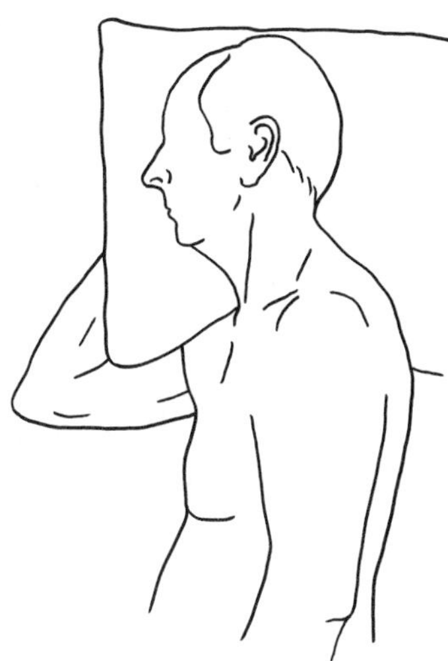

Figure 3.37 Sleeping with the arm under the pillow promotes trigger points by keeping the infraspinatus shortened.

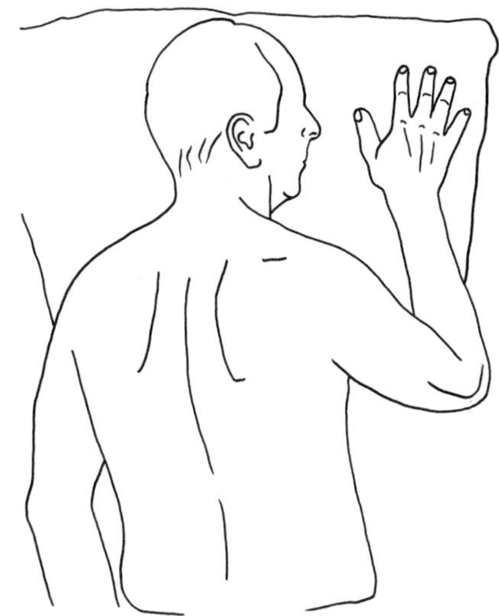

Figure 3.38 Sleeping on the stomach with the arm up promotes trigger points in the infraspinatus muscle.

the infraspinatus in a shortened state (Figures 3.37 and 3.38). This is a very serious issue and deserves all the time it takes to come up with some answers. You may have to change some treasured sleep habits, but it only takes about three days to drop an old habit and institute a new one. Plus, there's a good chance you may like the new one better.

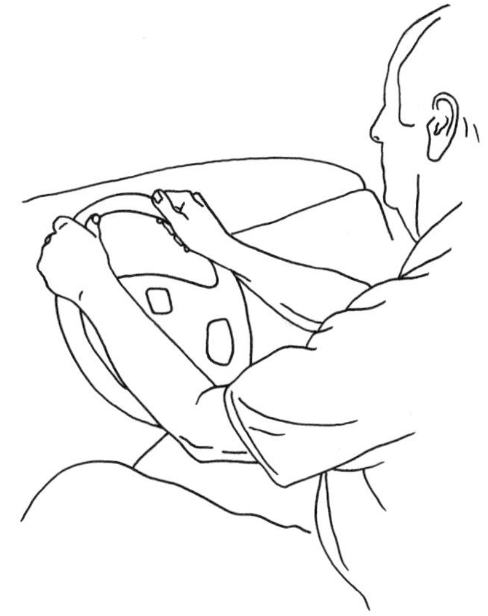

Figure 3.39 Driving with the hands high on the steering wheel can overtax the anterior deltoid, supraspinatus, and infraspinatus.

Long evenings sitting in front of the TV or driving long distances both have built-in dangers, mainly because of the immobility imposed on certain muscles. Immobility and inactivity foster trigger points in muscles. Driving can also put undue strain on the muscles of your right lower leg when they're overworked, even in normal use of the accelerator and brake pedals. Using the cruise control at every opportunity is a good way to keep this kind of trouble at bay. But even with cruise control, long trips are a hazard for shoulder muscles that have to stay continuously contracted to keep your hands up on the steering wheel (Figure 3.39). The anterior deltoid, infraspinatus, trapezius, and supraspinatus muscles are especially at risk. Trigger points in these muscles are specific causes of shoulder and neck pain. Trapezius trigger points are also a source of tension headaches.

Do you often reach behind you into the backseat for things? This is an extraordinarily bad idea because of the cramping effect this maneuver has on the rotator cuff muscles, the most vulnerable muscles in the shoulder complex. You'll notice a different feeling of strain depending whether your arm is rotated inward or outward. When reaching back, you're likely to severely overcontract either the subscapularis or the infraspinatus (Figures 3.40 and 3.41). For many people, this is exactly the movement that set them on the road to a frozen shoulder.

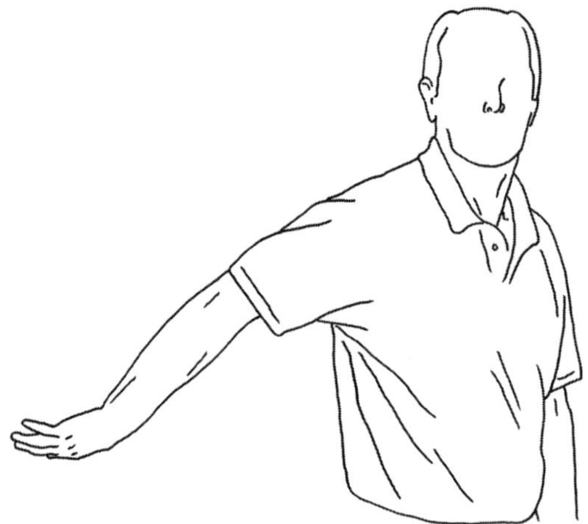

Figure 3.40 Reaching back with maximum inward rotation strongly contracts the subscapularis muscle.

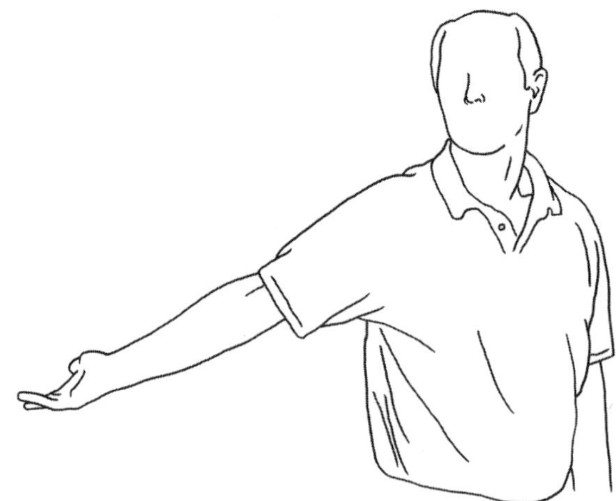

Figure 3.41 Reaching back with maximum outward rotation strongly contracts the infraspinatus muscle.

How about hobbies, household chores, and other day-to-day activities? Examine all of these activities just as you would the ergonomics of your job or your golf game. For instance, walking a dog who continuously pulls at the leash can put intolerable strain on your shoulder muscles. People get frozen shoulders from just this kind of trivial thing. Your shoulders will continue to pay the price for the dog's lack of self-control until you take the initiative and find a solution.

As you see, something very simple and mundane can underlie your shoulder trouble. Any regular or habitual activity can be full of unsuspected muscle abuse. Study how you may be running the vacuum cleaner, ironing shirts, shoveling snow, starting the lawn mower, washing windows, and lifting or carrying a child.

Be mindful regarding any household job that requires working with your hands above your head for a long period of time, such as painting or lifting things onto shelves (Figures 3.42 and 3.43). Assuming an unaccustomed posture for several hours can be particularly stressful, as many weekend gardeners can testify. Supporting your weight on one arm while

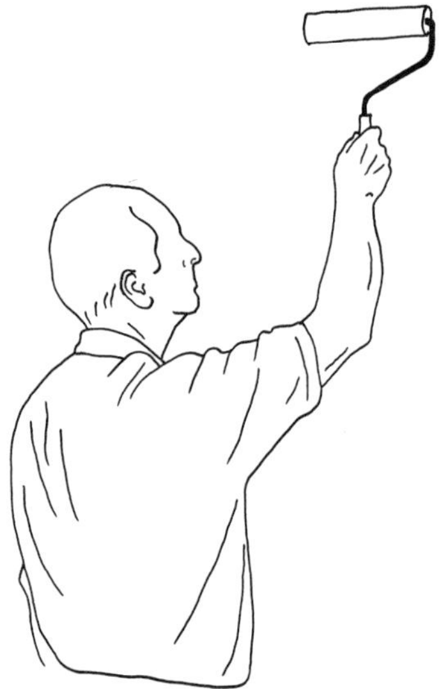

Figure 3.42 Painting overhead can strain the supraspinatus, trapezius, and deltoids.

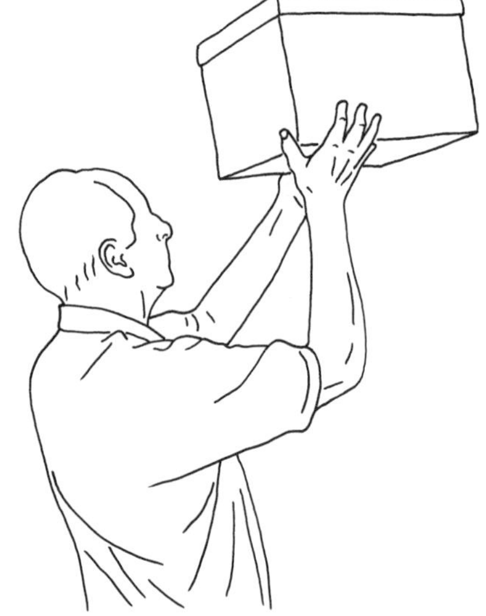

Figure 3.43 Lifting objects overhead can strain the deltoids, trapezius, and rotator cuff muscles.

on your hands and knees puts the subscapularis muscle under unusual strain (Figure 3.44). You may not recognize the abuse until it's too late and you have shoulder pain and reduced range of motion from subscapularis trigger points.

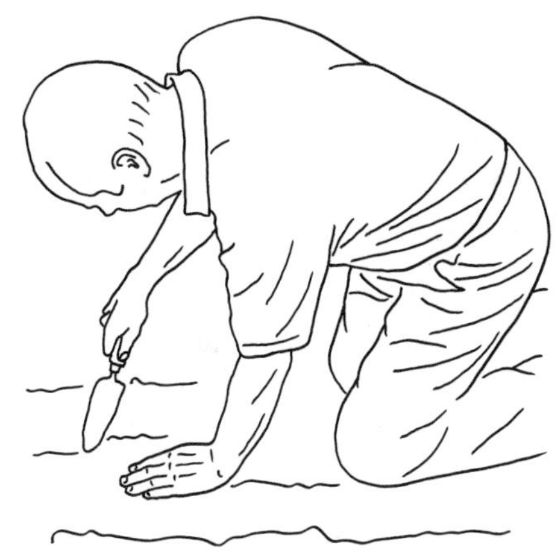

Figure 3.44 Supporting your weight on one arm can strain the subscapularis muscle.

Unavoidable Muscle Abuse

Muscles that suffer a direct impact in accidents such as falls and auto collisions are bound to be afflicted with trigger points afterward. Trigger points can also be expected to result from the wrenching movements that occur during these events, when muscles can be either overcontracted or overstretched. It's natural to thrust out an arm to catch yourself when you fall, but the subscapularis muscle very commonly undergoes a hard contraction during such an event, and trigger points are an inevitable result (Figures 3.45 and 3.46). If they go unrecognized and untreated, they can precipitate the development of a frozen shoulder.

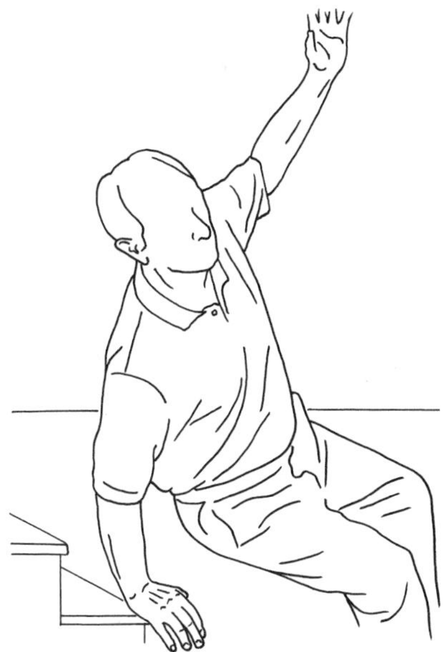

Figure 3.45 Catching yourself while falling can overcontract the subscapularis muscle.

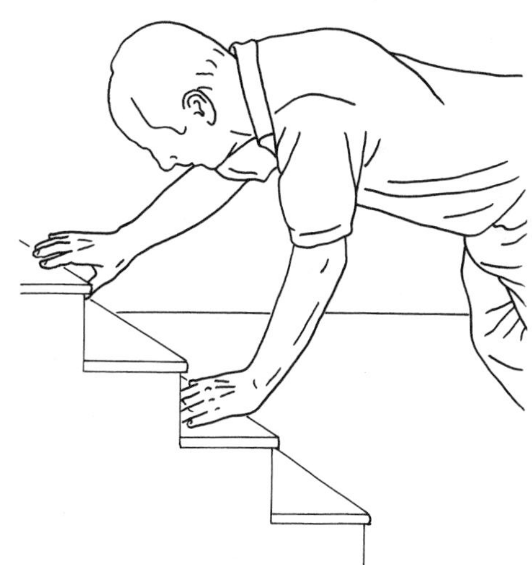

Figure 3.46 Catching yourself while falling forward can also overcontract the subscapularis muscle.

Myofascial trigger points are a major source of the pain of whiplash, though they too often go unsuspected and unaddressed. Also, any physical injury that entails a fracture, muscle tear, ligament sprain, or joint dislocation is likely to produce an accompanying insult to the muscles involved. Although the muscles may have no visible injury, they're certain to have trigger points.

Too often, health care practitioners are unaware of the effects of myofascial trigger points or discount them as trivial. Failure to recognize and treat trigger points as an inevitable part of any physical injury perpetuates needless pain and can defer complete recovery indefinitely. Falls or accidents that cause shoulder pain are of special concern, because pain from untreated trigger points in the shoulder area is the usual preamble to a frozen shoulder. In addition, muscle shortening and reduced range of motion from trigger points can leave you vulnerable to more serious injuries such as muscle and tendon tears (Simons, Travell, and Simons 1999, 437-439).

Unsuspected Muscle Abuse

According to Travell and Simons, many kinds of medical treatment can be an unrecognized cause of trigger points and myofascial pain. This is called *iatrogenic pain*, meaning that it's caused by medical treatment.

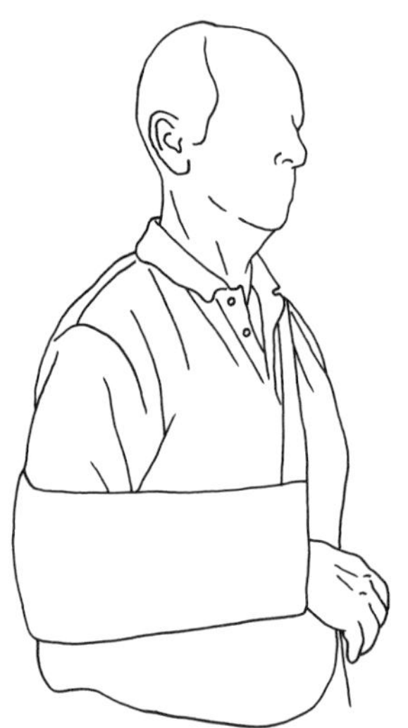

Figure 3.47 Carrying your arm in a sling can promote trigger points and sometimes lead to a frozen shoulder.

As an example, trigger points are frequently initiated by the immobility imposed by braces, slings, and casts. Indeed, the protective bracing that keeps you from moving an injured arm is a well-known beginning point for the development of frozen shoulder (Figure 3.47). Bed rest after suffering a stroke imposes a similar kind of inactivity on shoulder muscles. It's not a coincidence that stroke victims are frequently also the victims of frozen shoulder (Simons, Travell, and Simons 1999, 128).

When surgery leaves long-term residual pain, trigger points should be suspected in muscles that have been cut, stretched, bruised, or otherwise traumatized. Since these trigger points may send pain to places well away from the location of the surgery, physicians may persist in trying to treat the site of the pain, not recognizing it as referred myofascial pain. They may then overlook and fail to attend to the real cause, the trigger points associated with the surgical operation.

An ordinary injection in the buttocks can set up trigger points, particularly in the gluteus minimus, which can leave a patient with an agonizing case of sciatica that may last for months (Figure 3.48). Trigger points caused by an injection in the gluteus medius can leave you with low back pain that you didn't have before (Figure 3.49). An injection in the shoulder can leave deltoid trigger points (Figure 3.50).

Cortisone injected into painful shoulder joints, though seeming to bring relief, may not be an appropriate treatment when the pain is of myofascial origin. The trouble is that the patients may think they've been cured and unwittingly go on with the same stressful activity that caused the trigger points in the first place. The relief is only temporary anyway. When the trigger points go untreated, the pain usually returns unabated just as soon as the effects of the cortisone wear off. Also, overuse of cortisone and other steroids can seriously degrade the connective tissue of muscles, ligaments, and tendons, making them vulnerable to tears. Eventually, shoulder surgery may be needed to repair the damage. You can be fairly certain that a physician who uses steroids to get rid of your shoulder pain has never studied myofascial pain (Simons, Travell, and Simons 1999, 153).

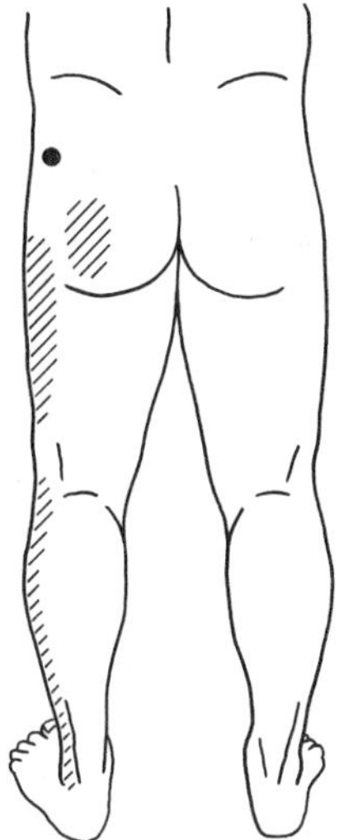

Figure 3.48 An injection in the buttocks can cause trigger points that produce sciatica.

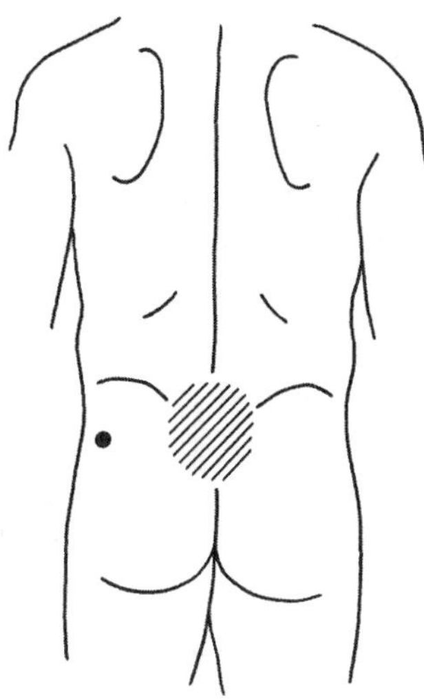

Figure 3.49 An injection in the buttocks can cause trigger points that produce low back pain.

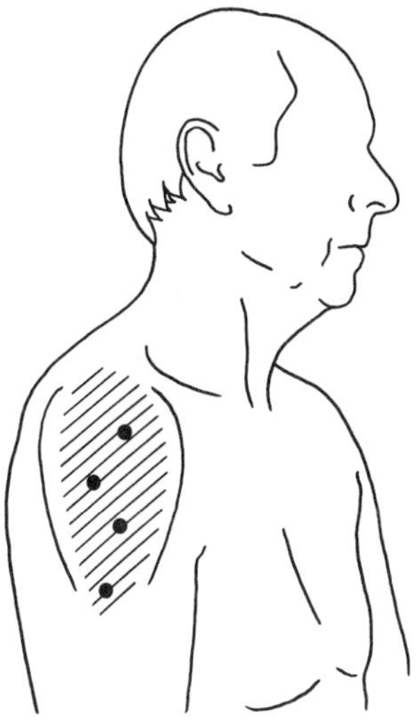

Figure 3.50 An injection in the deltoid can cause trigger points that produce shoulder

Pain medications continue to be the treatment of choice for pain because they work so well in reducing your awareness of it. But pain must always be viewed as a message that something is wrong and needs attention. It's not enough to kill the messenger with a pain pill and ignore the message. Many people concerned about side effects are becoming leery of all medications and remedies taken into the body. Tragically, medical history is full of examples of the truth about a prescription drug being revealed to the public only after horrifying damage has occurred.

It's not unreasonable to wonder whether a medication prescribed for pain, depression, anxiety, or such conditions as high blood pressure may cause more illness than it cures. As an example, Travell and Simons tell about research indicating that calcium channel blockers for hypertension appear to irritate and perpetuate trigger points. In other words, your high blood pressure medicine may be worsening your shoulder pain (Simons, Travell, and Simons 1999, 75). Doctor Sidney Wolfe, in *Worst Pills, Best Pills* (2005), lists scores of drugs known to potentially cause muscle pain as a side effect. If you take prescription drugs for any reason, it would be worth your while to look into natural therapies and changes in your lifestyle that would allow you to do without them. If you're taking painkillers, you may able to dispense with them by learning self-treatment of trigger points.

It's important to be aware that trigger points can also be activated by emotional distress, viral infections, diabetes, arthritis, joint dysfunction, or visceral disorders. Examples of visceral disease that can promote trigger points are angina, heart attacks, ulcers, gallstones, kidney disease, and cancer (Simons, Travell, and Simons 1999, 956-957). Viscerosomatic referral of pain from internal organs to muscles results in the formation of trigger points in the referral zone. Trigger points that form in response to systemic problems like viral infections, diabetes, and arthritis may be due to their effects on muscle metabolism. This may be the reason frozen shoulder affects as many as 20 percent of people with diabetes, compared to 5 percent of those without diabetes (Kordella 2002, 60-64; Bridgman 1972, 31-69; Cailliet 1991, 109).

Trigger Point Perpetuators

Sometimes trigger points can be very hard to subdue. After you seem to have successfully defeated them, you may find that they come right back. Also, it's easy to underestimate the influence of perpetuating factors on myofascial pain, even when you know about them. If you have a sense that some influence other than overuse is contributing to your problem, it's a valuable intuition, but only if you can figure out what it means. Hidden influences are likely to be chemical in nature and therefore rather subtle and generalized throughout your system, which makes them difficult to pin down.

Travell and Simons believe the management of perpetuating factors is the most important aspect of treating chronic trigger point pain. It can make a critical difference in whether trigger point therapy will succeed and whether its benefits will last. A perpetuating factor is sometimes so important that removing it allows a trigger point to resolve on its own. Some systemic factors, such as vitamin deficiency, can actually be the initiating circumstance in the creation of trigger points (Simons, Travell, and Simons 1999, 179).

The circumstances that make a frozen shoulder so persistent and long lasting may include factors that are far from obvious. Metabolic, genetic, and glandular disorders can perpetuate trigger points, as can psychological issues and numerous physical considerations.

Physical Factors

Some of the physical factors that can contribute to the perpetuation of trigger points are postural stress, poor work habits, repetitive strain, lack of exercise, and congenital irregularities in bone structure. All these factors except abnormal bone structure are largely under your own control, usually interrelated, and based essentially on habits that you've carelessly acquired. You may not be fully aware of how your personal habits are contributing to your shoulder trouble and other kinds of chronic pain. The next few pages will help you see whether you'd like to make some new decisions regarding how you go about your day. You may even be able to improve on some structural flaw that nature has bestowed on you.

Abnormal Bone Structure

Some people are born with a bone abnormality that can become a trigger point perpetuator. A short leg, an asymmetrical pelvis, short upper arms, and a long second metatarsal bone in the foot are often found to be the source of persistent problems with recurrent myofascial pain. Abnormal bone structure can make it necessary for the body to continuously compensate, resulting in perpetual strain on particular groups of muscles. Unequal leg length may create and maintain trigger points in the legs, buttocks, back, and neck. Unless corrected by a heel lift or other means, a short leg may cause persistent or recurrent pain in these areas. Using an appropriate heel lift has even been known to stop intractable headaches (Simons, Travell, and Simons 1999, 180-181). Unfortunately, leg length is difficult to measure accurately. Chronically tight muscles can add to the difficulty by drawing up one side of the body and causing the appearance of a short leg.

Sometimes, an entire side of the body is smaller than the other. In such cases, one side of the pelvis is likely to be smaller too, which makes your pelvis tilt while sitting. This causes the spine to curve abnormally, placing an extra load on the quadratus lumborum and other back muscles. The effect can be transmitted as far away as the sternocleidomastoid and scalene muscles of the neck. Crossing your legs with the same leg over the other all the time may indicate that you're compensating for an asymmetrical pelvis. Sitting on a pad or thin cushion under the smaller side of the pelvis can help remedy this condition (Simons, Travell, and Simons 1999, 930-932).

Short upper arms are more common than you might think, and they aren't usually recognized as a potential cause for lingering myofascial pain (Simons, Travell, and Simons 1999, 299-301). You should always have elbow support while sitting, even if your arms are of normal length. When you have short upper arms, you need higher arms on the chairs you sit in. Lack of support for your elbows causes continual strain on the trapezius and levator scapulae muscles, whose trigger points cause headaches and neck pain and contribute to shoulder problems (see Figures 3.25 and 3.26).

Morton's foot, an easily corrected disparity in the length of the first and second metatarsal bones of the foot, is known to be the origin of a variety of aches and pains. The instability in the foot and ankle caused by this condition can affect virtually the entire body and may often be the underlying cause of Achilles tendinitis. All disparities concerning the bones seem to ultimately affect the trapezius muscles of the neck, upper back, and shoulders. Bone abnormalities should always be considered when trying to resolve a frozen shoulder or even simple shoulder pain (Simons, Travell, and Simons 1999, 179-184).

Postural Stress

Strained or awkward positions in your work situation can not only cause trigger points but make them hard to get rid of. The apparent comfort and familiarity of a longtime habit can make you unaware of its effects on your muscles. It's wise to examine how you sit, stand, and work to find the ways in which you may be subjecting certain muscles to continuing tension and strain. See if you're keeping an arm or leg locked in a cramped position while you work. Observe whether you're keeping your head turned or cocked at an angle for long periods of time. Develop an awareness of unusual tightness in muscles that might indicate postural imbalance.

Badly designed seating is the source of much chronic back and neck pain and shouldn't be overlooked when working out a shoulder problem. Trigger points can be caused and perpetuated by misfitting furniture such as couches and chairs and the bucket seats in cars, all of which strain muscles by failing to properly support the body. You may be so accustomed to these strains that you don't notice them. One of Janet Travell's sidelines was redesigning various kinds of seating for manufacturers. She's the person who prescribed a rocking chair for President Kennedy (Travell 1968, 284-285).

Another factor that may perpetuate trigger points without ever rising to the level of consciousness is the constriction of muscles by a brassiere, necktie, purse strap, hat, belt, or even socks. Any muscle that's deprived of a free flow of blood and oxygen is apt to develop trigger points, and a continuing restriction will keep the trigger points going. You may have heard of the type of sciatica caused by carrying a fat wallet in the back pocket. This restricts circulation in certain buttock muscles and perpetuates trigger points that cause the muscles to pinch the sciatic nerve, causing pain and numbness in the leg. Trigger points generated in the trapezius muscle by a backpack or heavy purse on a shoulder strap can be the unsuspected source of chronic shoulder pain and headaches (Simons, Travell, and Simons 1999, 287).

The sedentary lifestyle so common in the world today is both a cause and a perpetuator of trigger points. Muscles need to work in order to stay healthy. Keeping them immobile or inactive encourages them to stiffen and shorten and makes their trigger points resistant to therapy. Shoulders are particularly at risk when you habitually go all day long without putting your arms through their normal range of motion. Poor posture in general, characterized by slumping with your head, neck, and shoulders hanging forward, is also a perpetuator, making it hard to resolve myofascial pain in these areas (Simons, Travell, and Simons 1999, 184-185).

Repetitive Movement

The seeming effortlessness of repetitive office work can have an insidious effect on large and small muscles alike. It can engage you in a continuing battle with myofascial pain. The small muscles of the forearms and hands have to slave away for hours at a time, contracting thousands of times a day. At the same time, larger muscles of the shoulders, upper back, and neck remain static and immobile but under continuous contraction to hold your head and arms in position. Even if you're very good at treating trigger points after the day is done, you won't achieve lasting relief unless you change your work habits.

The static posture and subtle but unrelieved strain of office work can perpetuate trigger points in any part of the upper body. Repetitive movement overloads muscles, even when it requires only minimal effort. Repetitive movement in more strenuous kinds of work can actually be healthier because you're more apt to be aware of when your muscles are growing tired. Even so, the repetitious nature of many jobs in industry makes it very difficult to permanently subdue myofascial problems. If the health of the workers is worth anything to the corporate bottom line, it would be much more cost-effective and productive to allow people to vary their tasks a number of times during the day (Simons, Travell, and Simons 1999, 185-186).

Vitamin and Mineral Inadequacies

Trigger points are aggravated by anything that cuts the supply of energy to your muscles, including deficiencies of essential vitamins and minerals. Travell and Simons were convinced that nearly half the patients they treated for chronic pain were lacking certain vitamins or minerals necessary for balanced muscle metabolism. These critical nutrients include the water-soluble vitamins B_1, B_6, B_{12}, C, and folic acid. Drinking excessive amounts of water can actually wash the soluble B vitamins out of your system, keeping you deprived of them even when your intake is presumably sufficient (Simons, Travell, and Simons 1999, 191).

The minerals calcium, iron, magnesium, and potassium are also critically important. Groups of people especially likely to be deficient in these minerals are the elderly, pregnant women, dieters, the economically disadvantaged, the emotionally depressed, and people who are seriously ill.

The problem in many cases is not inadequate intake of vitamins and minerals, but consuming other substances that cause their elimination. Smoking destroys vitamin C. Alcohol, antacids, and the tannin in tea impair absorption of B_1. Antacids can also affect absorption of folic acid. Oral contraceptives leave you short of vitamins C and B_6, as do antitubercular drugs and corticosteroids. Also be wary of overdoing a good thing. Too much vitamin C or folic acid can deplete your B_{12}.

Levels of the minerals calcium, magnesium, iron, and potassium must be adequate for muscles to function normally. The exchange of calcium ions is directly involved in the contraction and relaxation of muscle fibers. Magnesium is needed in conjunction with the body's use of calcium, and low levels of magnesium are associated with muscle hyperexcitability and weakness. Iron enables muscle tissue to use the nutrients and oxygen delivered by the blood. Iron also has a role in regulating body temperature. People with inadequate iron feel cold much of the time. Too much iron, however, is as bad as too little, sometimes leading to skin discoloration, heart disease, and slow recovery from stroke. Potassium deficiency affects the functioning of heart muscles and other smooth muscles.

Despite these concerns, Travell and Simons believe that it isn't necessary to conduct complete laboratory evaluations of your nutritional status. They believe that under normal conditions a good multivitamin with minerals should meet your needs (Simons, Travell, and Simons 1999, 186-213).

Metabolic Disorders

You're likely to have trouble getting rid of your trigger points when any chemical or glandular imbalance interferes with metabolism in the muscles. Some conditions to watch out for are thyroid inadequacy, hypoglycemia, anemia, and high levels of uric acid in the blood (uricemia). Nicotine, caffeine, and alcohol cause enough irregularity in metabolism to make it difficult to keep trigger points deactivated (Simons, Travell, and Simons 1999, 213-220).

Low output from the thyroid gland (hypothyroidism) can increase the irritability of muscles, predisposing them to development of trigger points and making relief from trigger point therapy very short-lived. Typical signs of hypothyroidism include muscle cramps, weakness, stiffness, and pain. Other symptoms are chronic fatigue, inability to tolerate cold, dry skin, hyperactivity, disturbed menstruation, and trouble losing weight. Thyroid inadequacy may also play a role in fibromyalgia. Lithium appears to lower thyroid secretion, while estrogen replacement increases it. This means that, indirectly, lithium may make your trigger points worse and estrogen may make them better (Simons, Travell, and Simons 1999, 214-218; Sonkin 1994, 45-60; Bochetta et al. 1991, 193-198).

Recurrent bouts with hypoglycemia (low blood sugar) tend to aggravate trigger points and decrease the effectiveness of trigger point therapy. Symptoms of hypoglycemia are a fast heartbeat, sweating, shaking, and increased anxiety. A more severe spell can bring visual disturbances, restlessness, trouble with thinking and speaking, and even fainting. Emotional distress makes you more susceptible to hypoglycemia. Caffeine and nicotine both accentuate the secretion of adrenaline, which can worsen this condition. Alcohol, even in moderate amounts, can keep your liver from producing glycogen and make you hypoglycemic while the alcohol is in your system and sometimes for a day or two afterward (Simons, Travell, and Simons 1999, 219-220; Foster and Rubenstein 1980, 1758-1762).

Uricemia can make your trigger points more troublesome. Gout, the deposit of urate crystals in the joints, is the extreme manifestation of this problem. A diet of too much meat and too little water is likely to promote uricemia. Vitamin C helps combat the problem (Simons, Travell, and Simons 1999, 220; Kelley 1980, 479-486).

Psychological Factors

Tension, anxiety, chronic depression, and common nervousness can make trigger point therapy ineffective. So can "good sport syndrome," wherein you insist on working or playing through the pain. On the other hand, hypochondria or a sense of hopelessness can handicap your immune system, lower your resistance, and make you unresponsive to trigger point therapy (Simons, Travell, and Simons 1999, 220).

Cultivate an awareness of when you're holding rigid postures and how this relates to your emotional state. Going around with hunched shoulders is a classic sign of excessive tension. You may breathe shallowly when things aren't going well. You may even hold your breath at times. If you tune in to your body during tense moments, you'll detect tightness in your chest and stomach. Emotional distress can often be reduced by simply relieving needless or excessive muscle tension. Don't be deceived into thinking that you can control muscle tension by turning on the TV, listening to music, smoking a cigarette, or taking a stiff drink. Amusements and indulgences such as these are good only as temporary distractions and are as likely to increase muscle tension as decrease it.

To cope effectively with habitual muscle tension, you have to take a decisive and organized approach. Make a decision to learn progressive muscle relaxation, a method for systematically relaxing your body one part at a time. It won't give you a quick fix for your frozen shoulder, but it will work toward preventing the next one. You can find out more about systematic muscle relaxation in chapter 12, Muscle Tension and Chronic Pain, in *The Trigger Point Therapy Workbook* (Davies 2004).

Other Factors

A number of other influences may affect your success with trigger point therapy. Chronic bacterial infections, including an abscessed tooth, sinusitis, and urinary infections, can keep trigger points going, as can viral diseases like influenza and herpes simplex virus type 1. Lack of sleep or sleep that isn't restful can also be a perpetuator of trigger points and the problems they cause.

An allergy to airborne irritants that causes respiratory distress can make it very difficult to keep up with trigger points in the neck, chest, and stomach. Food allergies can make all the body's muscles more vulnerable to stress. Parasitic infestation of the intestinal tract can perpetuate trigger points indirectly through depletion of essential nutrients. Infestations can be insidious and may be more common than you think (Simons, Travell, and Simons 1999, 220-226).

You can't depend solely on control of perpetuating factors to get rid of trigger points and myofascial pain. You may even find it hard to judge whether your work on perpetuating factors is having an effect. But keep an open mind and keep exploring. You may happen onto the one factor that makes all the difference.

Taking Action

There are many causes of trigger points that may be difficult to eliminate or change. The inescapable repetitive motion in a work situation is a perfect example. Be assured that regular self-treatment of trigger points can help keep the deleterious effects of repetitive motion at bay. You may have to massage certain muscles every hour or two, but it's well worth doing if it makes it possible to survive and prosper in a job you can't afford to lose. The next chapter will introduce you to the techniques of self-applied trigger point massage. You'll be astounded at how simple and effective trigger point massage can be if you do it right.

Chapter 4

Guidelines for Trigger Point Massage

The rubbing and kneading that you do intuitively on someone else's back or neck is exactly the right kind of therapy for trigger points. Massage seems to be something humans do by nature, for other humans and for themselves. But if extensive treatment is needed, massage can be extremely tiring for the hands. No one knows this better than a professional massage therapist who suffers from a repetitive strain injury from doing too much bodywork or going at it too hard. When doing anything with your hands, you should give due attention to ergonomics, safety, and efficiency.

Trigger points don't need a lot of hard rubbing, and you really don't have to make them hurt very much to do an effective treatment. If fact, you can easily overtreat a trigger point and leave it worse than when you started. You'll be surprised at how well trigger points respond to just the right amount of treatment—neither too much nor too little. Few things are more rewarding than trigger point massage, if you do it right.

The principles discussed in this chapter were worked out in self-treatment, which is really the best way to test their safety and effectiveness. By the same token, you should practice trigger point massage on yourself before attempting to apply it to a friend, family member, or client. A professional engaged in trigger point therapy, whether a physical therapist, physician, or massage therapist, should be a master of self-treatment. The guidelines are the same for ordinary citizens and for professional practitioners.

Self-Treatment

Although truly skillful professional massage is unquestionably the best method of trigger point therapy, there are many advantages to self-treatment. With self-treatment, you don't have to wait for an appointment, you can get help any time of the day or night, and it costs you nothing. Best of all, you don't have to rely on someone else knowing what's causing the pain in your shoulder, and you don't have to be dependent on someone else to "fix" you. No one can possibly have the connection with your pain that you have. You know exactly where it hurts and how much it hurts, and you know better than anyone else when a treatment is working and when it isn't. Most people feel a satisfying sense of empowerment when they learn how to get rid of their own pain.

Obviously, there will be some difficulties to surmount with self-treatment. You'll be able to make some kinds of pain go away very quickly, but a long-standing problem can take a while to clear up. Another reality is that trigger point massage can hurt a little, although if done correctly it will be a pleasant kind of pain at a level you can still relax into. If you're a person who reactively avoids all pain, trigger point massage may require an attitude adjustment. If you believe that all pain is bad and that it's a dumb idea to make yourself hurt, you may not be willing to do enough massage on yourself to solve your shoulder problems. On the other hand, if you try too hard to make massage work and do too much of it, your body will react against it and your pain may actually get worse.

When you work too long on your trigger points, you can also make yourself woozy or nauseous from the release of all the toxins in them. If you have widespread pain, you need to take a conservative approach. Don't try to fix everything at once. Work on your worst problems first and try to be patient with the method and with yourself.

Also, recognize that some of the trigger points related to ongoing stresses will tend to be recurrent. It's not reasonable to expect that you'll never have pain again. Nevertheless, with your new skills at trigger point massage, you'll be better equipped to cope with pain when it comes. Plan to be good at it. If you master the material in this book, you still may have to deal with shoulder pain from time to time, but it won't take long to get relief and it's very unlikely that you'll ever have another frozen shoulder.

Troubleshooting

Success with trigger point massage depends on understanding that most pain is referred pain and that the trigger points causing it can be found in surprising locations. Only by cultivating a methodical approach to troubleshooting can you become good at finding and deactivating trigger points. Blindly feeling around will only lead to frustration and failure.

It's too easy to get caught up in working on the place that hurts and never really solve the problem. With the shoulder, for example, it's quite natural to knead and rub the deltoid muscles, which are the superficial covering for the shoulder. This can seem to be the right thing to do because it feels so good. The deltoids often do indeed have trigger points, but they're rarely the primary cause of shoulder pain. About 90 percent of your shoulder pain is sent from somewhere else (Simons, Travell, and Simons 1999, 96).

The Trigger Point Guide at the beginning of chapter 5 or at the back of the book gives lists of muscles known to refer pain to specific places in the shoulder. To find the trigger point that's sending pain to a particular place, check the muscles on the appropriate list one at a time. The muscles are listed in order of greatest probability of causing the problem, the one at the top of the list being the most likely. Always allow for the possibility that a muscle lower on the list may be the main villain, and keep in mind that it's not unusual for several muscles to be contributing to the problem.

Muscle Names

It's important to know the right names for the muscles that are causing your shoulder trouble. It's an odd thing, but simply knowing the muscle's name makes it easier to find. The name gives it a separate identity and helps you zero in on it. You certainly have to be able to find the muscle before you can find its trigger points.

There are no other names for most of the muscles except their medical names, but don't let this intimidate you. You already know a lot more medical terminology than you may realize, thanks to drug company advertising and the medical dramas on TV. When it comes to muscles, most people have known about their biceps and triceps muscles since grade school. You also probably have a pretty good idea where your trapezius, deltoid, diaphragm, and pectoral muscles are. There are only a few muscles left to learn and you'll find their names really quite beautiful once you get them in your head.

With a little practice, you'll find that the words aren't as foreign as they seem. Many of the words we use every day are derived from Latin and Greek, and the English language has been enriched by them. Knowing the right words for your various shoulder muscles will enrich you, too. Sooner or later, you'll be telling people about trigger points and how you solved your shoulder problem. It's not enough to point and try to explain about "this thing here" and "that thing there." You really need to know the words for these things. If you need help with any of the muscle names, you'll find their pronunciations given in chapter 1, where the muscles are first introduced.

Each Muscle Has a Job

In the next three chapters, you'll learn exactly what each of the twenty-four muscles associated with the shoulder does. Understanding a muscle's mechanical function helps you find the trigger points that are causing your problem. It will also help you see what you can do to keep the problem from recurring. Simply getting rid of the pain is never enough. You need to know how to keep it from coming back.

A more intimate knowledge of your muscles also fosters an intuition about their trigger points. When you know exactly what your muscles do and have gained some experience treating them, you'll find your hands going right to the trigger points without having to consult the charts. Understanding how the muscles work also increases your awareness of problems when they're just starting up. This will enable you to nip trigger points in the bud, before they make real trouble.

Tracking Pain to Its Source

Pain referral is the essential fact about trigger points, and false assumptions about the source of your pain can defeat your every effort to get rid of it. Massage in the wrong place can feel good and yet have no effect whatever on the problem. Fortunately, patterns of pain referral are completely predictable, occurring in everyone with only small variations. The illustrations of the referred pain patterns for each muscle are the key to finding trigger points. Go back to these drawings every time you set out to deal with a pain problem.

You'll notice a tendency for trigger points to send their pain away from the center of the body, but the reverse is true too often for this to be a perfectly reliable guiding principle. Also, you'll often find that several different muscles send pain to exactly the same spot. As an example, trigger points in twelve different muscles are known to send pain to the front of the shoulder. Your pain may be coming from only one of them, or several may be contributing. The illustrations are absolutely vital for keeping it all sorted out.

To keep the illustrations simple, trigger points are usually shown on only one side of the body, but they can occur on either side or both. Referred pain typically occurs on the same side of the body as the trigger point. Only rarely will a trigger point send pain to the opposite side. Sometimes an illustration will put you exactly on target, and sometimes it will only get you in the ballpark. Ultimately you have to zero in on trigger points by feel. The aim is to get to the right area—usually a circle two or three inches in diameter, the size of a baseball—and then search for the spot of greatest tenderness.

Don't be discouraged if you can't feel the little nodules in the muscles. Some people never acquire that skill. Very experienced massage therapists are able to feel every little bump in muscles, and some can even find your trigger points with their fingertips without being told where you hurt. But when you work on yourself, you don't have to find them that way. The most reliable criterion for detecting a trigger point is its extreme tenderness (Simons, Travell, and Simons 1999, 117). Use the illustrations to get you in the ballpark, then just seek the spot that hurts the most when you press on it.

Obviously, there are medical conditions that can cause tenderness in muscles and other soft tissue. If you're in doubt, check with a physician, preferably one who's informed about trigger points and myofascial pain. It won't hurt to show physicians this book. It may be just the resource they've been needing.

The Trigger Point Massage Method

When it comes to doing trigger point massage the right way, there are two overriding issues: safety and effectiveness. You must be able to do massage without injuring your hands or the part of the body you're working on. You also have to work in a way that will actually have an effect on a trigger point.

Overuse injuries are a major issue with massage, whether it's self-applied or applied to others. Trouble stems mainly from not thinking about how you're using your hands. Massage is like any other hard physical labor. If you're not conditioned for it and go about it without any thought, you won't be able to do it very long. Even worse, you can end up with a serious, handicapping case of repetitive strain.

Doing too much massage on one spot in an effort to force a result can actually be counterproductive. Impatience will tempt you to try to kill the trigger point—to rub it out, to get rid of it right now. That's an understandable impulse, but it's generally very bad therapy because it can make things worse. It's not necessary to force a release. Trigger points release on their own when they get an appropriate level of treatment following the guidelines given in this chapter. The techniques presented here are simple and yet ergonomically sound, and you'll be pleased at how well they work. When treatment fails, it's usually the result of being too aggressive or simply treating the wrong spot.

The optimum treatment of an individual trigger point is actually quite brief, requiring no more than a dozen strokes. Then you need to leave it alone and let the body do its work. A basic tenet of good medicine is that you can only create conditions that promote healing. The body itself is the healer. You must trust your body's natural processes to respond and do their job.

Ischemic Compression

Established practice in therapeutic massage dictates that you press and hold a trigger point for a specified number of seconds, or until it presumably "releases." This is known as *ischemic compression*, meaning that you literally squeeze the blood out of the tissue. The trouble with pressing and holding a trigger point is that it can cause unnecessary pain in the muscles receiving the massage. It can be just as bad for the person doing the therapy. The press-and-hold technique requires a sustained contraction of the shoulders, arms, and hands—something you should avoid if you have any interest in working safely and efficiently.

Massage therapists who use press-and-hold as trigger point therapy very often have chronic pain in their forearms and hands. This is one of the serious ergonomic hazards that causes such a large turnover in the massage therapy profession. The burnout time for new massage therapists averages about three years. Whether you're treating yourself or someone else, you must do massage safely or you won't last very long. Fortunately, there's a much safer and more effective way to work on trigger points.

The Short, Repeated Stroke

Instead of the static pressure of ischemic compression, it's better to make a series of short, firm strokes across the trigger point nodule. This gets results quicker, with less damage to your hands, less irritation to the trigger point, and less risk of bruising the skin and muscle. In addition, a repeated moving stroke elicits a greater change in a trigger point than pressing and holding, no matter how hard you press or how long you hold.

Compressing the trigger point is the right idea, but a repeated "milking" action moves the blood and lymph fluid out more efficiently. Lymph fluid contains the accumulated waste that has been generated by the continuously contracted muscle fibers. Picture how you rinse out a dirty dishcloth. Wetting and wringing it out only once won't get it clean no matter how long and hard you twist it. You need to run fresh water through it over and over until the water wrings out of it clear and clean. A similar process works with a trigger point.

Increasing circulation in the trigger point tissue not only washes the lymph out, but also flushes out histamines and other sensitizing agents and brings in fresh blood, rich in oxygen and vital nutrients. The trigger point has been deprived of these essential substances because the knotted-up muscle fibers have been constricting the capillaries that supply them.

Another advantage of using the short, repeated stroke instead of static pressure is that intermittent pain is easier to tolerate than continuous pain. Intermittent moving pressure allows you to go deeper and evoke just a little more pain than you can stand with press and hold.

The Microstretch

Another benefit of the deep stroking technique is that it helps get the stretch back into the muscle fibers within the trigger point. Picture what would happen if you applied deep stroking massage to a ball of modeling clay: It would spread and lengthen in the direction you pushed it. The effect on muscle fibers in a trigger point is similar. Think of this as a *microstretch*, as opposed to the *macrostretch* of the whole muscle that's done in conventional stretching exercises. The microstretch is applied directly to the trigger point, right where it's needed. Done this way, there's little chance of overstretching the taut band of muscle fibers that lead from each side of the trigger point to the muscle's attachments at the bone. Abuse of this taut band risks irritating the trigger point and making it hold on tighter.

The short, repeated stroke is no more than an inch and a half long and moves slowly, a single stroke taking about two seconds—one thousand one, one thousand two. The stroke only needs to move from one side of the trigger point to the other. Stroke on one thousand one and reset on one thousand two. Also, rather than sliding your finger across the skin, move the skin with the fingers. This helps free up the underlying fascia, the thin membrane that envelops muscles. Tightness in the fascia is sometimes part of the problem. When you move the skin rather than sliding across it, you don't need oil or lotion as a lubricant.

Although you'll hear that you should always move the fluid toward the heart, it's not a critical issue here because so little fluid is being moved from an individual trigger point. It's best to stroke toward the heart if you can, but if it feels awkward, stroke in whatever direction feels easiest. If you don't make trigger point massage as easy as you can, it will wear you out and you won't want to do it. Apply pressure only as you stroke across the trigger point, taking the pressure off on the return. This gives your body a tiny but essential break between strokes and makes the work much easier.

One Kind of Stroke, Multiple Uses

This single, exceedingly simple therapeutic stroke is employed for trigger point massage everywhere in the body. It can be used not only for self-applied therapy, but also for massage between partners and for professional treatment. A physician would use exactly the same technique in palpating the muscles in search of a diagnosis. It's a technique that subjects the hands and fingers to the least strain.

Some of the methods of traditional Swedish massage are actually quite damaging to the hands when overused. One of the worst is *petrissage*, or deep kneading of the muscles with the fingers and opposing thumb, a popular and fundamental technique but one that can very quickly lead to overuse injuries. It's not unusual for massage therapists to graduate from school already disabled with chronic pain in their hands and forearms. The techniques shown in this chapter are intended to help keep this kind of thing from happening. Not only are they safer for the hands than generic massage techniques, they're also greatly more effective in treating trigger points and the pain they cause. The techniques are very efficient in terms of economy of motion, requiring much less effort than traditional methods.

Table 4.1 lists nine principles of safe, effective trigger point massage, whether self-applied or done by a professional. These rules define the basic massage stroke that is used everywhere on the body. The treatment of a given trigger point should be relatively brief, no more than fifteen or twenty seconds. When you've done that much, stop and move on. It's an adequate treatment.

Table 4.1: Massage Guidelines

1. For self-treatment, use a tool if possible and save your hands.
2. Use deep stroking massage, not static pressure.
3. Massage with short, repeated strokes.
4. Do the massage stroke in one direction only.
5. Do the massage slowly, about two seconds per complete stroke.
6. Aim for a pain level of seven or less on a scale of one to ten.
7. Limit massage to six to twelve strokes per trigger point.
8. Work a trigger point three to six times per day.
9. If you get no relief, you may be working the wrong spot.

A Pleasant Kind of Pain

Trigger points hurt when compressed, and you may be very reluctant to work them for fear of making your pain worse. You must understand that the moderate pain created by massage is actually beneficial. The electrical impulses of reasonable amounts of pain are therapeutic in that they disrupt the neurological feedback loop that maintains the trigger point. Furthermore, self-administered pain is usually self-limiting. Your natural defense mechanisms won't allow you to inflict more pain on yourself than you can stand. It's very unlikely that you'll do yourself real harm unless you try to massage too deeply with hard tools (Simons, Travell, and Simons 1999, 140-141).

The level of pain caused by massage is useful as a measure of its effectiveness. To gain maximum benefits, you should exert enough pressure to make it hurt in a good way. Aim at a pain level of seven on a scale of one to ten, where one is no pain and ten is intolerable. If a level seven seems too strong for you, pick a number you can live with. If you find yourself sputtering swear words and working with an agonized grimace on your face, you're using too much pressure.

Another positive effect of pain from massage is that it brings an immediate flood of painkilling endorphins. Interestingly, your naturally produced endorphins are chemically related to morphine but many times more powerful. If you have a really bad trigger point that you absolutely hate to work on, try giving it a good initial shot of pain, then back off and wait ten or fifteen seconds before going on. This gives the endorphins time to kick in and decrease your sensitivity. You'll then be able to work deeper with less discomfort.

If you're treating someone else, you need a way to determine the right amount of pressure to use. You can get a basic sense of this by practicing trigger point massage on yourself. When working on someone else, it's a good idea to begin with the trapezius muscles on top of the shoulders. The person's response to your pressure there is a good gauge of how much pressure to use elsewhere. Keep asking for numbers as a measure of the level of pain the person is feeling in the muscle you're working on. If you inadvertently evoke a severe level of pain, simply remove pressure from the trigger point and allow ten to fifteen seconds for the painkilling endorphins to take effect. You can often resume treatment with nearly the same pressure but with much less pain. Even so, resume cautiously.

With self-treatment, continue multiple daily treatments of the trigger point until your pressure on a trigger point elicits a pain level of only two or three. Don't expect to reach this goal in a single session. Normally, you should expect to continue massage for several more sessions after the trigger point has stopped actively referring pain.

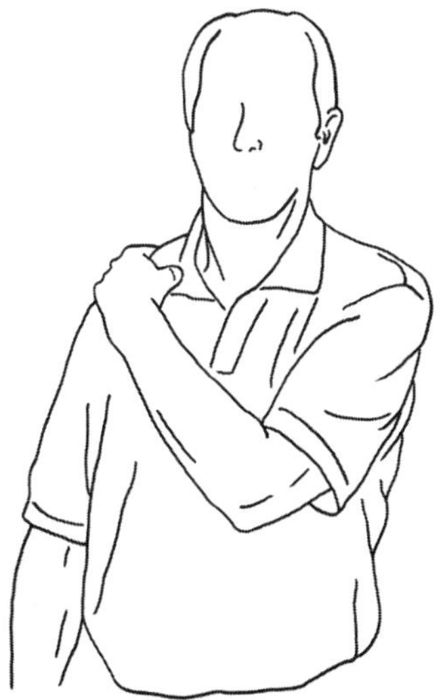

Figure 4.1 Avoid using the pincer grip for massage because it strains the fingers and thumb.

Tools for Self-Treatment

Considering the risks inherent in overworking your hands and fingers while doing self-applied massage, it's smart to avoid using them wherever possible. It seems natural, for instance, to massage your upper trapezius muscles by using a pincer grip and kneading them between your fingers and thumb (Figure 4.1). You'll find that your hand gets tired very quickly, however, without much benefit to the trapezius.

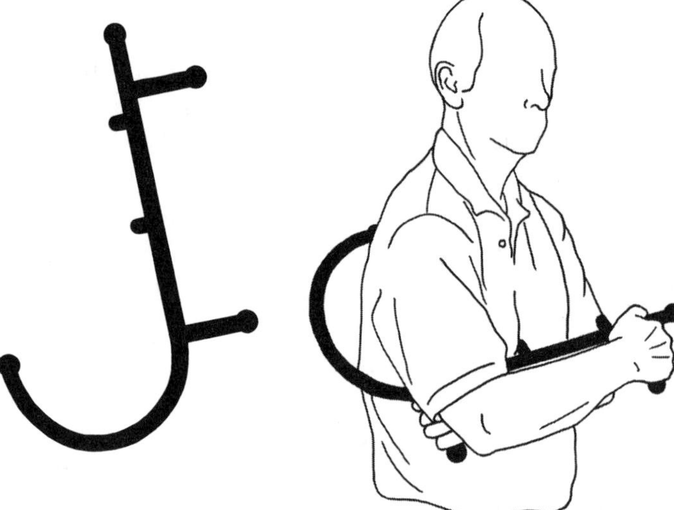

Figure 4.2 Thera Cane

Figure 4.3 Massage with crossed arms using the Thera Cane

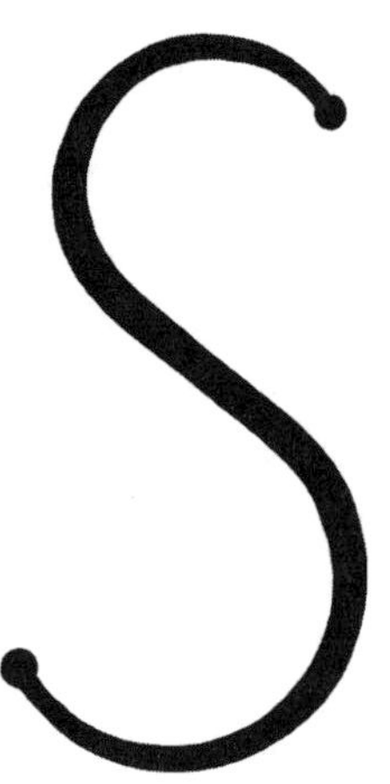

Figure 4.4 The Backnobber (comes apart in the middle for easy transport)

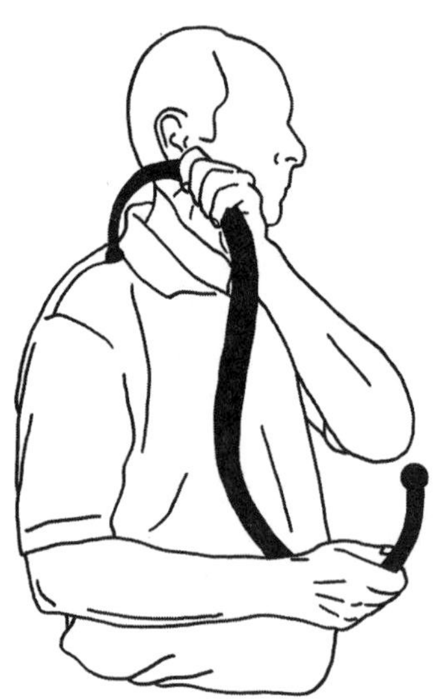

Figure 4.5 Using the Backnobber

A great variety of massage tools are available that will save your hands, amplify your strength, and let you reach difficult places. Four of the most versatile and well-designed tools are the Thera Cane (Figures 4.2 and 4.3), the Backnobber (Figures 4.4 and 4.5), the Knobble (Figures 4.6 and 4.7), and the Shemala (Figure 4.8). The Shemala is actually two tools, a rubber index finger and a rubber thumb, each with a wooden knob attached. These items, along with many other useful tools, are available through any massage therapist, massage school, or wellness center. You can also find them online.

For comfort and to avoid abrasion and bruising, massage tools should always be used through a layer of clothing. Also, notice that in using the Thera Cane or Backnobber you get better leverage by crossing your arms and reaching to the opposite side. This positioning also allows more relaxation in the muscles you're working on. The instructions that come with these tools may still advise using the press-and-hold technique on trigger points, but for all the reasons stated above, it's better to use the repeated stroke.

The simplest and least expensive tool for massaging anyplace on your back is a tennis ball pressed between your body and a wall. Putting the ball in a long sock (Figure 4.9) allows you to hang it down behind your back without the risk of dropping it and having to chase it all over the room. The sock is also a convenient handle that helps get the ball into position, which may be important if you have difficulty reaching behind your back. After you gain some experience and skill in controlling the ball and get some movement back in your arm, you can dispense with the sock (Figure 4.10).

High-bounce rubber balls give a deeper massage than tennis balls and can be found in well-stocked toy departments, often with several sizes in one package. The best size for use against a wall is the largest one, with a diameter of 60 millimeters or about $2\frac{5}{16}$ inches (Figure 4.11). High-bounce balls are firm and resilient without being too hard, and they make excellent massage tools. One problem with high-bounce balls is that they're seasonal toys and often can't be found in stores in the fall and winter. Another drawback is that they're cheaply made and are inclined to crack and break down with long-term daily use.

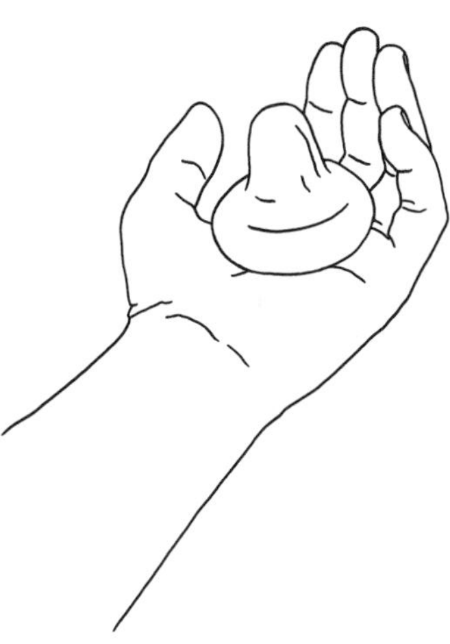

Figure 4.6 The Knobble massage tool

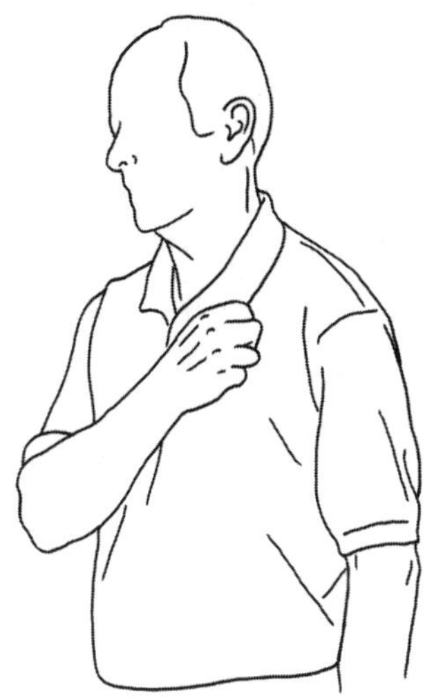

Figure 4.7 Pectoralis massage with the Knobble

A far more durable tool for massage against the wall is a lacrosse ball, which is the same diameter as a tennis ball, 64 millimeters or about 2½ inches (Figure 4.11). Lacrosse balls are harder than high-bounce balls and tennis balls, so they penetrate with less effort. They also don't slide around as much on the wall as tennis balls do. This adds up to finer, more sensitive control. For maximum effectiveness, you'll want to learn to use the lacrosse ball without the sock. Very thin people or those with very sore muscles may prefer a softer tool, such as a handball or racquetball.

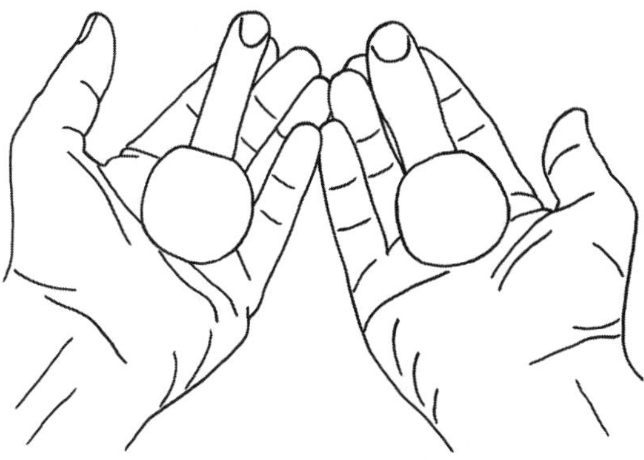

Figure 4.8 Shemala tools, the index finger shown on the left and the thumb on the right

A lacrosse ball is hard enough to dent drywall when used with sufficient force, particularly if you always use the same spot on the wall. Some people have skirted this issue by screwing a quarter sheet of half-inch plywood (two feet by four feet) to the wall to massage against. To keep the plywood from being obtrusive, install it behind an interior door that's usually kept open. Or you can put a polyurethane finish on an attractive piece of oak-veneered plywood and hang it in plain sight for all the world to see. You can invite visitors to try a little bodywork with your lacrosse ball against your "wall sculpture" while you proselytize about trigger points.

Lacrosse balls can be found in all seasons in large

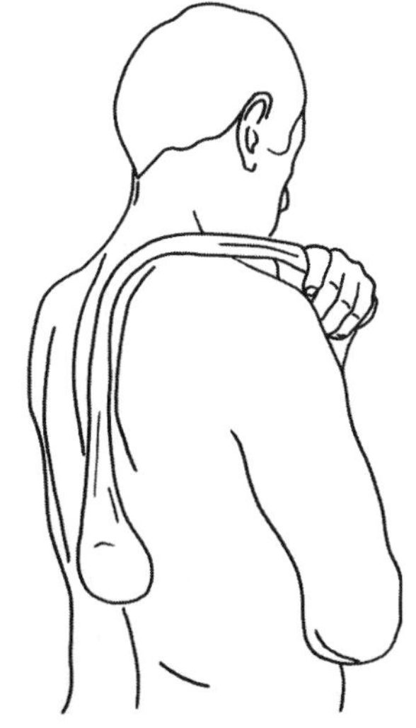

Figure 4.9 Back massage with a ball in a sock against the wall

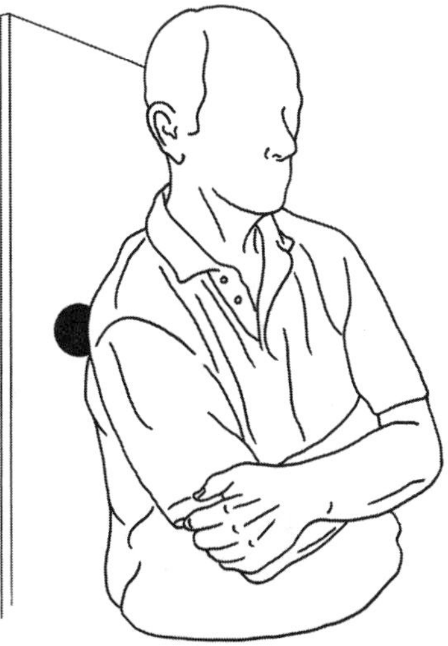

Figure 4.10 Massage with a lacrosse ball against the wall

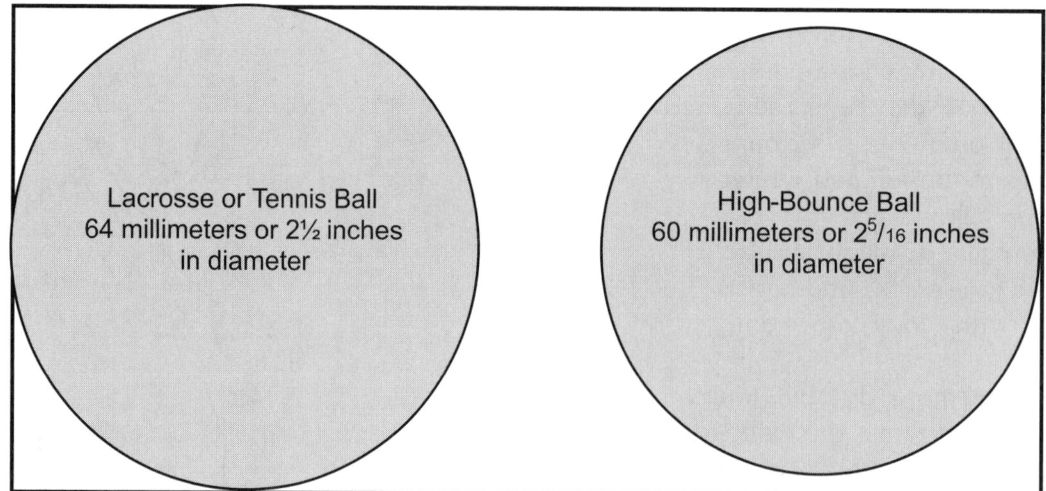

Figure 4.11 Balls used for massage against a wall, shown actual size for comparison

sporting goods stores or online. In a store, you can buy them singly. Online you may have to order a minimum of a dozen, but they're not expensive. Hand them out to friends and relatives to help spread the word on trigger points—as long as your supply of balls and receptive relatives and friends lasts.

It may occur to you to try lying on a ball on the floor to take advantage of the full weight of your body. This trick has been used for many years by people who favor the press-and-hold technique. However, you can also use your body weight with a ball against the wall if you simply move your feet away from the wall a little (Figure 4.10). When using a ball against the wall, you have more freedom to move around and execute the repeated stroke than when lying on the floor. Try it both ways and make your own choice.

A Stroke for Professional Treatment

In giving massage to someone else, it's generally not a good idea to use massage tools. To avoid unintentional injury, you really need to have the sensitive contact that you can have only with your hands and fingers. The basic principle in using your hands for massage is to apply adequate force with the least effort and strain. In treating trigger points, pair your hands whenever you can by using *supported fingers,* backing up the fingers that are doing the massage with the opposite hand (Figure 4.12). In this way, your hands can share the workload and minimize the effort and strain. This is an ideal way to make short, penetrating strokes in a safe, ergonomic fashion anywhere on the body.

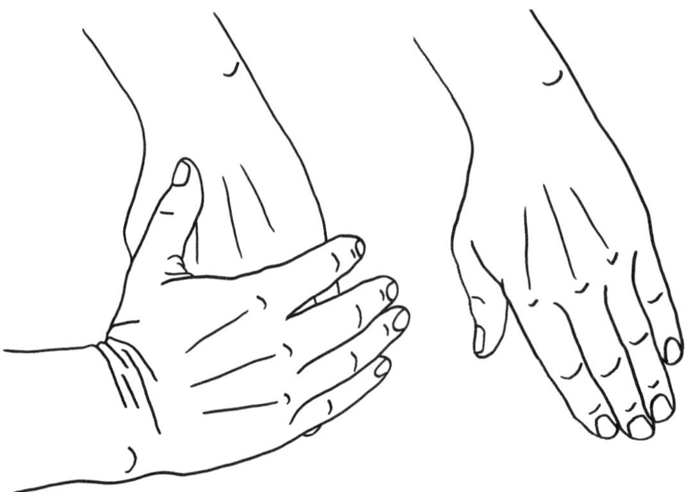

Figure 4.12 Massage with supported fingers. Note that the edge of the supporting hand covers the fingernails.

The single hand shown in Figure 4.12 illustrates how the wrist, hand, and fingers are kept straight and yet as relaxed as possible. This takes the hand and forearm muscles largely out of the equation and requires the force to come from larger muscles of the shoulders, chest, and upper back. Because of the unequal length of the fingers, focus the pressure on just two. Choose either the index finger and middle finger or the middle finger and fourth finger. Using just two strong fingers makes a very pointy tool that penetrates with minimal effort. Observe that the supporting hand completely covers the nails. The *ulnar* side (pinky side) of the hand should make contact with the skin in the area being worked on. The supporting hand actually does most of the work.

For the greatest mechanical advantage, the fingers should be held nearly vertical to the surface of the body (Figure 4.13). This allows the force to be directed in a straight line from the elbow down through the arm, wrist, and hand and out the ends of the fingers. An example of an appropriate use of supported fingers is shown in Figure 4.14.

You'll notice right away that if you have fingernails of even moderate length, they'll keep you from using your hands in this way. You'll only be able to use the flats or pads of your fingers. But massage done with the flats of the fingers is so poor ergonomically that you'll find your hands and fingers getting tired before you've gained any benefit. In some lines of work, the inefficiency imposed by long nails contributes significantly to formation of trigger points in the forearms and hands because the muscles have to work much harder to overcome the awkwardness.

If you feel that you can't do without your nails, try using *supported knuckles* (Figure 4.15). Note that the "door knocking knuckles" of your third and fourth fingers are the tool. Your wrist and "fighting knuckles" are kept straight to efficiently transfer force from the shoulders. The knuckles are a power tool and are rather blunt, unlike the fingers, whose best use is very precise massage requiring deep penetration.

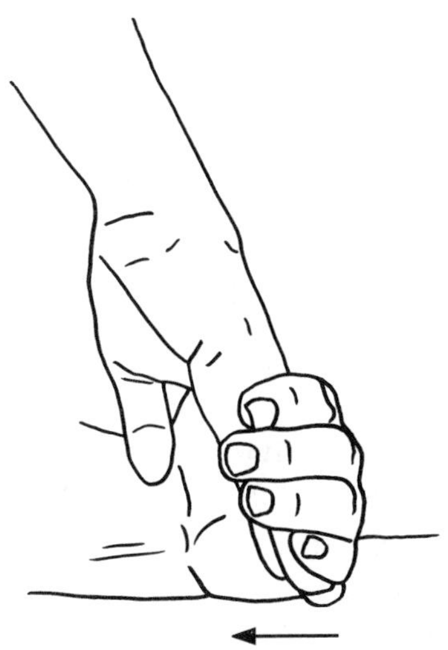

Figure 4.13 Supported fingers are used nearly vertical to the skin, pulling both hands toward you.

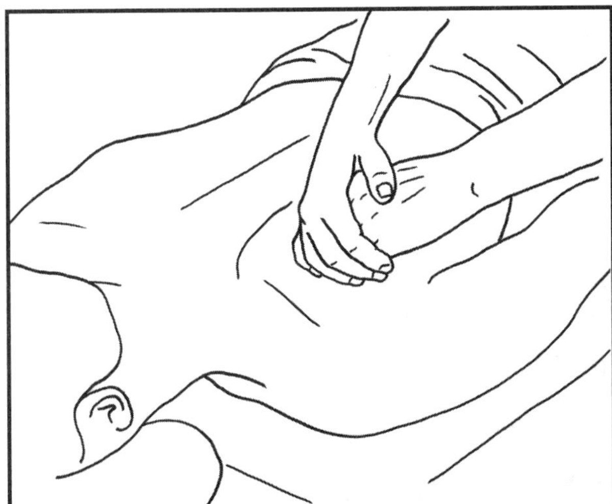

Figure 4.14 Clinical massage with supported fingers

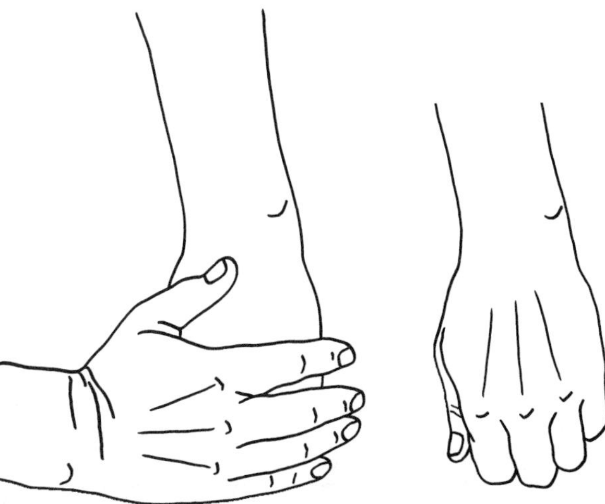

Figure 4.15 Massage with supported knuckles

Massage therapists who suffer from chronic pain in their hands, fingers, and thumbs can find full information on self-treatment in *The Trigger Point Therapy Workbook* (Davies 2004), which deals with myofascial pain throughout the body.

Massage Between Partners

There's something almost magical about the laying on of hands, even when the hands belong to someone with no particular talent or therapeutic gift. Everyone knows how pleasant a common neck rub can be. Simple human touch is extraordinarily calming and reassuring on some basic level. When the massage guidelines are understood and applied correctly, trigger point therapy can be exchanged between almost any two people, whether they be family members, domestic partners, or just good friends. A physician can use the same techniques for diagnosing trigger points. The illustrations in this section are of a father and daughter. Both, in this instance, are professional massage therapists, but partners really don't need such a high degree of skill. No degree or certification of any kind is required to do trigger point massage in an effective manner.

In the following three treatment chapters, techniques for "partner massage" will be presented for each of the twenty-four muscles that can be involved in your shoulder problem. It all comes down to being able to find the trigger points and then taking care to follow the massage guidelines.

Although it's not recommended to use a pincer grip on yourself—kneading a muscle between the fingers and opposing thumb—it can be used with discretion on someone else. But you must pair your hands to maximize the effect and minimize the risk to your hands, as shown in Figure 4.16. Note that the massage is being done from the front, which is a little counterintuitive but much more effective because trigger points in the trapezius on the top of the shoulder tend to be toward the front of the muscle. This technique works just as well with both people standing unless the disparity in height is too great. As an alternative, the point of the elbow makes an excellent tool for the top of the shoulders (Figure 4.17), but be careful to not apply too much pressure. Even in the thick trapezius muscles, the elbow can be a wicked implement. The knuckles of a loose fist make a good tool for any of the upper back muscles (Figures 4.18 and 4.19).

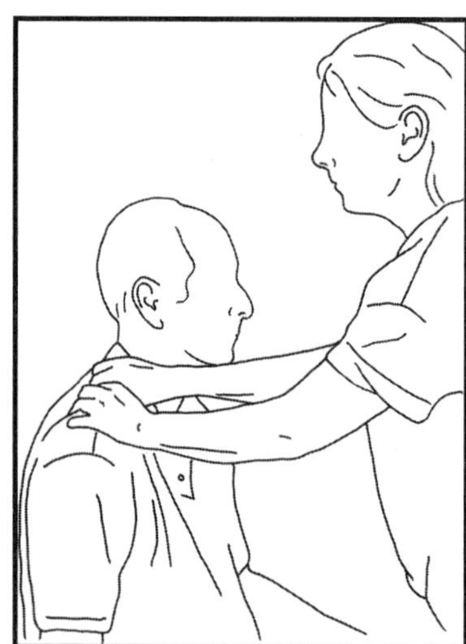

Figure 4.16 Massage using fingers and thumbs with paired hands

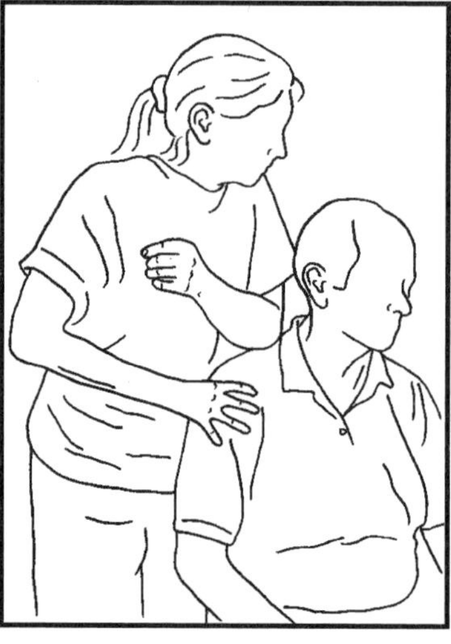

Figure 4.17 Massage with the point of an elbow

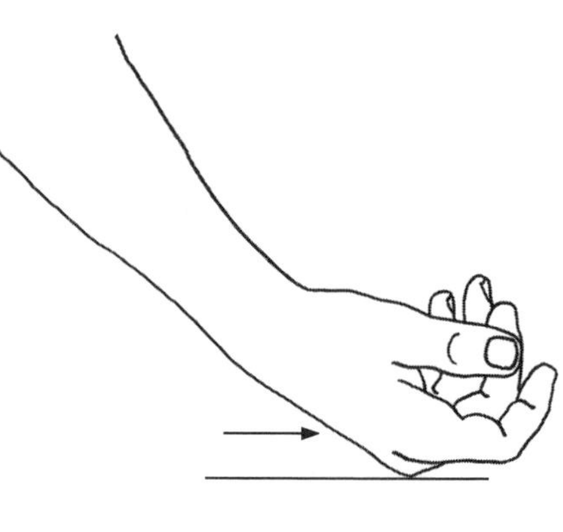

Figure 4.18 To save your fingers, use the knuckles of a loose fist for massage.

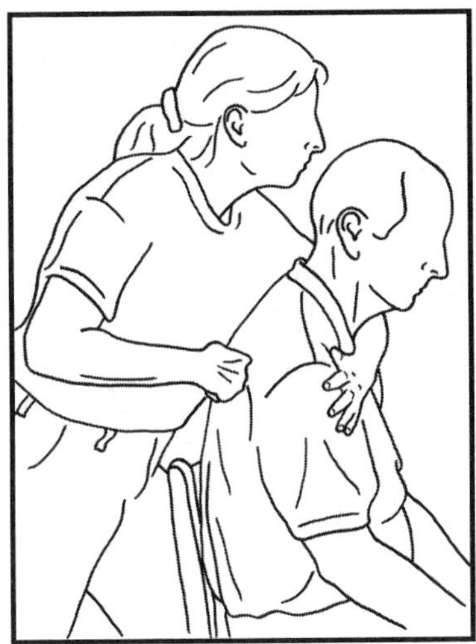

Figure 4.19 Massage with the knuckles of a loose fist

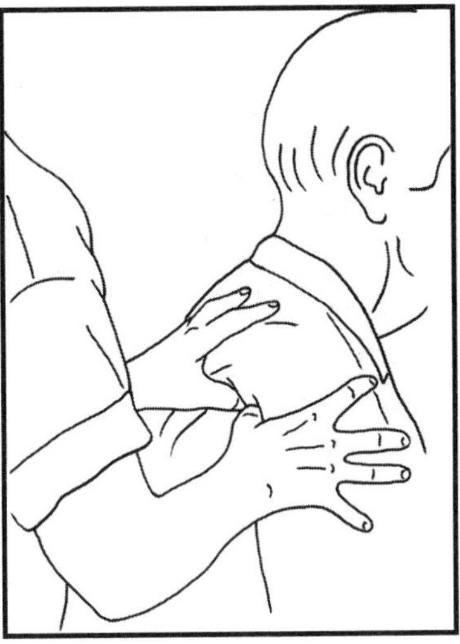

Figure 4.20 Unsupported thumbs tire too quickly.

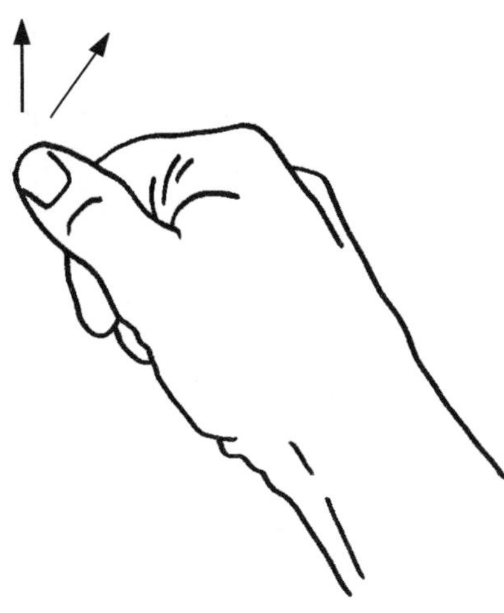

Figure 4.21 Supported thumb, the thumb resting on the index finger

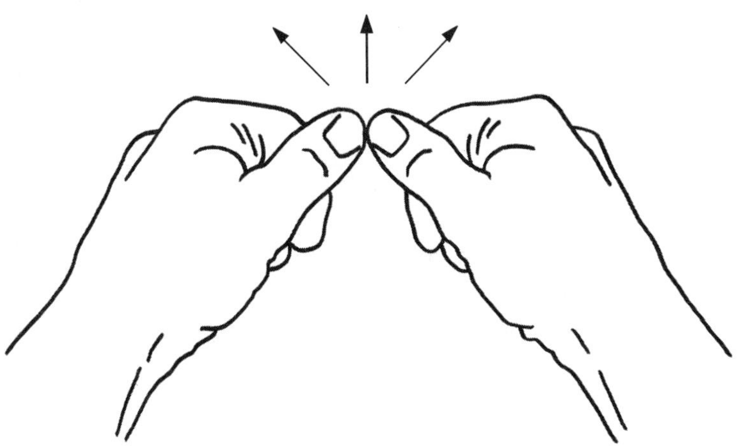

Figure 4.22 Paired supported thumbs stroking away from you or to the side

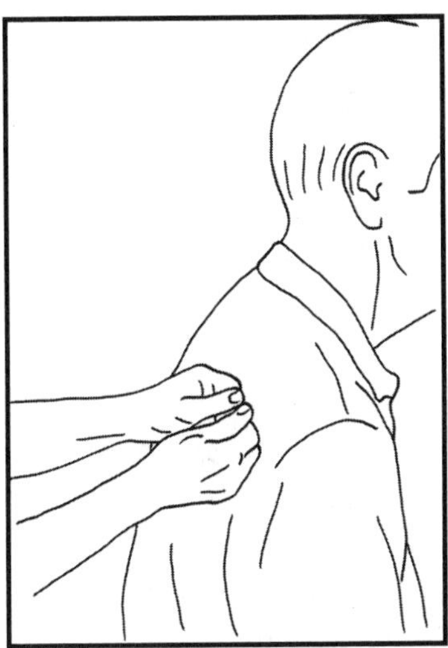

Figure 4.23 Massage is less tiring with supported thumbs.

Avoid using free or unsupported thumbs when applying massage to someone else (Figure 4.20). This overtaxes the muscles at the base of the thumb. When a thumb must be used as a massage tool, use a *supported thumb*, backing it up with the fingers (Figure 4.21). Note the direction to stroke with the thumb, as indicated by the arrows. As with the fingers, pair the thumbs whenever you can (Figures 4.22 and 4.23).

Making the Method Work

Even though trigger point massage works extremely well for getting rid of trigger points and referred pain, don't be surprised if you encounter some snags. It's like learning any new skill. You may need to do a little problem solving and refining of your techniques.

Dealing with Problems

Deep massage may occasionally cause bruising in tender areas. This is usually nothing to worry about, but you might want to use a bit less pressure. Bruising is most likely to occur when you're working the wrong place, evidenced by the fact that you're doing a lot of massage and getting no improvement.

Trigger points respond well to massage, and it ordinarily doesn't take long to feel a reduction in your pain. Most treatment failures are the result of working the wrong spot and never finding the right one. Keep checking the Trigger Point Guide at the beginning of chapter 5 or at the back of the book to keep track of all the possibilities for referral to a particular site. And remember that in some areas of the body, such as the shoulder, pain can be a composite of referral from several muscles.

A low level of enthusiasm and commitment can be an insidious problem. When treating yourself, halfhearted efforts won't get you very far. Once or twice a week simply won't do it. If you're not getting the results you think you should be getting, you may need to figure out a way to do treatments more often. You should treat especially bad trigger points at least three times a day. You'll be disappointed with the outcome if you do less. You can actually do as many as six treatments as long as you keep them short. Remember that treatment for a specific trigger point should take no more than fifteen or twenty seconds. This takes only a tiny snippet of time, not enough to slow you down or interfere with your day. You only need to do six to twelve strokes per session on any given trigger point to have a beneficial effect.

In addition to multiple treatments during the day, be sure to massage your most difficult trigger points just before going to bed and again when you get up in the morning. If pain wakes you up in the night, get up and have a treatment session. As a general rule, massaging often is much better than massaging long and hard.

Some people simply have trouble getting the hang of trigger point massage. You may find it hard to visualize the muscles or find trigger points, or you may feel clumsy and unsure with the tools and techniques. In such cases, you may benefit from a few sessions with a professional massage therapist who knows trigger points well. Be straightforward about it. Simply say that you want to learn how to treat your own trigger points. It's a life skill that everyone should possess.

Trigger point massage works extremely well for myofascial pain. Done correctly on the right trigger points, it usually shows clear results within a week, often in just a day or two. Don't forget that disease in an internal organ can promote and perpetuate trigger points in the skeletal musculature. The shoulder is frequently a site for this kind of thing. Pain that persists or keeps coming back could have an organic or systemic cause.

If your pain began with an accident or a fall, you may have hidden bone or tissue injuries that need medical attention. If you hurt all over and good massage isn't helping or seems to make the pain worse, you may be dealing with fibromyalgia or some other systemic problem and will have to seek other remedies.

Health Issues

If you're successful with deactivating your trigger points but your pain seems to come back after a short time, there may be health factors that predispose your muscles to the development and perpetuation of trigger points. Often these perpetuating factors can be controlled if you're aware of them and have the right remedies at hand. Consider whether you may be lacking B and C vitamins, calcium, magnesium, iron, or potassium. An inadequate intake any of these nutrients can make myofascial trigger points hard to get rid of. Smoking, excessive consumption of alcohol, birth control pills, and certain other drugs are all known to deplete vitamin C and some of the B vitamins.

If you can't subdue your trigger points, you may have a thyroid inadequacy. Hypoglycemia can also aggravate trigger points, and hyperuricemia, where you're not getting enough water or your kidneys aren't doing their job, can keep your trigger points going. Chronic infections or allergies may perpetuate trigger points. Prescription medications may be an issue in the perpetuation of trigger points. If a medication's listed side effects include muscle or joint pain, be suspicious.

Be aware that food allergies can play a major role in both myofascial pain and fibromyalgia. If you've had to deal with food allergies, you know they can be highly variable. Sometimes they go away, but often new ones take their place. In any case, be aware that food allergies affect muscle metabolism and can be central in your difficulty with trigger points and persistent shoulder pain.

Also be aware that caffeine, even in moderate amounts, can be an insidious perpetuator of trigger points. Caffeine is terribly addictive and weaning yourself from it can give you three or four days of unpleasant withdrawal symptoms. If you're having no luck at all with trigger point therapy, try avoiding caffeine from all sources and see what happens. If caffeine is your problem, you'll see an immediate improvement in your results.

Your Expectations

You may wonder what you should expect from trigger point massage. You may want to know how many treatment sessions will be needed to finally resolve this shoulder trouble that's been making you so miserable. Will your trigger points come back? Can you expect to be truly pain free? All of these things depend entirely on how much intelligence and commitment go into your efforts. With a reasonable amount of dedication, most people can learn to manage their trigger points quite effectively and use trigger point massage to cure a frozen shoulder.

Nevertheless, be realistic regarding your expectations. You may occasionally experience the much-desired one-shot fix with trigger point massage, but it's not wise to plan on it. Quick fixes are often illusory and can amount to nothing more than simply having swept the problem temporarily under the rug. This is what happens when you stop treatment too soon and merely convert active trigger points to latent trigger points, which can be revived by almost any kind of small strain.

Sometimes a permanent one-session triumph is genuine. The body can be very good about healing itself with the right stimulus. This happens most often with new pain. Long-standing trigger points can require considerable attention, sometimes taking several weeks to resolve. This will be true whether you do the massage yourself or seek help from a professional. If you're a professional massage therapist, you may experience frustration in getting clients to commit to the expense of an adequate number of treatments. This will change when insurance begins paying for trigger point massage.

People tend to quit too soon whether they're working on themselves or going to a professional. You'll be tempted to discontinue treatment as soon as you seem to be getting better. But remember, if the trigger point still hurts when you press on it, it has only been put into a latent state. Your massage program must continue until your trigger points no longer hurt when you press on them. Massage works miracles with trigger points and their pain, but only when done correctly and completely.

The Learning Curve

You'll be surprised at how quickly you can forget even your most useful discoveries about myofascial pain. It's useful to keep a journal about what you learn from day to day, making notes about the tricks and tools that work best. Then, if the problem comes up again, you'll find the solution already worked out in your journal and you won't have to reinvent the wheel.

To succeed in making trigger point massage work for you, the old rule applies: Just keep trying. For difficult problems, read, reread, and if necessary read again any passage in this book that may be relevant. Underline and make notes in the margins. Take time to study and think. All the anatomical detail and all the ramifications regarding myofascial pain are so new that it's not unusual to feel mystified and overwhelmed. Be assured that the treatment of trigger point pain is much simpler than it seems at first and it will eventually all come together. Don't give up! Keep trying! You're learning a new skill that can bring you relief from pain for the rest of your life.

There's a long learning curve to mastering everything in this book, but you can expect to see positive results from the very beginning. If you study this book on an ongoing basis and keep searching for solutions, you'll learn something useful almost daily. Work on knowing the muscles and bones. It's essential to understand what's beneath the surface of your skin. The bony landmarks that you can see or feel under the skin are particularly important.

To augment what you see in this book, you may want to get Frank Netter's *Atlas of Human Anatomy* (1989) and study his magnificent illustrations. If you've got the stomach to learn from dissected bodies, the six-part *Video Atlas of Human Anatomy* by Robert Acland (1995) will give you some unique insights. You'll only need the first one, titled *The Upper Extremity*, which is concerned only with the shoulder, arm, and hand. Dr. Acland uses a moving camera technique that effectively simulates a three-dimensional view that you can't get from a book, revealing usually hidden details of human anatomy and structure. In whatever way you can, keep exploring and learning. There are rewards in store that you can't imagine.

Hidden Benefits

When done by a professional, massage can be profoundly relaxing. Along with reducing muscle tension, a good massage reduces heart rate, blood pressure, and respiration rate. It may not be reasonable to hope for quite as much benefit from self-treatment, but the relaxing effect can still be considerable if you make conscious use of it. You can use your self-treatment sessions to slow down and calm down. Use it as a kind of meditation. Focus your mind on relaxing whatever muscle you're working on. When you're able to relax one muscle, your entire body tends to relax too.

The intentional reduction of tension in your muscles can also reduce the pain from trigger points. If you become good enough at progressive or systematic relaxation, you can achieve pain reduction nearly equal to that of a prescribed painkiller. Muscle relaxation won't get rid of trigger points, but it can make your pain more bearable until trigger point massage begins to succeed.

Some Words for Massage Therapists

When trigger point massage doesn't seem to be working for someone and pain continues to be a problem, it may not be your fault. The client may be involved in an ongoing activity that's unusually taxing or that involves a large amount of repetitive motion. If this activity created the problem in the first place, it's unreasonable to think it could do anything but bring the problem back and perpetuate it. Discuss these factors with the client and explore changes that could be made. The practical solution may be to help the person learn self-treatment skills that could be used intermittently during the troublesome activity to keep the recurrent trigger points at least partially subdued.

But don't overlook the possibility that you might need to improve your own skills as a professional therapist. If your therapy is less than successful with a particular client, don't waste time defending your approach. If the client says it isn't working, the client is absolutely right. It's the client's body and the client's pain. Janet Travell believed that our patients are our best teachers. When things don't go the way you thought they should, look at it as an opportunity to learn something new. Then beat the bushes till you find the answer.

The Stretching Issue

Be particularly alert for the complaint that you made someone's pain worse. There's a chance it may center around the issue of stretching. Many people can't be stretched at all without exacerbating their problem. Under many circumstances, stretching can be exactly the wrong thing to do, and the shoulder complex is a perfect example.

The muscles and tendons of the rotator cuff are extremely vulnerable to damage when the muscles have been shortened and stiffened by trigger points. People who promote stretching with no heed to the restrictions imposed by trigger points may be doing more harm than they know. Most therapists, particularly physical therapists, need to be much more circumspect about stretching. When someone says you've made their pain worse, consider whether you may have used stretching too soon or too aggressively. The safe approach is to defer stretching until you have deactivated all the trigger points. Even then, overly ambitious stretching can reactivate trigger points.

Stretching enthusiasts may find it hard to believe that properly executed trigger point massage works quite well without stretching. They should remember that, even with people who tolerate stretching well and benefit from it, trigger points are what keep muscles shortened and stiff. When trigger points are gone, muscles lengthen naturally and range of motion returns with normal activity. That's the stage at which stretching and exercise become safe and appropriate.

Specific Treatment for Specific Pain

The profession of therapeutic massage needs to take a much more objective approach to the treatment of pain. There's no denying that the standard Swedish-style, full-body massage delivered by a sensitive and skilled massage therapist is an unmatched experience that virtually everyone enjoys. This standard routine, however, is defined by the therapist and not necessarily by the needs of the client, and it rarely serves as adequate therapy for myofascial trigger points.

Most massage clients come for treatment with complaints about very specific kinds of pain. Therapists, however, too often seem to be more interested in doing their customary, one-hour massage than they are in taking a clinical approach to specific problems in limited areas. The focus in clinical massage therapy should be on solving the problem that the client comes in with. Truly effective clinical therapy requires a much greater facility in finding and treating trigger points than is currently being taught in most massage schools.

Massage therapy programs typically try to encompass too many modalities, each designed to approximately fill the time frame of the one-hour billing period. Trigger point massage is presented to students as just one of a dozen other treatment systems purportedly of equal value. The stated attitude of school administrators is that everything works, and criticism of a particular modality or of someone else's work is pointedly discouraged. This reveals a very shallow understanding of a fundamental aspect of myofascial pain, which is the absolute necessity of directly addressing trigger points as a first priority. Instead, a kind of political correctness seems to compel massage schools to give the student every weapon in the arsenal in the naive hope that something will hit the target.

A Sharper Focus

Trigger point massage is an extraordinarily practical and versatile approach to pain therapy. As a stand-alone therapy, it can be done anywhere, not necessarily requiring a massage table or massage chair. If need be, it can even be done quite effectively through clothing and without oil or lotion. Trigger point massage can be the sole therapy employed for a client, or it can be integrated with other massage modalities, greatly increasing their effectiveness. As a purely clinical modality, trigger point massage can be limited to specific problems and specific muscles and doesn't have to be part of a full-body treatment. When physicians and health insurance companies begin to see the potential in this unusually cost-effective treatment for pain, there will be a vastly increased need for massage therapists who are truly skilled in trigger point massage.

Trigger point therapy is not just another brand of alternative medicine. No one should view it as a fringe issue in the field of health care. Trigger points aren't merely one of the many causes of pain. They're perhaps the most frequent cause of pain, as Doctors Travell and Simons certainly believe they are (Simons, Travell, and Simons 1999, 12). Not only should trigger point massage become the primary method taught in massage schools, it should also be taught to students in all fields of health care, including medicine and nursing. Self-applied massage, in particular, should be taught as the best foundation for understanding and successfully treating trigger points. If practitioners can find and successfully treat their own trigger points, the pain problems of their clients will hold few mysteries.

Chapter 5

Shoulder Treatment, Part A

This chapter, along with chapters 6 and 7, will guide you through the process of identifying which muscles may be involved in your shoulder pain and help you learn how to find and treat their trigger points. The muscles are discussed in the approximate order of their importance, the most critical muscles being in chapter 5 and the others distributed through chapters 6 and 7 with less regard for their precise rank. If you have any difficulty locating a particular muscle on your body, just turn back to chapter 1 and review the relevant sections on anatomy.

Any of the muscles in these next three chapters can contribute to frozen shoulder. As you learn more about their trigger points, you'll also learn how each muscle works so that you can see what part it may have played in the origin of the problem. This will help make you more aware of activities that could tend to bring the problem back.

Trigger points do have a propensity for coming back, especially if you unthinkingly go right on doing things in the same old way. The reason for this is that chronic pain sensitizes the central nervous system by opening up large numbers of new synapses, the electrochemical switches that allow information to pass from one nerve cell to the next. Because of this, muscles that have had trigger points in the past are more likely to develop trigger points again. Also, the longer that trigger points have gone untreated, the quicker they'll reactivate under stress or stain. There's even evidence that permanent changes in the central nervous system made by widespread chronic trigger points may be a precursor to fibromyalgia (Mense and Simons 2001, 158-174, 186-187).

It's important to take steps to intervene in the process of trigger point reactivation. This is one of the best uses of trigger point therapy, which is not only good for fixing pain problems, but can also help keep them from cropping up again. If a particular activity has created the problem, brief sessions of self-applied trigger point massage before and after that activity will allow you to continue engaging in it with a greatly reduced risk of getting debilitating pain again. Trigger points don't need to make you quit your job or stop playing volleyball on weekends. Just figure out what you can do to keep previously overused muscles from becoming overused again. If a certain amount of overuse can't be avoided, you should plan to get very good at trigger point massage.

The Trigger Point Guide on the next two pages will help you organize your efforts to locate and treat the specific trigger points that are causing your pain. You'll also find these two pages at the end of the book. To make this book even more useful, you may want to have a coil binding put on it at a copy center, which will allow it to open flat at any page, leaving both hands free to do therapy.

Trigger Point Guide: Shoulder Pain

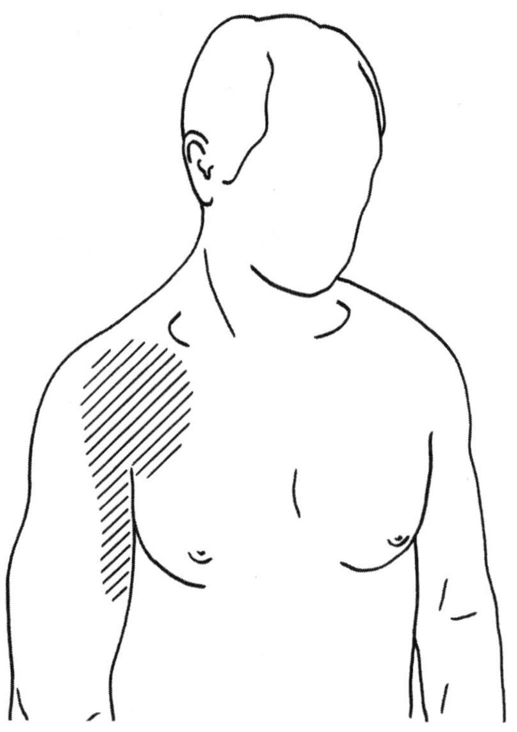

Front-of-Shoulder Pain

1. infraspinatus (135)
2. anterior deltoid (149)
3. scalenes (116)
4. supraspinatus (131)
5. pectoralis major (174)
6. pectoralis minor (180)
7. subscapularis (124)
8. biceps (189)
9. latissimus dorsi (143)
10. coracobrachiallis (197)
11. subclavius (179)
12. brachialis (191)

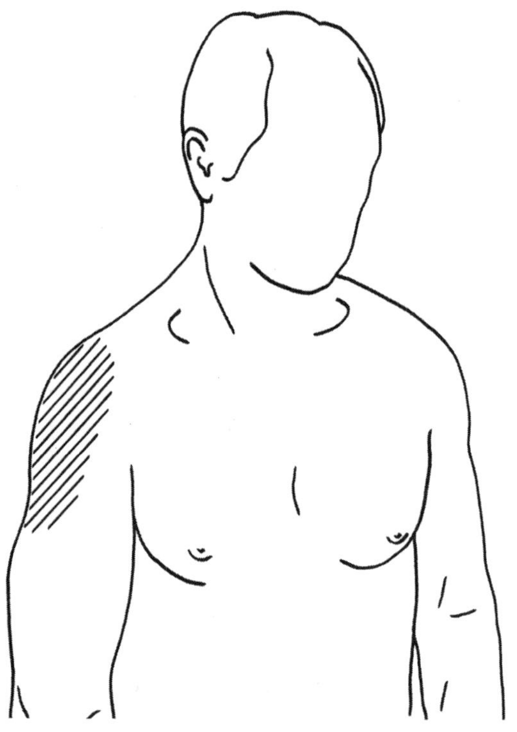

Side-of-Shoulder Pain

1. infraspinatus (135)
2. scalenes (116)
3. middle deltoid (149)
4. supraspinatus (131)

Trigger Point Guide: Shoulder Pain

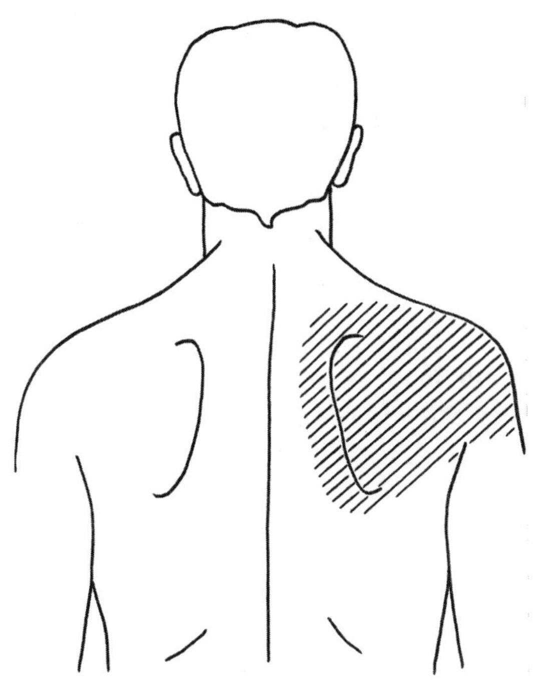

Back-of-Shoulder Pain

1. scalenes (116)
2. subscapularis (124)
3. teres minor (140)
4. trapezius (152)
5. levator scapulae (160)
6. posterior deltoid (149)
7. rhomboids (163)
8. serratus posterior superior (166)
9. supraspinatus (131)
10. teres major (147)
11. latissimus dorsi (143)
12. triceps (193)
13. iliocostalis thoracis (169)
14. serratus anterior (183)

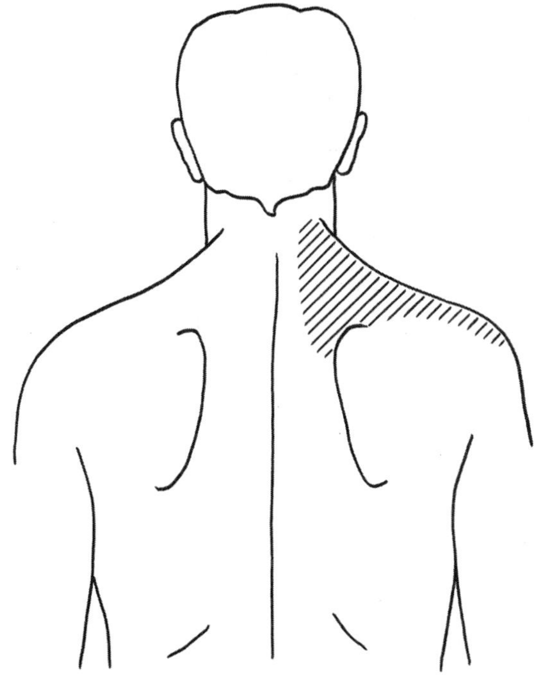

Top-of-Shoulder Pain

1. trapezius (152)
2. levator scapulae (160)
3. scalenes (116)
4. supraspinatus (131)
5. diaphragm (186)

Anterior Neck Muscles

Although the scalenes are muscles of the front and sides of the neck, their trigger points cause a surprising amount of pain in the upper back, shoulder, and upper arm. Note that the scalenes appear near the top of all four lists in the Trigger Point Guide. Scalene trigger points also contribute significantly to pain, numbness, tingling, and swelling in the forearm and hand. The scalenes are so important that they should always be among the first muscles to troubleshoot in your search for the cause of a shoulder problem.

Trigger points in the scalene muscles may sometimes actually precede trouble in the rotator cuff muscles. This is because scalene trigger points refer pain to almost all parts of the shoulder, tending to cause the formation of satellite trigger points in those areas. The infraspinatus, teres minor, triceps, deltoid, and pectoral muscles are particularly vulnerable to this effect.

For this reason, the scalene and sternocleidomastoid muscles will be discussed first in this chapter. The sternocleidomastoids don't send pain to the shoulder, but they can be very important in a shoulder problem because their trigger points tend to initiate and perpetuate trigger points in the scalenes. Also, you need to understand the structure of the sternocleidomastoids if you hope to successfully find and treat the underlying scalene muscles.

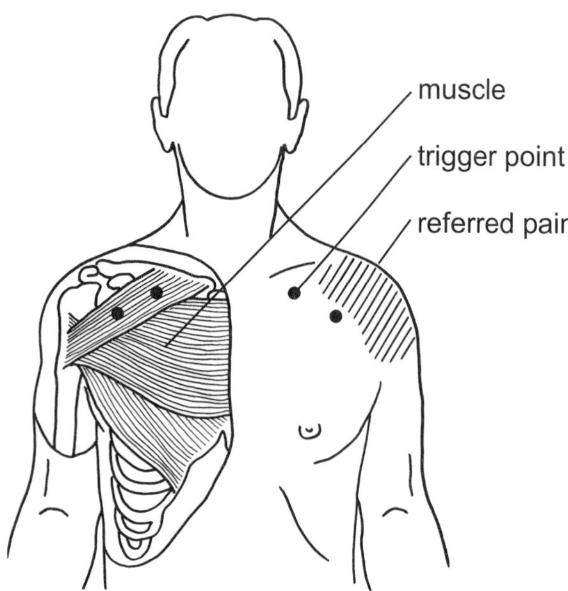

Figure 5.1 Key to pictorial devices

Figure 5.1 shows the graphic means of portraying the muscles, trigger points, and referred pain patterns in the following illustrations. An area of referred pain is represented by a group of parallel lines running diagonally from lower left to upper right. Parallel lines also represent a muscle, but the lines are always enclosed within the outline of the muscle. A black dot approximates the location of a trigger point and may stand for several trigger points in the muscle. To keep the illustrations simple, trigger points are sometimes shown on only one side of the body, but they can occur on either side or both.

Sternocleidomastoid

Note that the sternocleidomastoid isn't included in the twenty-four muscles associated with the shoulder that were discussed in chapter 1. Also, since sternocleidomastoid trigger points don't directly cause shoulder pain, the muscle doesn't appear in the Trigger Point Guide at the beginning of this chapter.

The sternocleidomastoid muscles on each side of your neck attach to three bones (Figure 5.2), the names of which give the muscle its name. "Sterno" is from the sternum, or breastbone, "cleido" refers to the clavicle, or collarbone, and "mastoid" denotes the mastoid process, the bony knob on the occipital bone behind the ear. The word "sternocleidomastoid" looks monstrously intimidating all put together, but if you break it into its three component pieces you'll find it very easy to say. You'd best make friends with your sternocleidomastoid muscles. They make more trouble than you can possibly imagine.

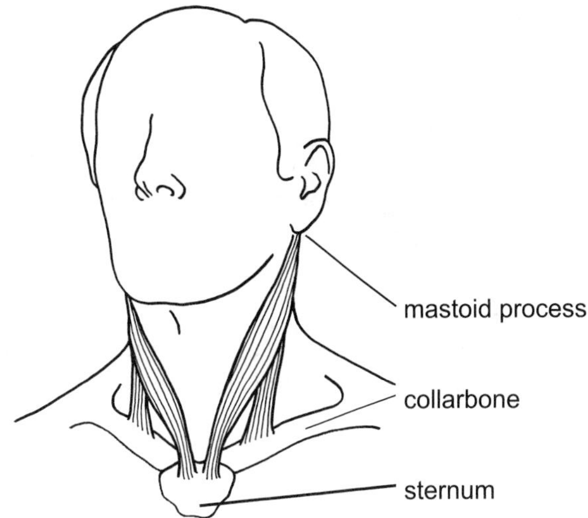

Figure 5.2 Sternocleidomastoid muscles and their attachments

Although the sternocleidomastoids, sometimes called "strap muscles," are in plain view on the front of your neck, you may never have paid much attention to them. That's because you usually don't get pain in the front of your neck; you get it in the back of your neck. Sternocleidomastoid trigger points actually cause an incredible amount of pain and other problems, but they're all sent upward to the jaws, head, and face. The sternocleidomastoids themselves rarely hurt, no matter how much trouble they're in or how much trouble they're causing (Simons, Travell, and Simons 1999, 308-311).

The case of Sally, age fifty-three, illustrates how difficult it can be to match certain symptoms to their cause unless you happen to know something about referred pain. Sally had been rear-ended by a semi on the interstate. No one was killed or seriously injured, but the accident gave everybody a few bruises and a good jarring.

By the next day, however, Sally had developed signs of whiplash. She had pain deep behind both eyes and a strong headache over both eyebrows and in the back of her head. Her doctor prescribed a narcotic for the pain and several sessions of physical therapy. The pills cut Sally's pain by about half, but it was still there. At the physical therapy clinic, they gave the muscles in her neck electrical stimulation treatments twice a week for three weeks. Although the treatments helped, the relief lasted for only a few hours. After that, she still needed the pills, but she was afraid of getting addicted. She felt as though she was getting nowhere.

Determined to find something that worked, Sally made an appointment with both a massage therapist and a chiropractor. The massage therapist had an earlier time, so she went there first. The therapist explained that whiplash could affect the front of the neck as much as it did the back. Checking, she found some very sore places in Sally's sternocleidomastoid and trapezius muscles. Firmly squeezing some of those spots reproduced all her pain exactly. Trigger point treatment left her with more relief than she'd had in almost a month. She made a follow-up appointment and cancelled her appointment with the chiropractor. Sally was lucky. It's not uncommon for relatively minor whiplash injuries like hers to progress to a frozen shoulder.

Symptoms

Sternocleidomastoid trigger points cause a large number of symptoms that can be amazingly varied and widespread. These symptoms fall into four categories: referred pain, balance problems, visual disturbances, and systemic symptoms. In addition, the production of satellite trigger points in other muscles by sternocleidomastoid trigger points extends their effect significantly.

Referred pain. Trigger points in the sternocleidomastoid don't cause pain in the muscle itself, but they can be so tender to pressure that they can be mistaken for swollen and sensitive lymph nodes (sometimes erroneously called "swollen glands"). They can be the source of a painless neck stiffness that keeps your head tilted to one side. Note that there are important differences in the referred pain patterns for the two branches of the sternocleidomastoid muscle (Figure 5.3). A headache in the top of the head or over an eyebrow is practically a signature of sternocleidomastoid trigger points.

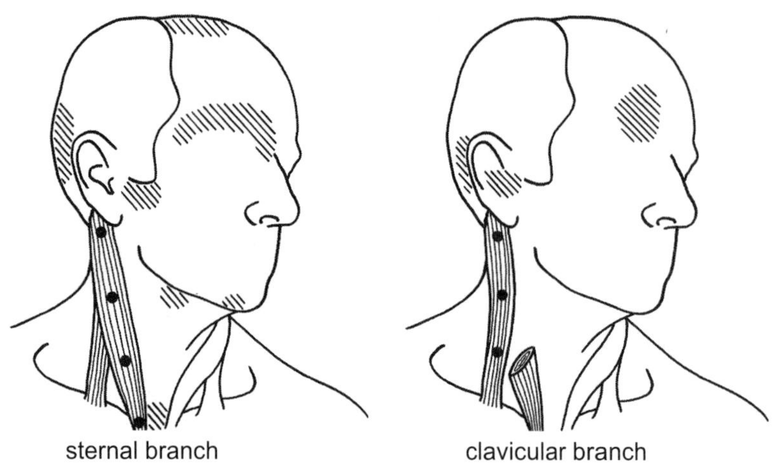

Figure 5.3 Sternocleidomastoid trigger points and referred pain pattern

Trigger points in the sternal branch can cause deep eye pain, tongue pain when swallowing, and headaches over the eye, behind the ear, and in the top of the head. They can contribute to temporomandibular joint (TMJ) pain, because their referral pattern tends to promote and perpetuate trigger points in the jaw muscles. Pain is also sometimes sent to the back of the neck. The only referral downward is to the top of the breastbone. Not shown in Figure 5.3 is an occasional spillover of pain in the side of the face, which mimics trigeminal neuralgia, a disorder characterized by brief attacks of pain caused by irritation of the trigeminal nerve. Pain in the face and over the eyebrows can also be mistaken for sinusitis.

Trigger points in the clavicular branch can cause a deep earache or a toothache in the back molars. An unusual feature of clavicular trigger points is that they can create a frontal headache that's cross-referred to the opposite side of the forehead (Simons, Travell, and Simons 1999, 308-318).

Balance problems. Another unusual trait of trigger points in the clavicular branch is that they're apt to affect your balance, making you dizzy, nauseous, and prone to lurching or falling. Fainting may even occur. This dizziness can last for minutes, hours, or days. These symptoms often lead to a mistaken diagnosis of vertigo or Ménière's disease. If the trigger points causing the symptoms remain unsuspected and untreated, the symptoms can become a lifelong recurrent condition, defying all medical treatments and medical explanations.

Chronic dizziness can be the result of confusing signals sent to the brain from the clavicular branch of the sternocleidomastoid. The changing tensions in this part of the muscle as you move around help your inner ear keep track of the position of your head. When trigger points cause aberrant tensions in the clavicular branch, false information is sent to the part of the brain that governs your balance. You then experience a kind of false vertigo that has nothing to do with the inner ear. Dr. Travell believed that the distorted perception caused by sternocleidomastoid trigger points could be a hidden cause of falls and motor vehicle accidents.

Trigger points in the clavicular branch of the sternocleidomastoid can also cause hearing loss on the side afflicted with trigger points. This is thought to be due to referred tension in the tiny stapedius and tensor tympani muscles that attach to the small bones of the middle ear. Tension in these little muscles could inhibit vibration in the inner ear and diminish perception of sound. Massage of the sternocleidomastoids and the jaw muscles has been known to bring back normal hearing when trigger points were to blame for the problem (Simons, Travell, and Simons 1999, 308-314).

Visual disturbances. Sternal branch trigger points can cause dimmed, blurred, or double vision. You may have reddening of your eyes and excessive tearing, along with a runny nose. These trigger points can also cause ptosis (a drooping eyelid) from a referred spasm in the orbicularis oculi muscle that encircles the eye. Referral to the orbicularis muscle can also cause twitching of the eyelid or make the print on the page seem to be jumping around when you read.

Systemic symptoms. A fourth group of possible symptoms from sternocleidomastoid trigger points includes disturbed weight perception, cold sweat on the forehead, and excess mucus in the sinuses, nasal cavities, and throat. These trigger points can be the simple explanation for sinus congestion, sinus drainage, phlegm in the throat, chronic cough, and continual hay fever or cold symptoms. Be especially suspicious if medications have no effect. A persistent dry cough can often be stopped with massage to the sternal branch near its attachment to the breastbone (Simons, Travell, and Simons 1999, 308-311).

Causes

A primary function of each sternocleidomastoid is to turn the head to the opposite side. The sternocleidomastoids also help maintain a stable position of the head during movements of the body. Trigger points can therefore be created by postures and activities that keep the sternocleidomastoids contracted to hold the head in position. Holding your head back in order to work overhead is particularly troublesome, and keeping your head turned to one side for long periods of time is also very abusive to these muscles (Simons, Travell, and Simons 1999, 314-316).

A single incident of heavy lifting can strain the sternocleidomastoids. Falls and whiplash accidents cause severe overstretching and overcontraction in all the muscles of the neck, including the sternocleidomastoids. Myofascial symptoms from whiplash injury to the sternocleidomastoid muscles can persist for years. Other conditions that encourage these trigger points are a tight collar, a short leg, an abnormal curvature of the spine, emphysema, asthma, a chronic cough, hyperventilation, emotional stress, and habitual muscle tension.

An auxiliary function of the sternocleidomastoids is to raise the breastbone when you inhale, so chest breathing can overwork them. Learn to breathe with your diaphragm, not with your chest. During normal breathing, your stomach should go in and out; your chest shouldn't expand and contract much at all.

To avoid unnecessary stress to the sternocleidomastoids, don't sit for long periods with your head turned to one side, don't read in bed, and don't sleep on your stomach. Don't slouch when sitting, don't hold the telephone to your ear with your shoulder, and don't sit in cold drafts. When you're having trouble with your sternocleidomastoids, you should avoid free-style swimming, which requires you to turn your head strongly for inhalation.

Self-Treatment

The good news about the confusing conglomeration of symptoms generated by sternocleidomastoid trigger points is that you can fix them yourself in the simplest imaginable way.

To massage the sternocleidomastoid, take all the soft tissue that you can between your fingers and thumb and knead firmly (Figure 5.4). Reach across with the opposite hand as shown in the drawings. Try to distinguish the two parts of the muscle, the sternal branch being in front of the clavicular branch. Visualize two long, fat fingers there on the side of your neck. If you pay close attention, you should be able to feel them separately. You really have to grasp a big handful of muscle to get hold of the very deep clavicular branch. Search for trigger points in each branch, starting up behind your earlobe and moving all the way down to your breastbone.

If your sternocleidomastoid muscles hurt when you squeeze them, trigger points are certain to be responsible for that chronic headache or whatever other symptom you may be having in your head, face, or jaws. When sternocleidomastoid trigger points are bad enough, a little squeeze will actually reproduce or accentuate a frontal headache, giving you a very convincing demonstration of pain referral.

Don't be afraid of the sternocleidomastoid muscles. Massaging them may hurt quite a bit in the beginning, but you can't do them any harm. These muscles respond unusually well to massage, and your symptoms may disappear in a short time. But continue working the trigger points repeatedly and patiently over several days until you can no longer find a place that hurts.

Sternocleidomastoid massage can make a frontal headache better almost immediately. The same is true for dizziness and many other sternocleidomastoid symptoms. Keep in mind, though, that overworking these muscles can irritate the trigger points and make the

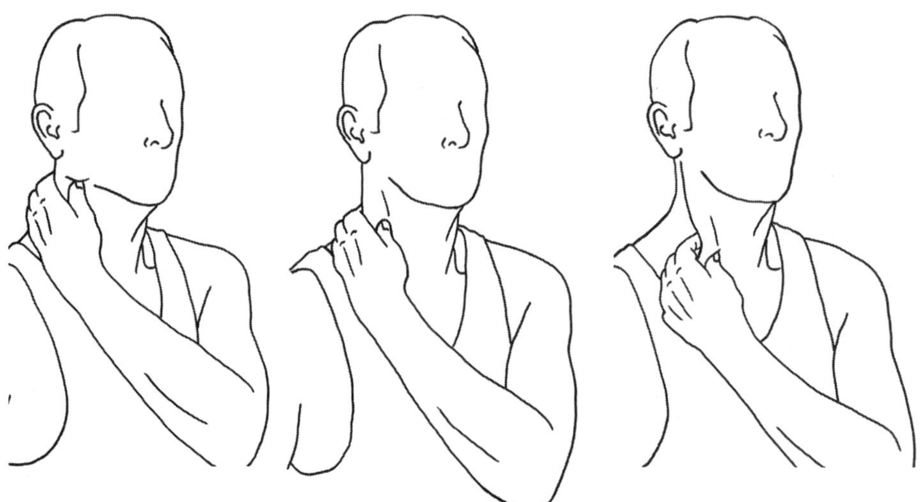

Figure 5.4 Sternocleidomastoid massage between fingers and thumb, one of the few places where the pincer grip should be used

symptoms worse for a while. A single session of sternocleidomastoid massage shouldn't last longer than a minute or two per side.

Physicians often warn that massaging the front of the neck can loosen plaque in the carotid arteries and cause a stroke, especially in the elderly. These fears can be laid to rest if you know where these arteries are and simply avoid them. The carotid arteries are where you feel your carotid pulse, high up under your chin alongside the windpipe. Proper execution of the techniques described here shouldn't endanger the carotids as long as you're mindful of not massaging the place where you feel your pulse. You can massage near a carotid artery, but not directly on it.

Partner Treatment

Evelyn, *age fifty-nine, had a frightening spell of dizziness one evening while sitting on her neighbor's porch. It took a long time to go away, and her neighbor finally had to help her back to her house. She was still feeling very unsteady the next day. A friend who had been studying about trigger points said she thought she knew what was wrong. She asked Evelyn if she could squeeze her neck. Skeptical and a bit apprehensive, Evelyn said okay.*

Her friend found excruciating tender spots in Evelyn's sternocleidomastoid, scalene, and upper trapezius muscles. She gave her an impromptu treatment and showed her how to massage some of the places herself. By the time her friend left, Evelyn's dizziness had disappeared.

Evelyn had been afraid she'd been having a stroke, and at her age that could certainly be a concern. Even so, spells of dizziness are much more common at any age than strokes. The reason for Evelyn's sudden onset of dizziness the night before was that she had been sitting and talking for two hours with her head turned in her neighbor's direction. Latent trigger points in her sternocleidomastoids had been activated by the unaccustomed strain.

To treat a friend, partner, or family member's sternocleidomastoids, simply stand face-to-face and massage the muscles as you would your own (Figure 5.5). Since you can't feel the other person's pain, be sure to keep asking for numbers rating their pain level so you can keep from hurting them. If they wince and draw away, you're overdoing it. If they slap you or punch you in the nose, you can be pretty sure they're dissatisfied.

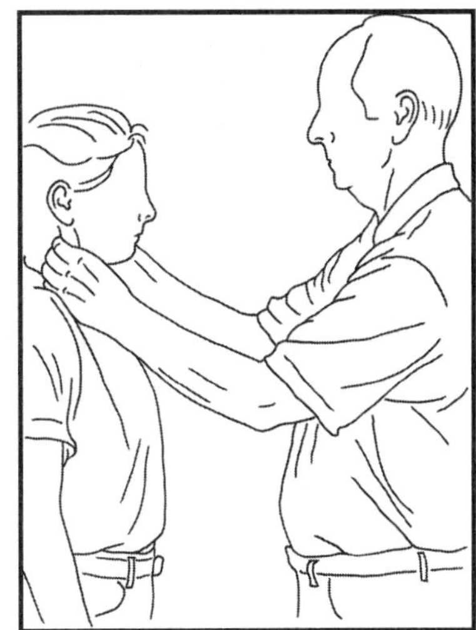

Figure 5.5 Partner massage of the sternocleidomastoid muscle, supporting the head and neck with the opposite hand

Clinical Treatment

If you're a massage therapist, you'll treat sternocleidomastoid trigger points with the client supine (faceup) on the massage table. Treat one side at a time by rolling the muscle between your fingers and thumb (Figure 5.6). Differentiate the sternal and clavicular branches by feeling for the narrow trough between them. The clavicular branch is deep to the sternal branch.

To be sure you're treating the clavicular branch, you must take all of the soft tissue on the side of the neck into your hand. Beginning just below the ear, slowly search the muscle along its entire length, treating trigger points in both branches as you come to them. It

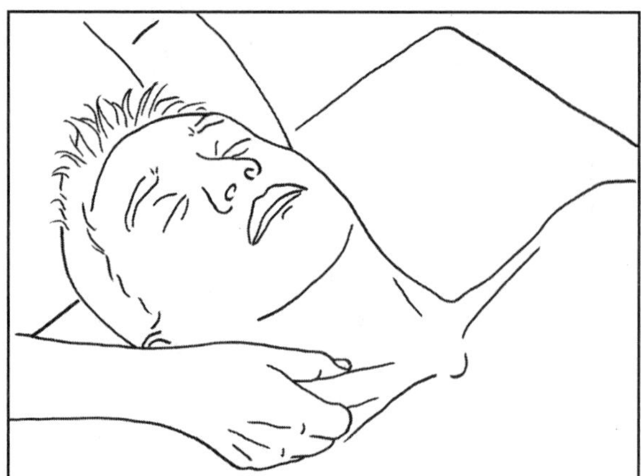

Figure 5.6 Sternocleidomastoid massage by kneading between the fingers and thumb, with the left hand supporting the back of the neck

doesn't require very much pressure, so use the flat pads of your fingers and thumb rather than the tips. The action of the treatment stroke should be like rolling a pea repeatedly between your fingers and thumb.

When the sternocleidomastoid is rigid with tension, the clavicular branch can be very difficult to grasp, particularly low on the neck where the two branches separate. You'll have more control of the sternocleidomastoids if you treat them without lotion. To make a tight sternocleidomastoid easier to treat, slacken it by bending the neck slightly toward that side. Unless the muscle has been injured, any pain caused by massage can be considered an indication of trigger points. Squeezing a healthy sternocleidomastoid doesn't hurt.

There should be little danger of inadvertently abusing the carotid arteries if you treat the sternocleidomastoids and scalenes as described in this book. It's wise, however, to know exactly where the carotid arteries are. They're what cause the pulse just above the Adam's apple on either side of the windpipe. This is where the carotids are the most vulnerable to direct pressure. The carotids are right beside the sternocleidomastoids in this area, but you'll be pressing or squeezing in the opposite direction, away from the carotids. When addressing any of the anterior neck muscles, simply move away from any pulsing that you feel under your fingers.

It's unfortunate that so many therapists have been taught to stay away from the front of the neck, because it makes them ineffective in treating whiplash, carpal tunnel syndrome, and other distressing problems caused by trigger points in this area. Your understanding of the sternocleidomastoids will be greatly increased by mastering self-treatment.

Scalenes

The scalenes are a group of three or, in some people, four small muscles in each side of the neck. The word "scalene" comes from a Greek word meaning "uneven." Each scalene muscle attaches to several vertebrae, resulting in sets of muscle fibers of uneven lengths. Since trigger points typically occur midway in muscle fibers, the scalenes can have many trigger points in many different locations. The following case histories are a sampling of the broad diversity of problems that can originate in the scalene muscles. In each case, self-applied trigger point massage solved the problem, after treatment and instruction by a massage therapist. In any of these cases, the scalene trouble could have led eventually to a shoulder problem.

> Betsy, *age thirty-two, had worked for the post office until someone rear-ended the vehicle she was driving. It was only a minor accident, but it left her with periodic disabling spasms in the right side of her neck. Almost any little strain would set it off. When she had a flare-up, recovery typically took several days, and during that time she was unable to work.*

Hong Sun, *a thirty-one-year-old professional ballet dancer, complained of a constant ache in his upper back between his spine and left shoulder blade. It felt good to reach over his shoulder and massage the place with his fingers, but it didn't stop the pain. He'd had the pain for several years, and it made him not want to raise his arm. He was thinking of looking for a less strenuous way to make a living.*

Amy, *age seventeen, had been a serious student of the cello but she'd had to quit playing because of weakness and numbness in her shoulders, arms, and hands. Her parents believed the problem might be related to a diving accident in which her head had hit the bottom of the pool, but thousands of dollars of medical tests had turned up nothing.*

Gerhardt, *age fifty-six, had suffered shooting pains in his left shoulder and upper arm ever since falling on the back of his neck a year and a half earlier. The pain increased when he carried or tried to lift anything. Chiropractic treatments and physical therapy exercises made the pain worse. Numbness in his fingers convinced his doctor that he needed carpal tunnel surgery.*

Connie, *a forty-nine-year-old potter, had pain in her shoulder and all down her right arm. It was always worse in the morning, and it often awakened her at night. Her forearm and hand were vaguely numb most of the time and her hand often felt swollen. She was concerned that she wouldn't be able to continue her work and support herself if the trouble got any worse.*

Symptoms

Scalene trigger points are among the most common sources of shoulder and upper back pain. Unfortunately, the scalenes are easily ignored and neglected because they're difficult to visualize and are almost entirely hidden by the sternocleidomastoid muscles (Figure 5.7). Since the sternocleidomastoids and scalenes have overlapping functions, trouble in one typically provokes trouble in the other.

Pain is hardly ever felt in the scalenes themselves, but their trigger points can be the primary cause of pain in their referral areas. They're likely to create satellite trigger points in their referral areas, so scalene trigger points are quite frequently the ultimate source of pain, numbness, and other abnormal sensations in the chest, upper back, shoulder, arm, and hand. Unsuspected scalene trigger points are often the critical element in the failure of conventional therapies for conditions such as frozen shoulder, thoracic outlet syndrome, and carpal tunnel syndrome (Simons, Travell, and Simons 1999, 504-506, 514-525; Hawley 1996, 254-256).

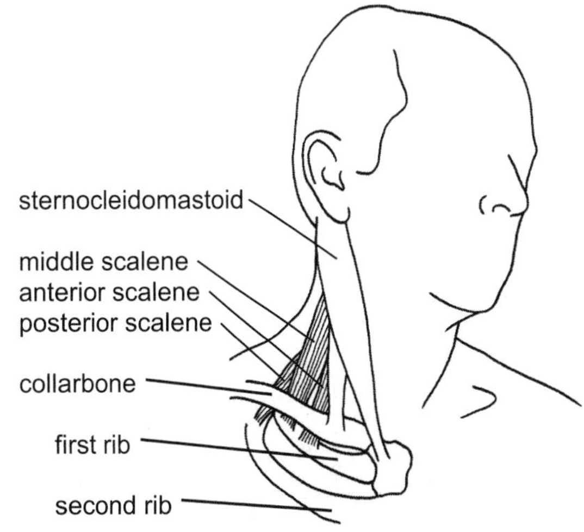

Figure 5.7 Location of anterior, middle, and posterior scalene muscles behind the sternocleidomastoid muscle

Given what small muscles the scalenes are, their trigger points cause an impressively wide distribution of pain (Figures 5.8, 5.9, and 5.10). Any of the trigger points in the scalene muscles can cause symptoms in any part of the referral areas, though certain trigger points may favor certain areas. For example, trigger points in the lower parts of

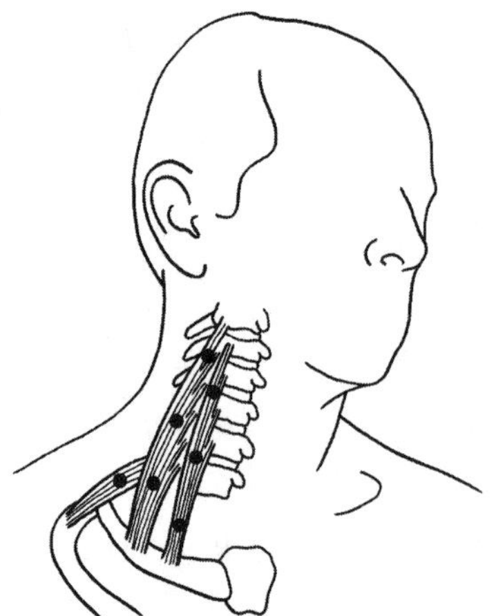
Figure 5.8 Scalene trigger points

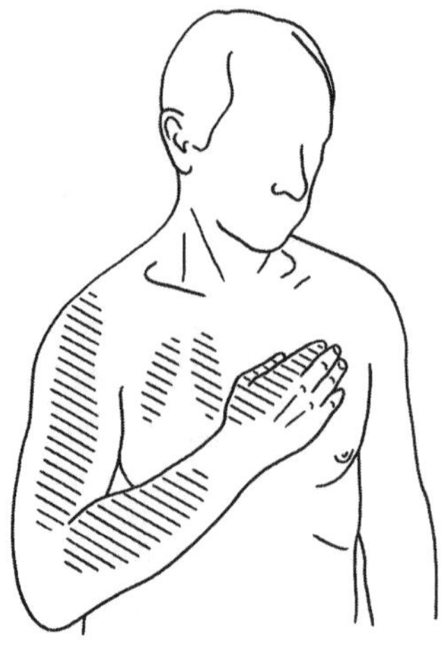
Figure 5.9 Scalene referred pain pattern, front view

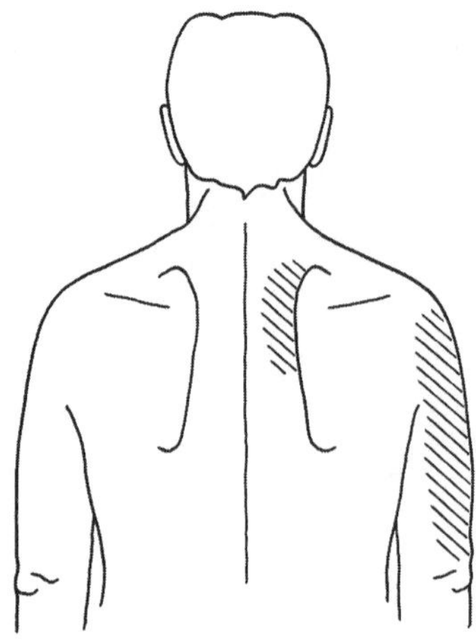
Figure 5.10 Scalene referred pain pattern, back view

the middle and posterior scalenes cause chest pain. Trigger points high in the middle and anterior scalenes cause pain in the upper arm and shoulder.

Symptoms created by the scalenes are frequently misdiagnosed. Upper back pain evoked by scalene trigger points is almost always wrongly blamed on the rhomboid muscles or a vertebra out of place. Restlessness in the neck and shoulder, a classic sign of scalene trigger points, is often written off as a nervous tic. Pain referred from the scalenes to the chest can be especially worrisome because it's easily mistaken for angina. Pain sent to the shoulder is almost universally mislabeled bursitis or tendinitis. Referred pain down the front and back of the upper arm can be mistaken for muscle strain.

The pattern of scalene pain referral in the shoulder, arm, and hand may make a physician believe that a herniated cervical disk is causing compression of a nerve root. Sometimes this is the case, but scalene trigger points are more likely to be the cause of the symptoms and an examination should be done for them before prescribing an expensive battery of unnecessary tests (Simons, Travell, and Simons 1999, 509-511; Long 1956, 22-28).

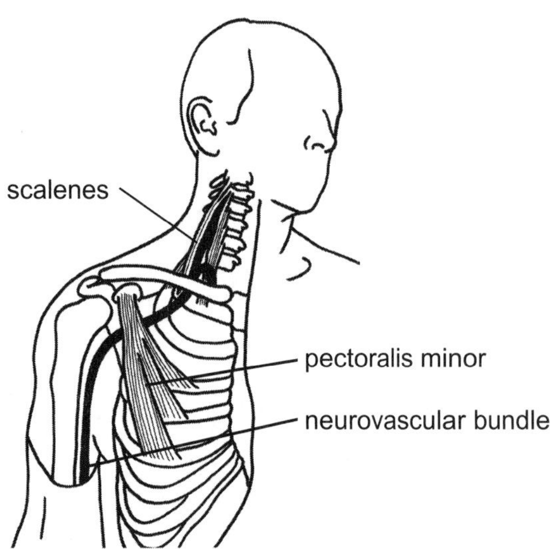

Figure 5.11 The neurovascular bundle includes the nerves, blood vessels, and lymphatic ducts that serve the arm and hand.

When trigger points shorten the scalene muscles, they tend to keep the first rib pulled up against the collarbone, squeezing the blood vessels, lymphatic ducts, and nerves (collectively the neurovascular bundle) as they pass through the area on their way to the arm (Figure 5.11). This entrapment impedes blood flow and disturbs nerve impulses, causing pain, swelling, numbness, tingling, and burning in the arm and hand. If your hands are often uncomfortably puffy, making rings tight on your fingers, look for scalene trigger points, especially in the anterior scalenes.

The collection of symptoms caused by compression of the nerves and blood vessels in this region is properly termed *thoracic outlet syndrome*, although it's very often incorrectly diagnosed as carpal tunnel syndrome. Travell and Simons make the point that both of these syndromes are heavily overdiagnosed, leading to a great number of unneeded surgical operations (Simons, Travell, and Simons 1999, 515-525).

Scalene-induced weakness in the forearms and hands can make you unexpectedly drop things. This is likely to be mistakenly ascribed to a neurological defect. The mysterious phenomenon of phantom pain that feels as though it's coming from an amputated arm or hand can actually be created by scalene trigger points (Simons, Travell, and Simons 1999, 505; Sherman 1980, 232-244).

When conventional treatments fail to improve symptoms created by scalene trigger points, it's not unusual to be told it's all in your head. This is especially apt to happen when the unremitting discomfort created by the scalenes makes you sleepless, irritable, and depressed. Given that scalene symptoms can occur so far from their source and are so variable, it's no wonder that their cause is misunderstood. Fortunately, once you do understand that all of these symptoms can be coming from the scalene muscles, the solution is remarkably simple and quick (Simons, Travell, and Simons 1999, 504-525).

Causes

The scalene muscles attach to the sides of your neck vertebrae and to your top two ribs. Although the scalenes help stabilize and flex the neck, their main job is to raise the upper two ribs on each side to give your lungs greater capacity when you inhale. The scalenes are active to some degree in every inhalation, and they work extremely hard when your breathing is labored during vigorous activity.

Habitually breathing with the chest instead of the diaphragm severely overtaxes the scalene muscles. Simple nervous hyperventilation stresses them too. People who are prone to emotional tension should expect to find terrible trigger points in their scalene muscles. When people who suffer from asthma or emphysema struggle for breath, this can promote scalene trigger points, as can a bad cough from pneumonia, bronchitis, allergies, or a common cold. Playing a musical wind instrument is famous for fostering scalene trouble (Simons, Travell, and Simons 1999, 510-511).

Many ordinary activities cause scalene trouble when overdone to the point of strain. Working for long hours with the arms out in front of the body can be very stressful for the scalenes. Pulling, lifting, and carrying heavy loads can also be bad. Carrying a heavy backpack is especially rough for the scalenes as well as several other muscles not designed for mule duty, such as the trapezius, pectoralis minor, and sternocleidomastoid. The scalenes are among the muscles most abused in activities like running and swimming, which demand a lot of strenuous breathing. Scalene trigger points are prone to initiating and perpetuating satellite trigger points in other muscles (Simons, Travell, and Simons 1999, 510-511).

You can expect violent movement of the head during a fall or an auto accident to bring about trigger points in the scalenes. Both the scalenes and the sternocleidomastoids are severely affected by whiplash, and both are easily overlooked in the treatment of pain from this type of injury. Apparent neurological symptoms in the upper back, shoulder, arms, and hands that mysteriously persist after an auto accident can often be traced to the scalenes. One study found scalene trigger points in 81 percent of whiplash patients (Simons, Travell, and Simons 1999, 511).

Scalene muscles help manage the weight of the head, and anything that creates an imbalance in this regard puts an additional burden on them. For this reason, it's wise to be aware of postures that may be holding your head off center. Slouching or habitually carrying your head forward are both sure to keep trigger points going in all of the muscles in the anterior neck (Simons, Travell, and Simons 1999, 510-511).

Self-Treatment

Success in finding and dealing with the scalenes depends on your understanding of their relationship to the sternocleidomastoid muscle, illustrated in Figure 5.7. The anterior scalene, the front-most scalene muscle, lies between the sternocleidomastoid and the neck vertebrae and is almost completely hidden. You have to move the sternocleidomastoid aside to get to the anterior scalene.

The middle scalene is behind the anterior scalene, more on the side of the neck, with its lower half free of the sternocleidomastoid. The posterior scalene lies almost horizontally behind the middle scalene in the soft triangular depression just above the collarbone and below the front edge of the trapezius, the thick roll of muscle on top of your shoulder. A fourth scalene muscle, the vertically oriented scalenus minimus, is found behind the anterior scalene (not shown). Not everyone has scalenus minimus muscles; it's a normal human anatomical variation.

The scalenes cling closely to the neck and feel much firmer than the soft, loose, mushy sternocleidomastoids. Think of what a turkey neck looks like. When massaging the scalenes, you'll be pressing them against the bony vertebrae underneath.

Scalene massage won't hurt unless you encounter a trigger point, in which case it can be painful indeed. Pressure on a scalene trigger point evokes a spooky kind of pain that will make you duck and cringe. It can actually feel like you're pressing on a nerve. At the same time, you may feel the referred pain or other symptoms being reproduced or accentuated in the upper back, shoulder, or chest. This can be a very convincing demonstration of the reality of referred myofascial pain. If your scalenes are really bad, you'll want to begin with light pressure.

To massage the anterior scalene, which is the chief troublemaker, you have to get your fingers behind the sternocleidomastoid or move it out of the way. To do this, orient yourself by first gripping the sternocleidomastoid between your fingers and thumb as if you were going to massage it. Then let go with your thumb and use your fingers to pull the entire sternocleidomastoid toward your windpipe. Pull hard. These are not delicate muscles. The idea is to get your fingertips as far around in front of the vertebral column as you can, with the sternocleidomastoid pulled out of the way. In this position, you can press the anterior scalene back against the vertebral column with the tips of your fingers. Note that you have to pull the sternocleidomastoid aside to begin each stroke (Figure 5.12). The middle finger does most of the work, assisted by the ring finger.

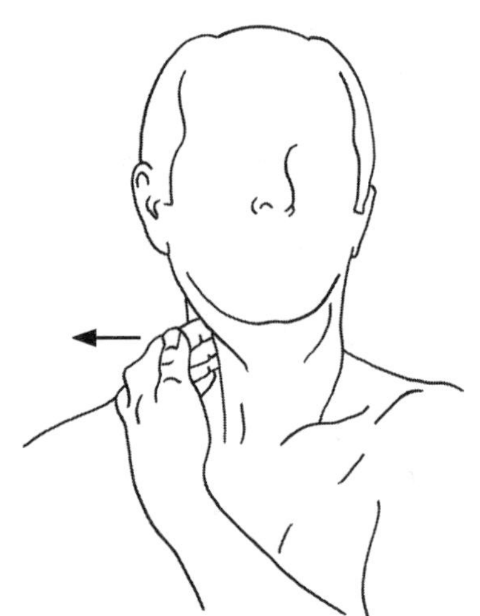

Figure 5.12 Anterior scalene massage. Before each stroke, pull the sternocleidomastoid out of the way toward the windpipe, then stroke back across the scalene as shown by the arrow.

The massage stroke is executed by pressing with your fingertips as you stroke across the muscle toward the side of the neck. The skin of the neck should move with the fingers. At the end of the

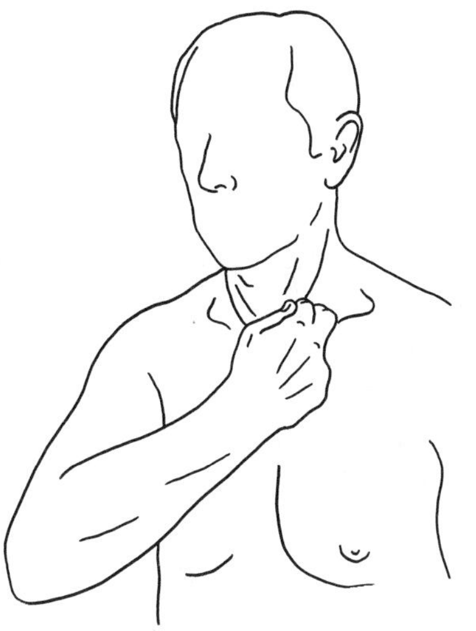

Figure 5.13 Scalene massage behind the sternocleidomastoid attachment to the collarbone

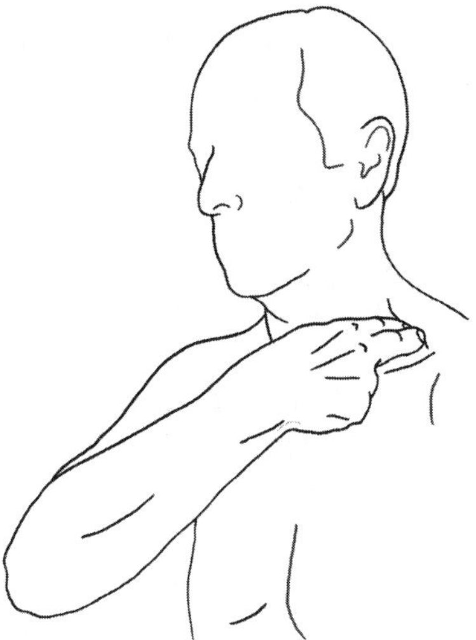

Figure 5.14 Posterior scalene massage in front of where the trapezius attaches to the collarbone

stroke, which will be only an inch long, let up on the pressure, move your fingers back where you began the stroke and repeat several times. This procedure should be carried out all along the back edge of the sternocleidomastoid, from up under your ear clear down to the collarbone. You'll find some of your worst scalene trigger points behind the sternocleidomastoid where it attaches to the collarbone (Figure 5.13). You may even find a trigger point hiding deep down behind the collarbone at that spot.

To massage the middle scalene, use this same stroke on the side of the neck. Six strokes on each scalene trigger point are enough for one session. Come back to them three to six times a day. You may find as many as five spots of exquisite tenderness in your scalenes.

To massage the posterior scalene, push your middle finger under the front edge of the trapezius muscle near where it attaches to the collarbone (Figure 5.14). Exert downward pressure and drag your finger toward your throat, parallel to the collarbone. This stroke is also about an inch long and should move the skin with it. The boniness you may feel under your finger as you do this stroke is the top of your first rib. Don't neglect the posterior scalene. It can have trigger points when the other scalene muscles don't, and it can cause any of the scalene symptoms.

To massage the scalenes effectively and without damaging the skin, your fingernails must be cut and filed to the quick. Your scalenes will be among the most difficult muscles to understand, locate, and treat, but any success you have with them will be well worth the effort. The scalenes are likely to be involved in any myofascial pain problem in the upper body and are sure to be involved in your frozen shoulder.

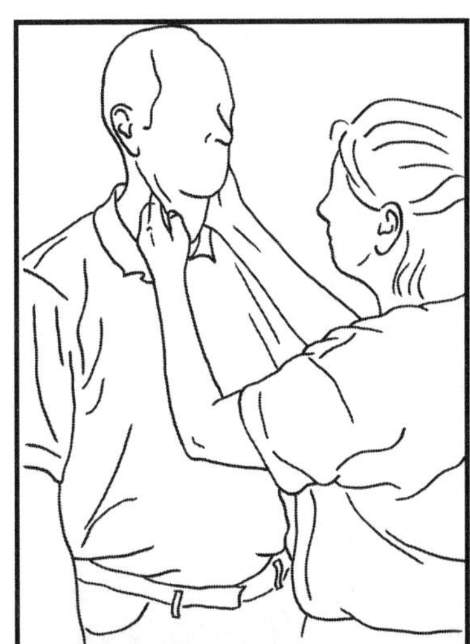

Figure 5.15 Partner massage of the anterior and middle scalene muscles

Partner Treatment

You can massage your partner's scalenes while standing face-to-face (Figure 5.15). Press against the vertebrae either with your thumb or with paired index and middle fingers. Make the same short, repeated stroke away from the windpipe. Six strokes are enough for any trigger point that you find. Don't neglect the posterior scalenes. Find and treat them with two fingers paired. Go very, very lightly at first. Even with minimal pressure, scalene massage can be very unpleasant. For this reason, anyone planning to massage others should first practice self-treatment of their own scalenes to appreciate the danger of overdoing scalene massage on other people.

Clinical Treatment

To effectively treat the scalenes, you must have a clear mental picture of their location relative to the sternocleidomastoid muscles. The anterior scalene may be the most difficult to treat, since it's entirely hidden behind the sternocleidomastoid. Excessive tightness in the sternocleidomastoids due to trigger points can make the anterior scalene even harder to access. Address the anterior scalene by moving the sternocleidomastoid firmly toward the windpipe with the backs of the index and middle fingers (Figure 5.16). In the correct position, the fingers will be partly covered by the sternocleidomastoid.

Press the anterior scalene downward, toward the table and against the vertebrae, searching its length all the way down to the collarbone. Treat each trigger point with the usual short, repeated treatment stroke, moving the fingers cross-fiber away from the windpipe. Note that it's necessary to push the sternocleidomastoid aside to begin each stroke. Scalene massage often reproduces the client's particular referred pain or numbness pattern. Pressure on scalene trigger points can also produce an unpleasant electrical sensation that feels like you're pressing on a nerve. This doesn't happen after trigger points have been deactivated.

The middle scalene covers the side of the neck just behind the sternocleidomastoid. With two fingers or your thumb, stroke either along the fibers or across them repeatedly, all the way down to the collarbone. The posterior scalene can be found just above the collarbone at the angle it makes with the thick roll of trapezius muscle on top of the shoulder. Pressure for the treatment stroke should be toward the client's feet, but stroke in the direction of the throat with the middle finger (supported by the index finger) along the top of the collarbone (Figure 5.17). When the client takes a deep breath, you may feel the posterior scalene contracting and the first rib rising against your fingers. Don't be concerned about the scalenus minimus, the fourth scalene muscle that's present in only part of the population. The pressure from anterior scalene massage will project through to any scalenus minimus trigger points that may be hiding there.

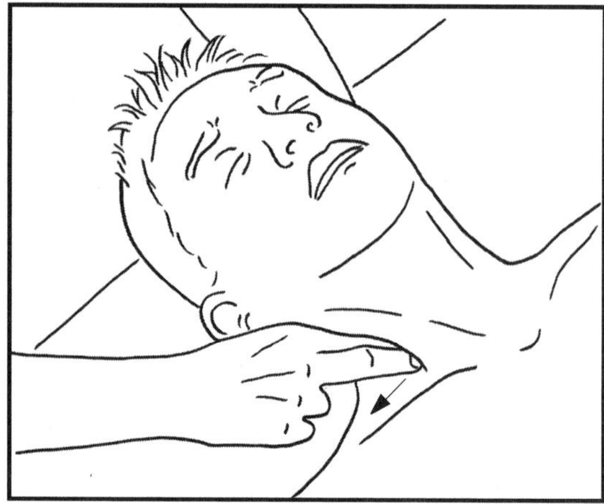

Figure 5.16 Anterior scalene massage. To begin each stroke, push the sternocleidomastoid toward the windpipe, then stroke as shown by the arrow.

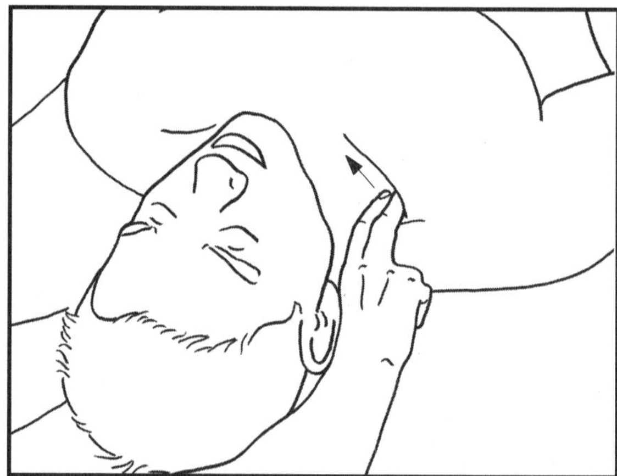

Figure 5.17 Posterior scalene massage just above the collarbone with the middle finger, making very short, deep strokes as shown by the small arrow

If you're unsure of the location of the individual scalene muscles, palpate them while having the client repeatedly sniff through the nose while taking air into the chest (as opposed to abdominal breathing). This causes the scalenes to contract more strongly so they can be felt more clearly.

Rotator Cuff Muscles

Jeanie, *age forty-five, developed chronic pain in both shoulders after trying to catch herself during a fall on the stairs where she worked. Doctors had offered only two options: cortisone shots or exploratory surgery, both of which she declined. She went through two ineffective courses of physical therapy and then settled into getting professional massage once a month. The "feel-good" massage was relaxing but did little to relieve her chronic shoulder pain. She lived with her shoulder trouble for the next fifteen years.*

In a class on self-treatment of pain, trigger points were discovered in all of Jeanie's rotator cuff muscles. She said the massage techniques she learned the first night in class brought more relief of her shoulder pain than she'd had from any previous treatment. She had spent thousands of dollars on therapy and evidently had suffered unnecessarily for fifteen years.

The most frequent cause of shoulder pain, loss of upper arm motion, and clicking or catching in the shoulder joint is trigger points in the four rotator cuff muscles: the subscapularis, supraspinatus, infraspinatus, and teres minor. When you're able to treat these trigger points yourself, you may be able to avoid forced manipulation of the shoulder, steroid injections, and harsh physical therapy. The safest and most direct and effective therapy for shoulder pain is specific trigger point massage of the rotator muscles. Even when surgery is required to correct a genuine structural problem, the trigger points in the rotator cuff muscles should be given attention to ensure you don't have unnecessary residual pain (Simons, Travell, and Simons 1999, 141-142, 542, 556, 599; Danneskiold-Samoe et al. 1983, 17-20).

In order to successfully locate and treat the shoulder muscles, it's very important that you become familiar with the shoulder blade as a bony structure. If you can't find all seven of the shoulder blade's bony landmarks, you may not have much luck finding the muscles. Before you go on reading this chapter, it would be a good idea to review the material on the shoulder blade in "Bones of the Shoulder" and Figures 1.1 to 1.9 in chapter 1. The seven parts of the shoulder blade you should be able to find are the superior angle, medial (inner) border, lateral (outer) border, inferior angle, acromion, coracoid process, and scapular spine.

The four rotator cuff muscles attach the shoulder blade to the top of the humerus, or upper arm bone. These important muscles operate separately to rotate the arm, and they work together to hold the ball-and-socket joint together. Trigger points in the rotator cuff muscles cause a major portion of the pain in your shoulder, along with loss of mobility and annoying clicks and grinding noises in the joint. These trigger points are believed to be responsible for many kinds of deterioration of the shoulder joint itself in terms of inflammation, arthritic growth, and any adhesions that do develop. Trigger points that maintain shoulder muscles in a shortened state also predispose the shoulder to serious physical injury, including rotator cuff tears, muscle tears, ligament sprains, and joint dislocation (Simons, Travell, and Simons 1999, 538-571, 596-607).

Supraspinatus and subscapularis trigger points are the primary factor in the development of true adhesive capsulitis. This begins when muscle stiffening caused by trigger points irritates their attachments and bursas, which promotes inflammation. The overgrowth of connective tissue that results from this inflammation is the essence of adhesive capsulitis. The development of these fibrotic adhesions could be prevented with early treatment of trigger points, specifically in the four rotator muscles.

Supraspinatus trigger points cause *enthesitis*, or inflammation of the muscle's tendinous attachments to the head of the humerus, making them very tender to the touch. Enthesitis has a strong tendency toward fibrosis, calcification, and the development of arthritic spurs. In this way, supraspinatus trigger points may be more of a factor in the development of true adhesive capsulitis than trigger points in the other rotators. *Impingement syndrome*, in which the head of the humerus is drawn up tightly against the acromion, is also thought to be due to shortening of the supraspinatus by trigger points.

A troubled subscapularis muscle is of paramount importance, because it plays a consistent role in the frozen shoulder phenomenon from the very beginning. Although it's important to treat all other muscles whose trigger points are contributing to your pain, a frozen shoulder will persist until the subscapularis trigger points are addressed (Simons, Travell, and Simons 1999, 605; Lewit 1991, 204-205).

Because trigger points in the rotator muscles keep the shoulder stiff and immoveable, they imitate true adhesive capsulitis. The two conditions can generally be distinguished, however, because trigger points create a painful condition, whereas true adhesive capsulitis is characterized by a more or less painless rigidity. So it may not be a good sign when after a year or more your shoulder pain finally abates but none of your range of motion has returned (Simons, Travell, and Simons 1999, 488, 685).

The two remaining rotator cuff muscles, the infraspinatus and teres minor, contribute to the stiffening of the shoulder when trigger points inhibit their lengthening. They also promote trouble in the subscapularis by causing it to work harder to overcome this limitation. It's important to remember that the infraspinatus and subscapularis have opposite actions. Each must relax and lengthen to allow the other to contract freely and easily. Freedom in this reciprocal action is fundamental to the healthy operation of the shoulder. When either of these primary muscles is in difficulty, all the finely coordinated movements of the arm are thrown out of kilter. This is where a frozen shoulder begins.

Subscapularis

The subscapularis is an exceptionally powerful muscle lining the front side of the shoulder blade (Figure 5.18). Visualize it sandwiched between the shoulder blade and the ribs. (In the illustration, the chest ribs have been removed so that you're looking through the body to the subscapularis muscle, which covers the front side of the shoulder blade.) The subscapularis's attachment to the head of the humerus allows it to rotate the arm inward, or medially. It also enables the subscapularis to help keep the joint together and keep the head of the humerus centered in its socket. When the subscapularis is weakened by trigger points, it allows the supraspinatus to pull the humeral head up against the bony acromion, causing impingement of the supraspinatus tendon and bursa.

You'd think that the subscapularis muscle would be unreachable and untreatable, buried as it is between the shoulder blade and chest wall. Actually, it's surprisingly accessible if you go about it the right way. With a frozen shoulder in particular, knowing how to treat subscapularis trigger points can be the key to a timely recovery (Simons, Travell, and Simons 1999, 599, 603-607; Cantu and Grodin 1992, 154-155).

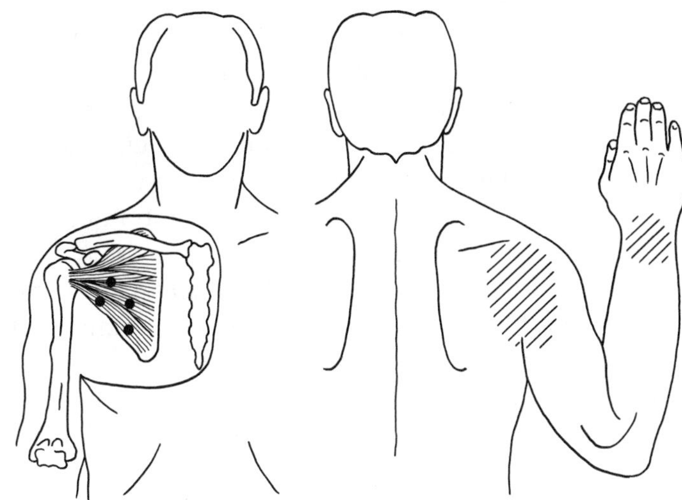

Figure 5.18 Subscapularis trigger points and referred pain pattern. The ribs have been removed to show the muscle on the front side of the shoulder blade.

Bernie, *age forty-eight, had endured pain in his left shoulder for several months. The problem began when he fell and jammed his arm while picking up broken branches after a storm. His shoulder ached all the time and woke him repeatedly at night. He'd stopped even trying to raise his arm, and he dreaded putting on his shirt in the morning. He hated the idea of going to the doctor, but the problem wasn't getting any better.*

Bernie's wife gave him a gift certificate for a massage, and to her great surprise he went. The therapist worked on an extremely painful place under his arm and then showed him how to massage the spot himself. His shoulder was better right away, which encouraged him to continue working on it on his own. When asked three months later how his shoulder was doing, he realized he'd had no pain in quite a while. To test it, he raised his arm all the way up. "I'd forgotten about it," he said. "I don't even think about it anymore."

Ruth's *shoulder trouble came about in a very different way. At age sixty-seven, she had decided to pursue her lifelong dream of learning to play the banjo. But soon after her first lessons, she began having pain behind her left shoulder whenever she began to practice. It hurt just to stick her arm out to hold the neck of the instrument. Luckily, her teacher knew something about trigger points, having had problems of his own.*

He explained that the left hand position for playing a banjo, a guitar, or even a violin requires maximum outward rotation of the left arm. To permit this, the subscapularis muscle has to lengthen all the way, which can be a terrific strain if you try to practice too long and the muscle isn't strong and resilient. "And then you get trigger points," he told her. After he showed Ruth how to do self-applied subscapularis massage, she was able to continue playing her banjo pain free as long as she didn't overdo it.

Symptoms

The main symptom of subscapularis trigger points is severe pain deep in the back of the shoulder (Figure 5.18). An ache in the back of the wrist is almost always present and should be seen as a sure sign of subscapularis trigger points. Sometimes the shoulder pain extends down the back of the upper arm (not shown). You may also have an extremely tender spot on the front of your shoulder where the troubled subscapularis has been continuously pulling and jerking on its attachment to the humerus (Simons, Travell, and Simons 1999, 556, 600).

A clicking or popping noise when you move your shoulder indicates probable trigger points in the subscapularis or the supraspinatus, or both. This is an indication that the joint isn't articulating correctly, in which case you may be at greater risk of rotator cuff tears and chronic shoulder instability (Simons, Travell, and Simons 1999, 545-546, 599).

Subscapularis trigger points also keep the muscle from lengthening, reducing the shoulder's range of motion and restricting rotation of the arm in either direction. This makes it difficult to reach above your head, across your body, or up behind your back. When you reach forward, it's impossible to fully turn your hand over with the palm up. The disabling pain and stiffness caused by subscapularis trigger points are commonly mistaken for bursitis, arthritis, bicipital tendinitis, rotator cuff injury, and adhesive capsulitis. A subscapularis muscle handicapped by trigger points promotes the development of trigger points in other important muscles, including the pectoralis major, teres major, latissimus dorsi, triceps, and anterior deltoid (Simons, Travell, and Simons 1999, 596-607).

Causes

A sudden unprepared overloading of the shoulder muscles, such as might occur when you catch yourself during a fall, is especially likely to make trouble for the subscapularis. Your shoulders are more vulnerable to this kind of accident when you're an older person, overweight, or simply out of shape. Another common cause for the development of subscapularis trigger points is prolonged immobilization of the shoulder for healing of a broken arm. Stroke victims who have lost the use of an arm often develop subscapularis trigger points because of inactivity. Similarly, when chest surgery, a case of shingles, or trigger points in the intercostal muscles between the ribs restrict movement of the arm, they too can initiate subscapularis trigger points (Simons, Travell, and Simons 1999, 878).

Trigger points commonly develop in the subscapularis when you overexert yourself during exercise or sports activity without proper conditioning. Fitness enthusiasts, swimmers, tennis players, and anyone who throws a ball as part of their game are in special danger of abusing their subscapularis muscles. Pitchers who have to retire prematurely because of "pitcher's arm" or chronic shoulder pain might well have been able to continue playing if their subscapularis and other rotator muscles had gotten appropriate trigger point therapy.

Self-Treatment

Luckily, the most troublesome subscapularis trigger points occur near its accessible outer edge. They can easily be reached for massage if you position your arm in a way that will move the shoulder blade forward and around the side of the body. Figures 5.19 and 5.20 show how the fingers or thumb should be placed in the slot between the shoulder blade and the chest wall. The arm is raised in these two drawings only to show how to get to the muscle. For the actual work with either the thumb or the fingers, the elbow needs to be down. Put your hand on your opposite shoulder if you can (Figure 5.21). This pulls the shoulder blade around the body and exposes a good bit of its front side.

Figure 5.22 shows the position of the thumb when it contacts the muscle. If you find it difficult to visualize how this image of the shoulder blade is oriented in regard to the body, look again at Figure 5.18. With your thumb in place, you should be able to wrap your hand around and touch the back side of the shoulder blade with your fingers. Figure 5.23 shows the fingers touching the subscapularis. The pads of the fingers should be tight against the ribs with the fingertips pressing very deeply into the back wall of the armpit.

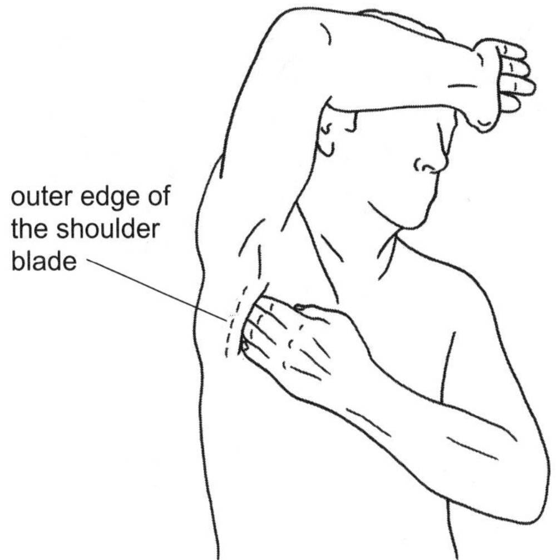

Figure 5.19 Position of the fingers for subscapularis massage. The arm is up for clarity. Keep the arm down for massage.

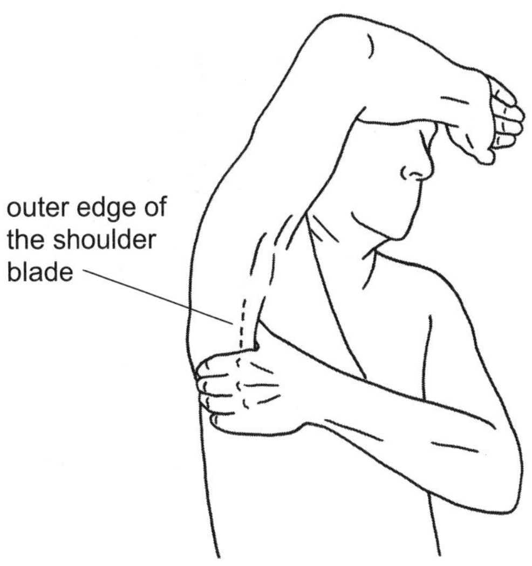

Figure 5.20 Position of the thumb for subscapularis massage. The arm is up for clarity. Keep the arm down for massage.

With the arm across the body, you can massage the subscapularis muscle sitting, standing, or lying on your back. You'll quickly discover that long fingernails will keep you from effectively self-treating your subscapularis muscles. You may be able to feel even very short nails, so your skin will probably be happier if you wear a light shirt when you work on your subscapularis. The massage techniques are shown on bare skin, not only to display the splendor of the model's physique, but also to show more clearly what is being done. If nails continue to be a problem or your hands and fingers hurt too much from overuse to self-treat your subscapularis, try one of the Shemala tools (see Figure 4.8).

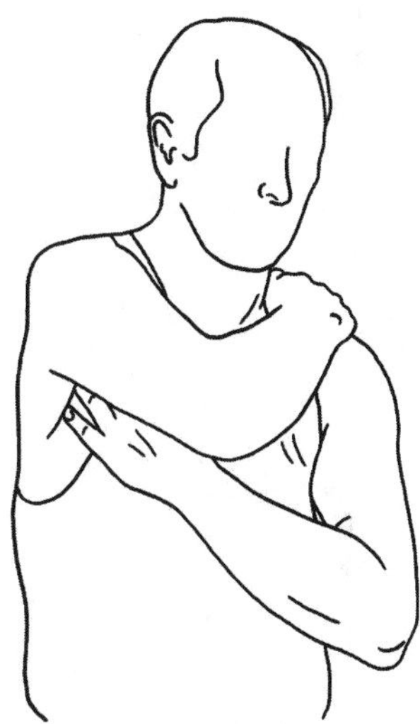

Figure 5.21 Position of the arms for subscapularis massage. Stroke away from the ribs and toward the outer edge of the shoulder blade.

Note that the fingers are not prodding the armpit but are inserted behind it. Also, you should not be massaging the thick web of muscle that defines the back of the armpit. For the subscapularis, your fingers (or thumb) need to be between this web of muscle and your ribs, as tight against your ribs as you can get. You must be able to feel and visualize the outer edge (lateral border) of the shoulder blade. Remember that the subscapularis muscle covers the front side of the shoulder blade between its outer and inner edges. The subscapularis lies between the bony outer edge and the ribs. If you're working anywhere else, you're missing it.

By far the best technique for gaining maximum access to the subscapularis is to sit with your arm hanging down between your legs (Figure 5.24). This position allows the shoulder muscles to relax and the weight of your arm to bring even more of the shoulder blade around the body. With the flats of your fingers firmly against your ribs, push deep into the pocket between the ribs and the roll of muscle that defines the back of the armpit.

If your hand and fingers are tight against your ribs, your fingertips will bump right into the subscapularis if you press deeply enough. The thumb also works for this. This technique was the primary therapy the author used to successfully treat his own frozen shoulder, as

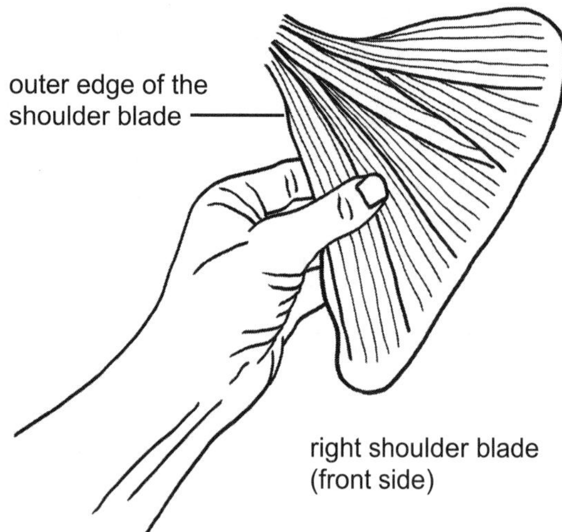

Figure 5.22 Subscapularis muscle with the thumb in place for self-treatment, stroking toward the outer edge of the shoulder blade

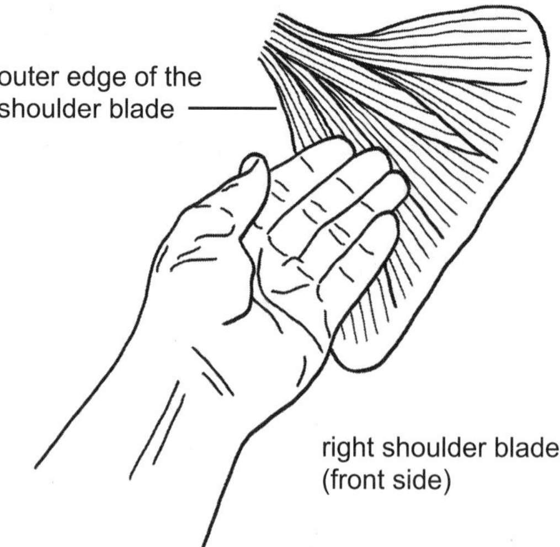

Figure 5.23 Subscapularis muscle with the fingers in position for self-treatment, stroking toward the outer edge of the shoulder blade

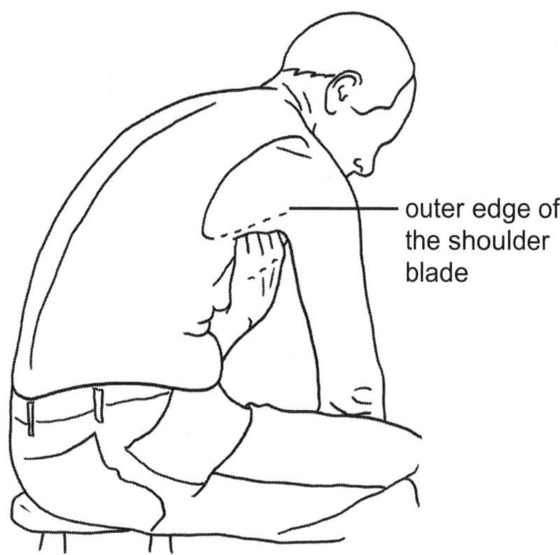

Figure 5.24 Subscapularis massage with the arm hanging down between the legs, stroking toward the outer edge of the shoulder blade

described in the introduction. Although many other muscles were involved, the subscapularis was the heart of the problem.

If massage in this position is too tiring for your neck, rest your forehead on a table with a folded towel as a pad. If you're unsure whether you're touching the subscapularis, contract it by strongly rotating your arm inward. Inward rotation, also called medial rotation, is when you turn your elbow outward.

Search for exquisitely tender spots all along inside the edge of the shoulder blade. For the uppermost ones you'll be poking very high back of the armpit and aiming at the ball-and-socket joint itself. Don't overlook trigger points in the lower part of the subscapularis as you approach the shoulder blade's inferior angle. When you find a trigger point, treat it with slow, one-inch strokes from the ribs outward. Keep your hand and fingers stiff like a board. The movement is in the wrist. Give your subscapularis trigger points six to twelve strokes several times a day. If pain wakes you up in the night, get up and have another massage session. It should cut the pain enough to let you get back to sleep.

Continue daily massage until you can no longer find trigger points. Significant relief can come right away, but complete deactivation may take as long as six weeks. Trigger points that have been in place for months or years will require a great deal of attention. Subscapularis trigger points can be horribly painful, but don't let this discourage you. Just lighten up to a pressure you can tolerate, do only a reasonable amount of massage, and keep coming back to it. If you don't master the subscapularis, your trouble will probably continue.

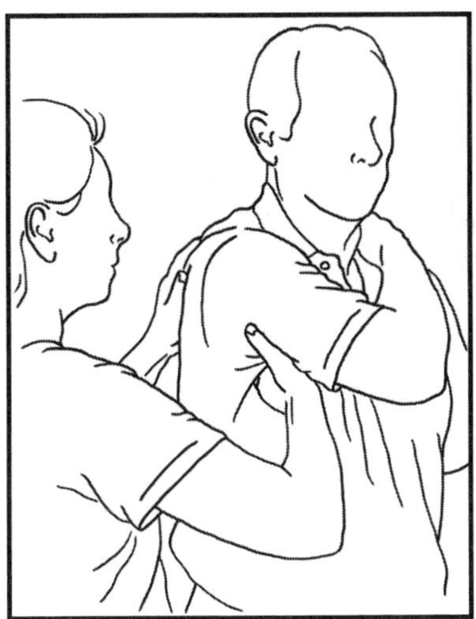

Figure 5.25 Partner massage of the subscapularis with the fingertips just inside the outer border of the shoulder blade

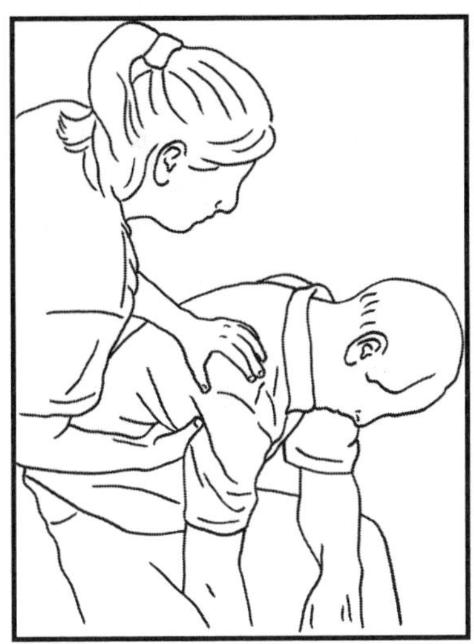

Figure 5.26 Partner massage of the subscapularis with the arm hanging down between the legs

Partner Treatment

A gentle, conscientious partner can often be of immense aid to someone who is too handicapped by pain to do their own massage or who can't comprehend the mechanics of the whole thing. Nurses, physicians' assistants, and occupational therapists skilled in trigger point massage can do a lot of good with elderly patients or those who have suffered strokes. Capable family members can also learn to provide treatments to those who aren't able to care for themselves.

Before working on someone else's subscapularis muscles, it's absolutely necessary that you rehearse the techniques on yourself. If you don't take the time to do this, it's fairly certain that you'll give the person a very unpleasant experience. There's no place on someone else's body where you must work with such care, caution, and intelligence, except perhaps the abdomen. Study the techniques on yourself beforehand and make sure you know what you're doing.

You can massage a partner's subscapularis standing at the side (Figure 5.25). In this case, it's helpful to pull on the inner (medial) edge of their shoulder blade with your other hand to help expose the front side of the shoulder blade and thus the muscle. However, the technique with the partner's arm hanging down between their legs may be even more effective (Figure 5.26). Take a look at Figure 5.27, which shows a partner's fingers on the muscle itself. It's difficult to illustrate exactly what's going on, but if you've done the therapy on yourself you'll get the idea.

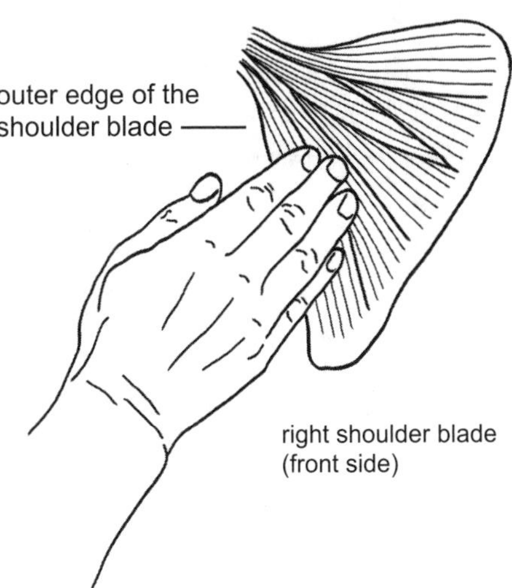

Figure 5.27 Subscapularis massage with the fingers in position for massage, stroking toward the outer edge of the shoulder blade

Clinical Treatment

Jessica, *age fifty-eight, had suffered from pain in her right shoulder for close to ten years. At one point she had gone through the additional agony of having adhesions broken under anesthesia. Although she got back her range of motion for a while, the pain had never gone away. She had gone to physical therapy several times, but it never seemed very effective.*

In the past year, she'd tried a chiropractor and had also bought a set of magnets to wear over her shoulder. She took ibuprofen and slept with an ice bag. Despite all of this, she couldn't remember the last time she'd been able to put her arm up behind her back to zip a

dress. She had stopped wearing clothing that zipped in back and only wore bras that fastened in front.

Trigger point massage was a revelation to Jessica. After her first treatment, she said, "There must be something to this. I feel better already." A week later, the therapist commented on how much better she looked—happier, more hopeful. After another week, she reported she was sleeping through the night. In two more months, after half a dozen more treatments, her pain was essentially gone.

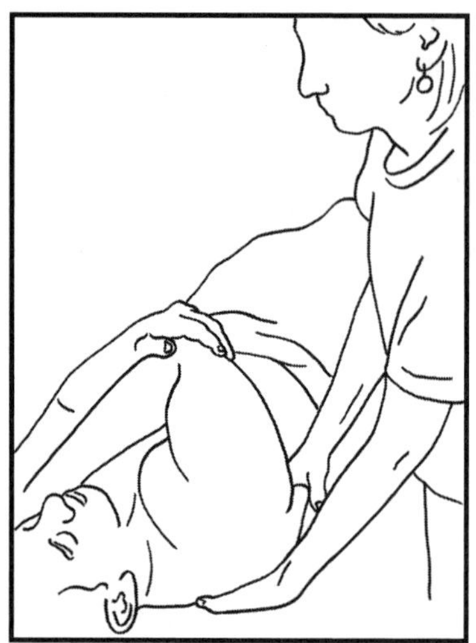

Figure 5.28 Subscapularis massage, starting with the backs of the nails tight against the ribs and stroking toward the therapist

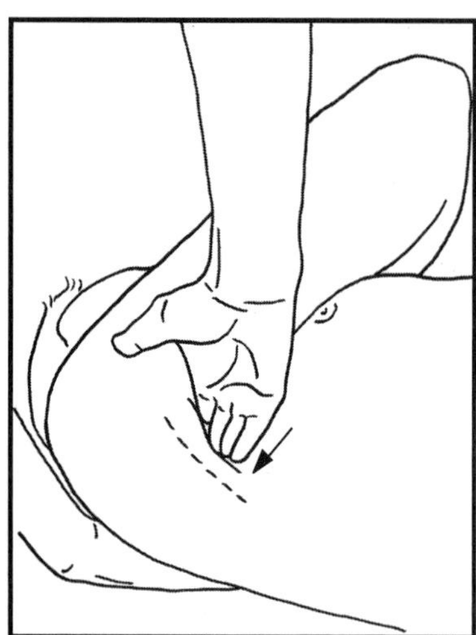

Figure 5.29 Subscapularis massage with the fingers in the slot between the shoulder blade and the ribs

To treat the subscapularis, place the supine client's hand on the opposite shoulder to move the shoulder blade around the body and forward (Figure 5.28). The client should use the other hand to press the elbow gently down against the chest. This creates a larger space for your treatment hand. A client with a truly frozen shoulder may not be able to reach the opposite shoulder, so be extremely gentle. This will improve with time as treatment goes along. To avoid abrading the client's skin, use plenty of lotion in the armpit and make sure your fingernails are very short. If the client can still feel your nails, do the massage through the sheet.

Reach under the client's shoulder with one hand, curl your fingertips around the medial border of the shoulder blade, and gently pull it toward you. Place your other hand one inch below the armpit with the palm toward you. In the correct position, your fingers will be in the slot between the shoulder blade and the chest wall, and your fingertips will be touching the subscapularis muscle. The backs of your nails should be firmly against the client's ribs. Exert pressure down toward the hand that's underneath the shoulder blade (Figure 5.29). Proceed slowly and with caution. Even light pressure on active subscapularis trigger points can be quite intolerable. Keep asking for numbers estimating the level of pain. Encourage the client to focus on relaxing the area you're working on, as this can help reduce the pain.

Two directions are possible for the treatment stroke. You can stroke with the fibers of the muscle down along the edge of the scapula, or you can stroke in a very short, cross-fiber scooping motion toward you. The cross-fiber strokes are indicated by the arrow in Figure 5.29. When you use the cross-fiber stroke, you can readily feel the tendonlike tautness of the muscle. Work your way up toward the head of the humerus where the subscapularis attaches, and then down to the inferior angle of the scapula. Sometimes trigger points are worse in this lower part of the muscle.

Although treatment would ordinarily call for six to twelve strokes for each trigger point, it's wise to use fewer strokes with the subscapularis and undertreat it during the first couple of sessions. Be aware that in this position you can inadvertently exert pressure on the serratus anterior with the back of your fingers. Pain evoked in this way from active serratus anterior trigger points can easily be mistaken for a subscapularis problem.

Some massage therapists have been taught that the proper way to treat the subscapularis muscle is to reach under the shoulder blade at its inner edge (Figure 5.30). This may be a helpful auxiliary technique for subscapularis attachment trigger points, but it can't replace working from the outer edge of the shoulder blade. Tenderness encountered under the inner edge is just as likely to be from trigger points in the trapezius, rhomboids, or serratus anterior, since you have to work through those muscles in this location to get to the subscapularis. Note that in order to get under the shoulder blade you must make it wing out by placing the client's hand in the small of the back. Tightness in the rhomboids may prevent this.

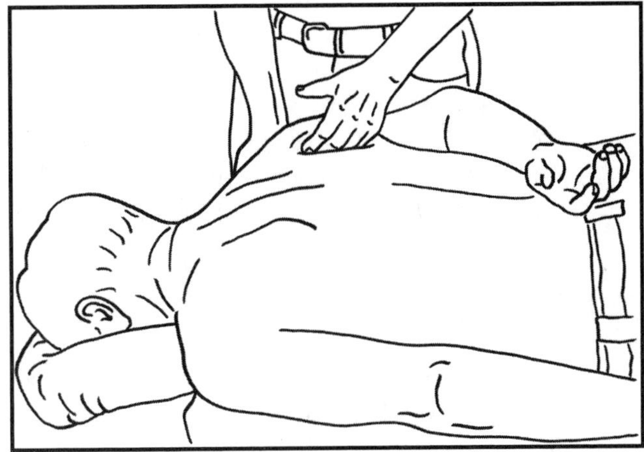

Figure 5.30 Subscapularis massage under the inner edge of the shoulder blade

Supraspinatus

The supraspinatus is buried in a pocket in the top of the shoulder blade above the scapular spine (Figure 5.31). At its outer end, the muscle passes under the acromion and crosses over to attach to the outer side of the head of the humerus. This attachment gives the supraspinatus great leverage for helping raise the arm. It also allows the muscle to help the other rotators hold the ball-and-socket joint together.

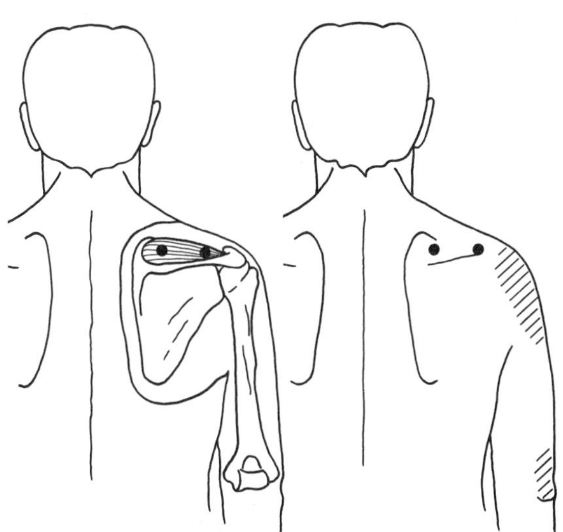

Figure 5.31 Supraspinatus trigger points and referred pain pattern

The supraspinatus is not the easiest muscle to find, and it's not the easiest to massage. Many massage therapists, even quite good ones, don't even try. Nevertheless, this muscle is too important a part of common shoulder problems to ignore. Therapists will actually find the supraspinatus easy to treat if they use the right technique. The muscle can even be self-treated if you understand it well enough and are determined to take it on. This is important, because supraspinatus trigger points can be at the heart of an otherwise unexplainable shoulder problem.

Erik, *age fifty-five, had a bad fall while skiing. Eighteen months later, he still felt the effects in the outside of his left shoulder and in his left elbow. He couldn't raise his arm without the most excruciating pain, and sometimes it hurt just to walk across the room with his arm hanging at his side. He had played the piano on weekends for many years for extra income, but even that had become an unpleasant ordeal. The doctor thought Erik had probably torn his rotator cuff, but an MRI revealed no problem of that sort.*

Pressure applied to an extremely tender spot in Erik's left supraspinatus muscle accentuated the pain in his elbow and shoulder. He was shown how to massage the muscle himself with a Backnobber. After a year and a half of misery, his pain was finally gone within just three weeks and by his own efforts.

Symptoms

Pain from supraspinatus trigger points is felt primarily as a deep ache in the middle deltoid muscle on the outer side of the shoulder (Figure 5.31). The pain isn't felt in the shoulder joint, as is the case with infraspinatus trigger points. The outer elbow also very often hurts, and pain occasionally spreads to the outer side of the upper arm, forearm, and wrist (not shown).

Pain is experienced both at rest and throughout any movement that raises the arm. Because trigger points can keep a muscle from lengthening, which the supraspinatus must do when you reach back or put your arm behind you, these movements can also cause pain. Washing, combing, or styling your hair becomes a problem, and men have trouble shaving. Playing tennis or painting the ceiling is out of the question. These difficulties and the pain causing them are frequently misdiagnosed as subdeltoid or subacromial bursitis (Simons, Travell, and Simons 1999, 538-546; Bonica and Sola 1990, 947-958).

Other common misdiagnoses include supraspinatus tendinitis, brachial neuritis, rotator cuff injury, and impingement syndrome. Rotator cuff tears do happen, but not as often as you might have been led to believe. When they do occur, they usually cause pain only in a limited part of the arm's upward movement. Trigger points give you pain all the way up (Simons, Travell, and Simons 1999, 542).

Rotator cuff damage, even when verified by an MRI, doesn't necessarily require surgery. Trigger point massage actually promotes the healing of small tears because it relieves the constant pulling of the muscle on the tendon. Furthermore, it's possible that tension in the muscle from trigger points could well have instigated the tear in the first place. Stretching should never be part of therapy when a rotator cuff tear is suspected (Simons, Travell, and Simons 1999, 545).

Strain induced by trigger points can also cause calcium deposits to form in the rotator cuff at the supraspinatus attachments to the head of the humerus. Interestingly, these deposits have been known to disappear after trigger point therapy, evidently because of the relief of strain (Simons, Travell, and Simons 1999, 542-543).

Supraspinatus trigger points are to blame for the clicking or popping that is sometimes felt or heard in the shoulder joint. This happens because the muscle is kept so tight that the head of the humerus is prevented from gliding smoothly in its socket. The popping stops when supraspinatus trigger points are deactivated. The balance of tension in the rotator muscles has to be very finely tuned to maintain the correct position of the ball in the socket. Any catching in the joint is likely due to an imbalance of muscle strength from the effects of trigger points (Simons, Travell, and Simons 1999, 542-546).

The supraspinatus is also one of many sources of the pain in the lateral epicondyle (outer elbow) known as "tennis elbow." Although commonly given such catchall diagnoses as arthritis, bursitis, tendinitis, or inflammation, tennis elbow is often nothing more complicated than referred pain from myofascial trigger points, which can be treated very effectively with massage. Trigger points in forearm and triceps muscles are the most common cause of tennis elbow, but supraspinatus trigger points can also be part of the problem. Unfortunately, they're generally overlooked as a source of this common pain (Simons, Travell, and Simons 1999, 538-546).

Causes

The supraspinatus is easily overloaded during a one-time incident of extreme exertion, such as moving a large couch or carrying things like heavy boxes or suitcases. People often get supraspinatus trigger points from dragging heavy suitcases through an airline terminal. The supraspinatus muscles have to work extraordinarily hard to keep the shoulder joint from pulling apart, especially when you carry something heavy with your arm hanging straight down.

Repetitive strain such as working with the arms overhead for long periods of time or typing at a computer keyboard with no elbow support can also exhaust supraspinatus muscles. The simple act of swinging your arms while walking can add an intolerable degree of strain on the supraspinatus when it's already in trouble. Catching yourself to prevent a fall can initiate supraspinatus trigger points. So can a large, strong, eager dog who can't be broken of pulling on the leash (Simons, Travell, and Simons 1999, 542; Hagberg 1981, 111-121).

Self-Treatment

You'll find the supraspinatus muscle at the top of the shoulder blade, immediately behind the thick roll of the trapezius muscle that lies on top of the shoulder. Place your fingers between the scapular spine and the superior angle of the shoulder blade. (Figure 5.32 shows how to find the superior angle.) If your hand is in the right place, your fingertips will be contacting the top edge of the scapular spine and the heel of your hand will be resting on your collarbone. To use isolated contraction to verify that you're touching the supraspinatus, begin to raise your arm forward and a little to the side. Just as your arm starts to move, you should feel the muscle contract and bulge up under your fingers.

Trigger points occur in two places in the supraspinatus (Figure 5.31). One is in the belly of the muscle, just below the superior angle of the shoulder blade. The other is an inch or two further out, near where the muscle dives under the acromion, the bony point of the shoulder. It's right in the bony V formed by the scapular spine and the collarbone, which come together at this spot. There will also be an attachment trigger point in the supraspinatus tendon under the outer edge of the acromion on top of the ball of the humerus. This can be an exceedingly tender spot that may lead a doctor to diagnose as bursitis or impingement syndrome, but it can be expected to resolve on its own without treatment after you've deactivated the two primary trigger points in the muscle.

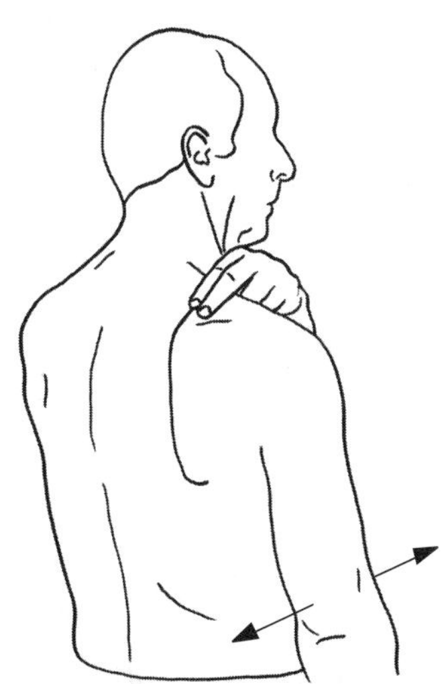

Figure 5.32 Swing the arm forward and back to move the superior angle under your fingers.

The sensitivity of the fingers is helpful for locating trigger points in the supraspinatus, but massage with the fingers is very hard to sustain here. It's also difficult to get

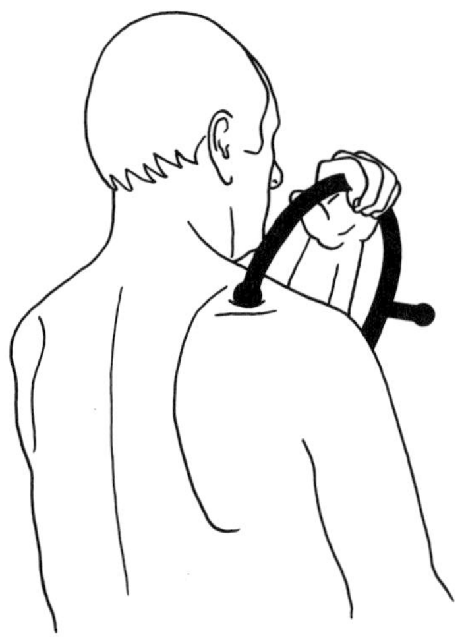

Figure 5.33 Supraspinatus massage with the Thera Cane (opposite hand is in the bow)

the pressure needed to go deep enough. Not only can the supraspinatus be quite thick, it's also covered by a thick part of the trapezius. The Thera Cane or Backnobber are better tools, at least for saving your fingers (Figure 5.33). It helps to first guide the knob carefully into place with your fingers, feeling for the superior angle of the shoulder blade and the scapular spine. The smaller knob on one end of the Backnobber probably makes it the better tool for this job. With either tool, placing the opposite hand high up in the bow gives you the greatest leverage for digging into this deeply situated muscle. As usual, use the short, repeated stroke.

The supraspinatus creates satellite trigger points in the middle deltoid. They will need some attention too, but don't be misled. Pain in the middle deltoid will tempt you to expend all of your energy massaging that location. Deltoid massage is easy, feels great, and may even do some good, but it won't fix your shoulder pain if the problem is originating in the supraspinatus.

Partner Treatment

You can massage someone else's supraspinatus muscle through a shirt if the cloth isn't too thick (Figure 5.34). The person must be seated with you standing behind so that you can get enough pressure to penetrate to the trigger points. When working with a thin person who has extreme tenderness in the muscle, use the fingers of one hand, as shown in the drawing. For a heavier person, use supported fingers.

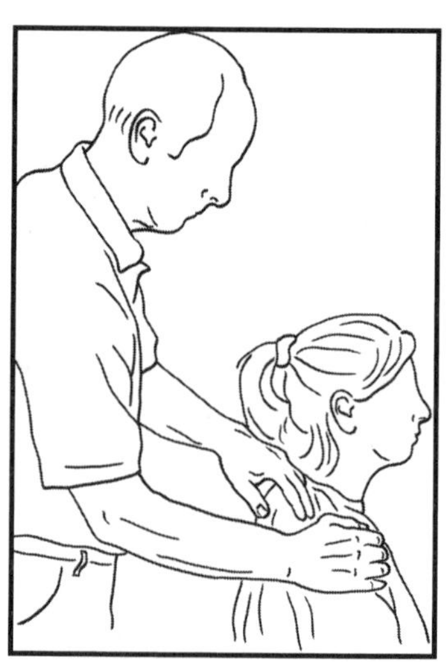

Figure 5.34 Partner massage of the supraspinatus with two fingers of one hand

Clinical Treatment

Jack, *age sixty-five, felt he was handicapped by weak upper body strength when doing work around the house. Yard work made him feel like an old man. He couldn't reach up behind to scratch his back without causing pain in his shoulder. He said he'd had a bike accident when he was nineteen that crushed his left shoulder, and he'd been in a body cast for weeks. He'd favored his left side ever since to avoid reactivating the pain he'd had way back then. It turned out that the bike accident and his present pain were just a coincidence.*

The therapist found excruciatingly tender spots in Jack's left supraspinatus and scalene muscles. Three treatments in two weeks left him pain free. He called later to say he was working with great freedom and self-confidence in the yard. He said he was feeling strong and empowered and was impressed at how simple the solution had been.

A massage therapist should treat supraspinatus trigger points with paired supported thumbs from the head of the table (Figure 5.35). The thumbs should be facing one another with the nails touching. This makes a very strong, pointed tool capable of penetrating through the trapezius, which can be very thick and muscular where it overlies the supraspinatus. Keep your wrists and elbows straight, then simply lean in, using your weight for the pressure.

If you implement this technique exactly as described, you'll find it surprisingly effortless and effective. Focus on the small triangular space between the superior angle and spine of the shoulder blade. Use six to twelve short strokes toward the outer shoulder to treat this deep central trigger point, then move a short distance further out to where the muscle dives under the acromion. If this outer trigger point is present, it will feel highly sensitive, very much like a bruise. Treat this thin part of the muscle gently. The supraspinatus is one of the most critical muscles in a shoulder problem. You should make a commitment to master it.

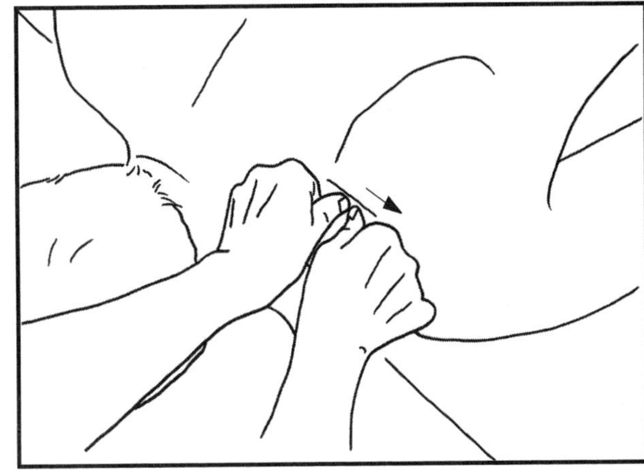

Figure 5.35 Supraspinatus massage just above the spine of the shoulder blade with paired supported thumbs

Infraspinatus

The infraspinatus covers essentially the entire shoulder blade below the scapular spine (Figure 5.36). The infraspinatus attaches to the back of the head of the humerus, giving it the ability to rotate the arm outward (see Figures 1.41 and 1.42). This is the motion you make in preparing to throw a ball or to make a forehand stroke with a tennis racket. Without outward rotation, the arm can't be raised above the level of the shoulder. The infraspinatus is also a strong participant in keeping the head of the humerus in its socket.

Among the four rotator cuff muscles, the infraspinatus is usually the first to develop trigger points. In fact, it's one of the most frequently afflicted muscles of the body. Infraspinatus trigger points that cause recurrent pain and keep the muscle stiff and weak can endanger an athletic career.

> Kim *was a thirty-two-year-old professional tennis coach who had lived with pain in both shoulders ever since she began playing tennis as a child. Diagnosed with rotator cuff tendinitis, Kim had had numerous steroid injections and was going for physical therapy almost weekly. Despite the treatments, pain kept her from playing much of the time. She was concerned that several of her young players were developing shoulder pain very similar to her own. "I make them play through the pain just like I was told to do at their age," she said, "but I'm afraid they'll end up as tennis cripples like me. I don't know what else to do. They want to play so badly."*
>
> *After a massage therapist showed Kim how to self-treat her shoulder with a tennis ball against the wall, she became free of shoulder pain for the first time since the age of fourteen. She felt that the best part of the new therapy was in being able to teach it to her students.*
>
> *Heather, age twelve, one of Kim's students, seemed to be needing more help than the others. She was small for her age and had started getting severe pain in the front of her right shoulder and down the outside of her arm after getting a full-sized tennis racket for Christmas. The pain increased sharply when drawing back the racket for a forehand stroke and again when the racket struck the ball.*

A sports orthopedist had diagnosed rotator cuff tendinitis and prescribed exercise, stretching, and a steroid patch for her shoulder. Heather complained to her mother that the stretching and the exercises left her with even more pain and refused to do them. She said the tennis ball against the wall was the only thing that helped. But she felt that something else was wrong. "Aren't there more muscles than just this one?" she asked.

On Kim's advice, Heather's mother took her to Kim's massage therapist, who discovered and treated trigger points in a number of other muscles. All four of the girl's rotator cuff muscles were in trouble, along with her scalenes and most of the muscles in her forearm. The therapist showed her how to self-treat her shoulder and arm. He further suggested that she put her new long-handled tennis racket away for a couple more years.

Symptoms

You'll remember from chapter 2 that Janet Travell was also kept from playing tennis by infraspinatus trigger points. It was the very thing that had introduced her to the phenomenon of referred myofascial pain. Dr. Travell was impressed by the strange paradox of infraspinatus trigger points causing pain in the front of her shoulder, though the muscle itself was behind the shoulder (Figures 5.36 and 5.37).

Infraspinatus pain usually feels like it's deep in the joint, which is what misleads physicians into diagnosing arthritis or a rotator cuff injury. Infraspinatus trigger points actually do a very good job of mimicking true arthritis. Pain may also travel some distance down the biceps and shoot down the outer side of the shoulder. Tenderness in the anterior deltoid and the bicipital groove in the head of the humerus can lead to an erroneous diagnosis of bicipital tendinitis.

Occasionally, pain is referred to the back of the neck, the inner border of the shoulder blade, all the way down the upper arm and forearm, and into the thumb side of the hand (not shown). When pain is referred to the forearm, it tends to promote formation of satellite trigger points in the extensor muscles, compounding pain and other symptoms in the hand. Many hours can be wasted rubbing all these places when you don't realize that the problem originates in the infraspinatus (Simons, Travell, and Simons 1999, 552-554).

Other symptoms of infraspinatus trigger points include weakness and stiffness in the shoulder and arm, which can make your shoulder and arm tire easily. Both inward and

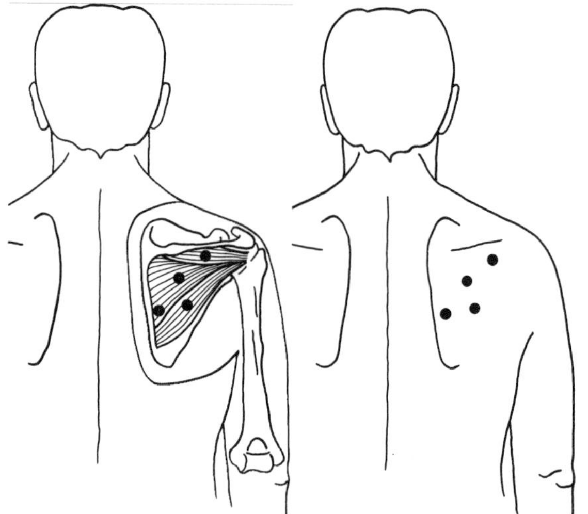

Figure 5.36 Infraspinatus trigger points

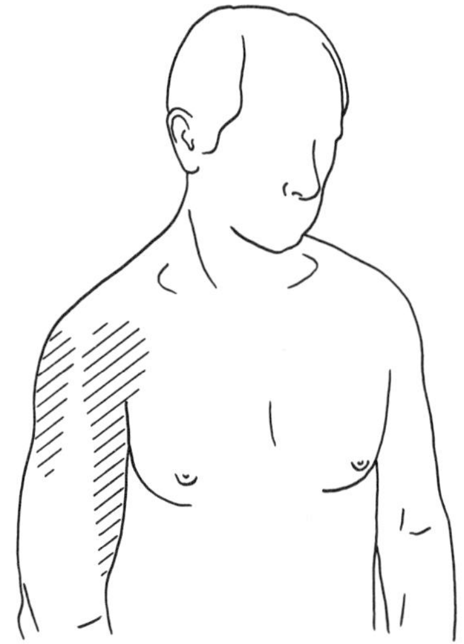

Figure 5.37 Infraspinatus referred pain pattern

outward rotation of the arm are restricted, making it difficult to move the arm in any direction. Since inward rotation is necessary for reaching behind you, it becomes impossible to reach up behind your back. You struggle getting your jacket on or off. Lying on the afflicted shoulder is painful, but lying on the opposite side is painful as well, because the weight of the arm pulls on the infraspinatus. You may only be able to sleep in a recliner or propped up with pillows in bed (Simons, Travell, and Simons 1999, 556; Sola and Williams 1956, 91-95).

Dysfunction of the infraspinatus typically causes the other rotators to tighten up in an effort to compensate, which tends to overload them too. All four rotators end up with trigger points, and soon you're unable to move your arm at all. This rigidity can give your doctor the idea that you have adhesions in the joint, which can lead to a recommendation for forced manipulation under anesthesia. However, this kind of restricted motion can usually be treated very successfully with trigger point massage of the rotator cuff muscles (Simons, Travell, and Simons 1999, 552-558).

Causes

Any type of work that requires keeping your arms overhead or out in front of you for long periods of time abuses the infraspinatus muscles because they have to hold a contraction to keep the arms up. Repeatedly reaching backward can also leave the infraspinatus in a tight contraction and full of trigger points. Accidents, falls, and many sports can overload the infraspinatus. Ball throwing and racket sports are especially taxing.

Driving with your hands on the top of the wheel puts continuous strain on both the infraspinatus and supraspinatus, since they work together to keep the arms up. For the same reason, working at a computer keyboard without elbow support exhausts both muscles. Keeping your hand on the mouse out to one side can be the cause of chronic shoulder pain on that side, since this position requires nearly maximum outward rotation of the arm and constant contraction of the infraspinatus.

Study your activities to discover other ways an infraspinatus muscle may be habitually overloaded in relation to its function in outward rotation of the arm. As an example, it might be worth the trouble to learn to use the mouse with your left hand. Since the right side of the keyboard has so many extra keys, positioning the mouse to the left of the keyboard brings your hand closer to center and requires less outward rotation.

Self-Treatment

Since the infraspinatus is fully exposed on the outside of the shoulder blade, it's easy to treat with self-applied massage. Confirm its location by feeling it contract and bulge as you put the arm into outward rotation (Figure 5.38). The Thera Cane works well for infraspinatus massage (Figures 5.39 and 5.40), as does the Backnobber. You may like a ball against the wall even better (Figure 5.41). As shown in the drawing, it's important that you stand not with your back flat to the wall, but rather at about a 45 degree angle.

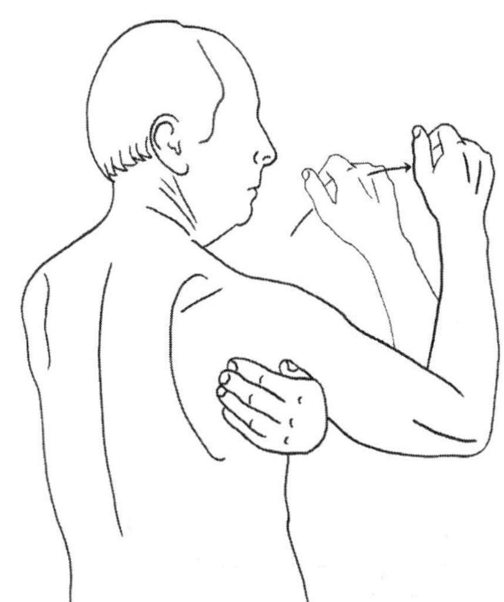

Figure 5.38 The arrow shows outward rotation for locating the infraspinatus with isolated contraction.

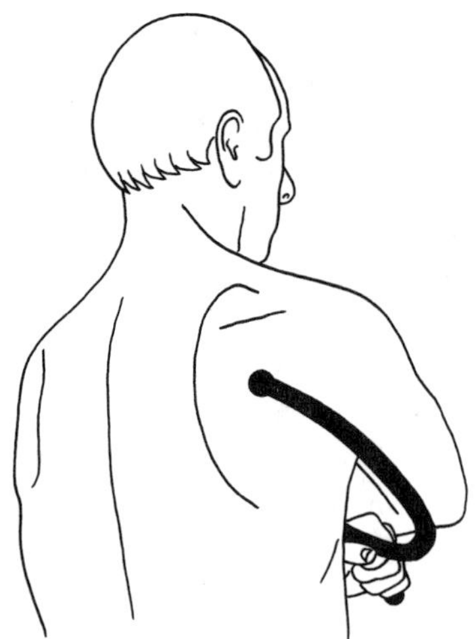

Figure 5.39 Infraspinatus massage with a Thera Cane

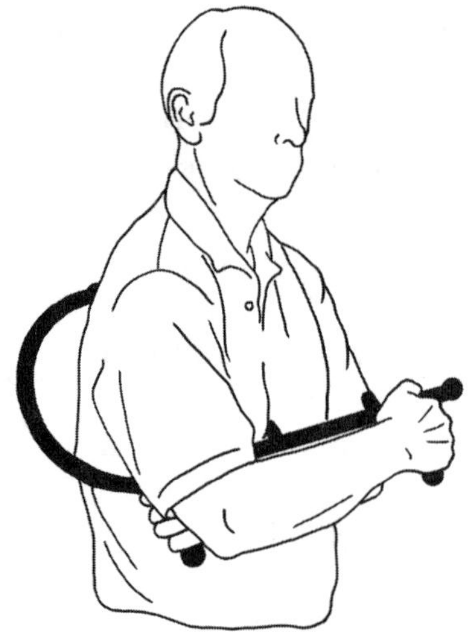

Figure 5.40 Thera Cane massage through a layer of cloth

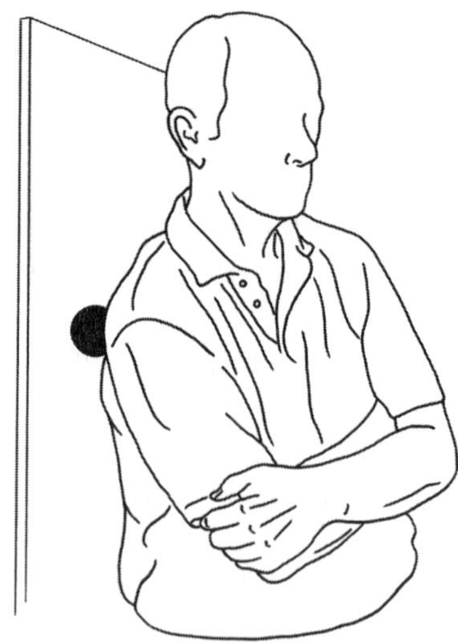

Figure 5.41 Infraspinatus massage with a lacrosse ball against the wall

in the drawing, it's important that you stand not with your back flat to the wall, but rather at about a 45 degree angle.

When you exert pressure on infraspinatus trigger points, the pain reaction takes a while to wake up, so don't conclude too quickly that you don't have a problem there. It may take several strokes before you feel the characteristic exquisite tenderness. Six to twelve massage strokes constitute a treatment, but come back to it several times a day.

The infraspinatus is an especially sneaky muscle. You'll rarely experience pain in the infraspinatus itself. You'll find yourself rubbing away at the front or outer side of your shoulder, forgetting that infraspinatus trigger points are almost always the cause of pain felt there. You won't know the infraspinatus is the culprit until you press on it.

Be wary of exercising and stretching the infraspinatus or any of the other shoulder muscles until the trigger points have been taken care of. Trigger points in the infraspinatus are unusually irritable, making stretching counterproductive as therapy. A physical therapist may insist on the need for exercising the shoulder, but the weakness and stiffness that seem to be the problem are actually part of the protection the trigger points are trying to provide. Muscle strength comes back quickly when trigger points are deactivated, at which point exercise and stretching are helpful for getting your range of motion back. Keep in mind that if there's any chance that a muscle or its tendon has a tear in it, stretching is exactly the wrong thing to do.

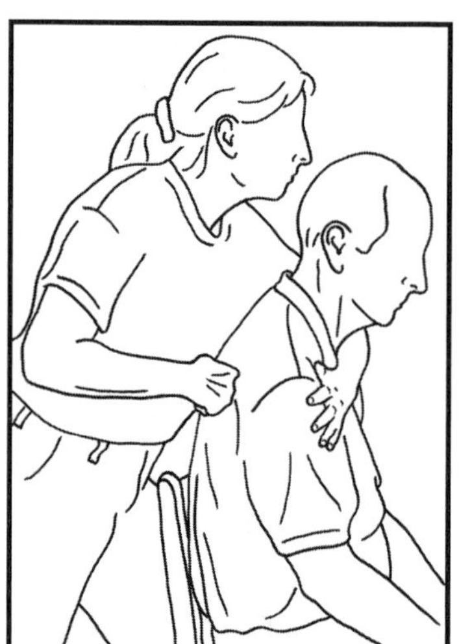

Figure 5.42 Partner massage of the infraspinatus and teres minor with the knuckles of a loose fist

Partner Treatment

The infraspinatus isn't difficult to treat on someone else if you get a little bit above the muscle so you can use your weight to exert pressure. Use a loose fist with the person seated while you stand behind (Figure 5.42). It also works to use paired supported thumbs with both people standing

(Figure 5.43), but you may have to work harder, particularly if the person is taller than you.

In working the infraspinatus, a common mistake is to get off the shoulder blade and get lost massaging the rhomboid area between the shoulder blade and the spine. This always feels great and it may seem just the thing to do, but you won't be treating the infraspinatus and you won't be solving any of its problems. If you're working on an especially well-fed or muscular person, you may have difficulty feeling the bony landmarks, but you can at least try to visualize them.

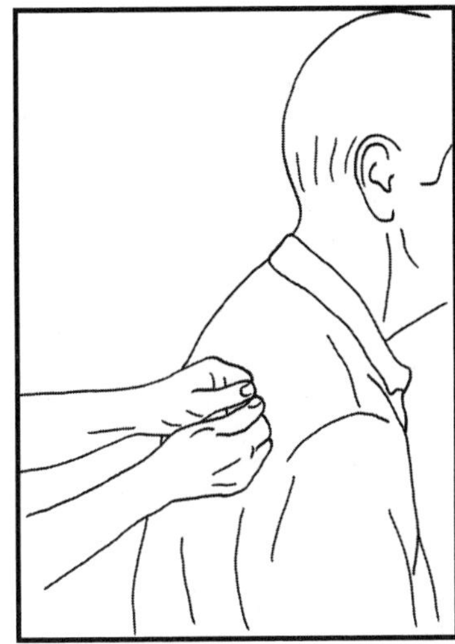

Figure 5.43 Partner massage of the infraspinatus with supported thumbs

You should search out the more or less horizontal scapular spine above the muscle and the medial and lateral borders of the shoulder blade on either side. These three landmarks form a rough triangle. The shoulder blade isn't right on the flat of the back, but rather a little to the side. Look for opportunities to practice on someone slender so you can get a clear idea of where these bony ridges lie and how they feel under your fingers. On really skinny people, you can often see and feel the outlines of the shoulder blades quite plainly through a thin shirt.

The most active infraspinatus trigger point is usually in the thickest, most muscular part of the muscle. You'll ordinarily be able to feel it if you're in the right place. If in doubt, have the person briefly contract the muscle a few times with outward rotation of the arm. Treat the trigger points, as usual, with six to twelve short strokes.

Clinical Treatment

To treat infraspinatus trigger points use supported fingers (Figure 5.44). Infraspinatus trigger points can be present in several places below the spine of the scapula between the medial and lateral borders. The infraspinatus often needs multiple deep strokes before trigger points begin to produce the familiar sense of exquisite tenderness. It may take ten or fifteen seconds before the client can give you a number high enough to indicate the need for treatment. This is a good place to practice good body mechanics while you work by keeping your neck and spine straight and using your body weight instead of muscle action to exert pressure.

The infraspinatus is also a good place to learn the supported fingers technique if you don't already use it. You'll want to keep the fingers on the massaging hand straight and nearly vertical to the client's body. In this position, all four fingers won't touch. Concentrate on having the middle and ring fingers do the work. Let the pinky and index fingers just be there for moral support. Keep the strokes short enough to move the skin with your fingers. This helps you focus on the trigger point, where the work is needed. It's not necessary to

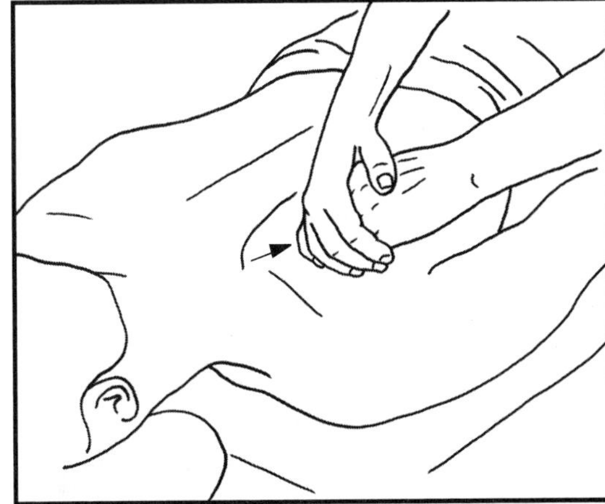

Figure 5.44 Infraspinatus massage with the edge of the right hand on the body pulling the fingertips of the left hand toward the therapist

massage the whole muscle, except for a few warming strokes before and after you address the trigger points.

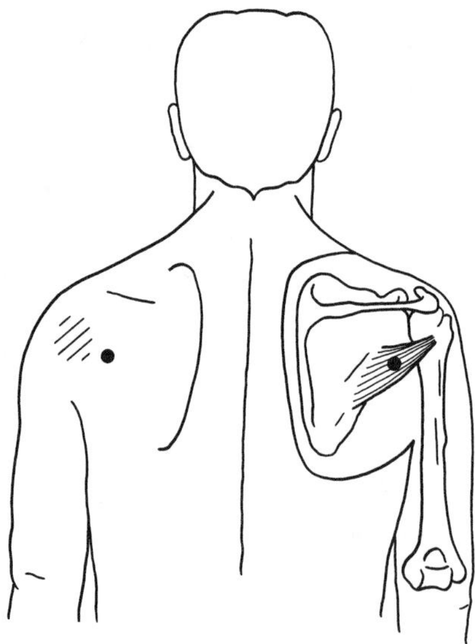

Figure 5.45 Teres minor trigger points and referred pain pattern

Teres Minor

The teres minor muscle lies right below the infraspinatus where it crosses the outer edge of the shoulder blade, and it has a similar attachment to the back of the head of the humerus (Figure 5.45). The teres minor helps the infraspinatus rotate the arm outward. The two muscles could be considered different heads of one muscle except that they're served by different nerves. The suprascapular nerve supplies the infraspinatus; the axillary nerve supplies the teres minor.

Symptoms

Compression of the axillary nerve, which serves the teres minor, can cause quadrilateral space syndrome, which is marked by pain in the shoulder and atrophy of the teres minor muscle. This compression can be the result of either trigger points or an anatomical abnormality. Fortunately, the condition is rare (Simons, Travell, and Simons 1999, 568-569).

The pain pattern for the teres minor is quite different from that of the infraspinatus. It refers pain primarily to a very confined spot on the back of the shoulder in the area of its attachment to the humerus. Pain from trigger points in the teres minor may not be noticed until after more oppressive problems with other shoulder muscles are dealt with. As with all of the rotator muscles, if the teres minor is in trouble, the others probably are too (Simons, Travell, and Simons 1999, 564-569).

Myofascial knots in the teres minor can feel like a lump the size of a prune behind the shoulder. This can be grounds for a mistaken belief that you have subdeltoid bursitis, which is actually quite unlikely, since there are no bursas under or near the teres minor.

Teres minor trigger points can also be the cause of a worrisome *dysesthesia* (abnormal sensation), which in this case is a feeling of numbness or tingling in the fourth and fifth fingers. This is almost as common as the pain behind the shoulder and is easily misconstrued as ulnar neuropathy or evidence of a pinched nerve in the neck. Note that a comparable pattern of finger numbness can also come from trigger points in the pectoralis minor. Pain, rather than numbness, in these two fingers suggests latissimus dorsi trigger points (Simons, Travell, and Simons 1999, 564, 572).

Causes

The same kinds of abuse and overuse that adversely affect the infraspinatus can get the teres minor into trouble with trigger points. Repeatedly reaching behind you with the arm outwardly rotated can be especially damaging. Tennis is one activity that can overwork the teres minor. Interestingly, volleyball can also tire this muscle excessively because of the way the ball is struck with the heels of the hands, which puts both arms into extreme outward rotation.

Self-Treatment

As with the other rotator cuff muscles, no attempt should be made to stretch the teres minor until its trigger points have been deactivated. If any small tears are present in the muscle or its tendinous attachments to the humeral head, stretching can aggravate them (Simons, Travell, and Simons 1999, 569).

Teres minor trigger points are found high on the outer edge of the shoulder blade. Feel the muscle bulge up at this spot as you rotate your arm outward, just as you did with the infraspinatus (see Figure 5.38). Teres minor trigger points are only an inch or so away from those in the infraspinatus and can be massaged at the same time with the same techniques. A tennis ball or lacrosse ball is a perfect tool for rolling repeatedly across the teres minor against a wall (Figure 5.46). Notice in the illustration that the body is at an angle to the wall. Be sure to check the posterior deltoid and triceps muscles for satellite trigger points created by the teres minor in its referral zone. All of these trigger points will be within an inch or two of one another.

Partner Treatment

When people begin to experience pain relief from self-applied trigger point massage, they often feel compelled to spread the good word, making a wild-eyed nuisance of themselves among friends and relatives. Sadly, you'll discover that even the people closest to you will be very skeptical of your effusive claims about how well trigger point therapy works. They probably won't have heard of it anywhere else, and their snake oil detector will be turned on.

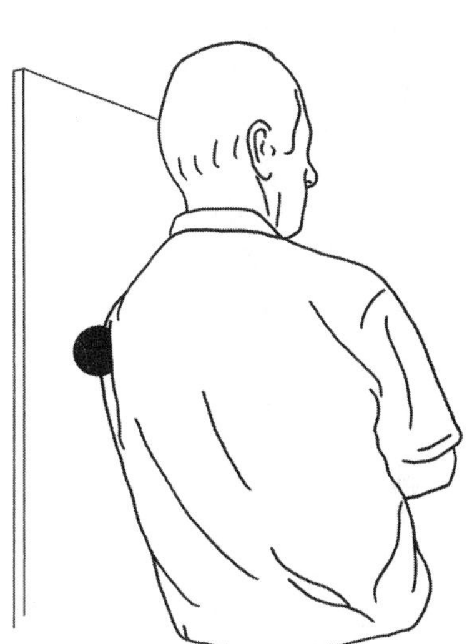

Figure 5.46 Teres minor massage with a lacrosse ball against the wall

Instead of letting your enthusiasm bubble over (you'll just get your feelings hurt), wait patiently for opportunities to be helpful. Look for instances where a person is having a kind of pain that you've already successfully self-treated. It's a chance to help someone have the same experience you've had, which is far more convincing than mere words. Just take care to get permission to go "hands-on" and don't make extravagant promises. If you can find a specific trigger point on yourself, you shouldn't have trouble finding it on someone else. The first-time experience of pressure on an exquisitely painful but unsuspected trigger point is often enough to make a person sit up and take notice, and want to know more.

Theresa, *age twenty, had chronic pain in the front of her right shoulder. She was a flute major at the university and the pain increased when she played or practiced. It looked as though she was going to have to change her course of study to another field.*

The problem was the arm position for holding the flute. Her right arm had to be cocked so far back that the muscles behind her shoulder were in a continuous contraction the entire time she was playing. Theresa was fortunate to have a roommate who was interested in trigger points. Working together, they discovered viciously tender spots in Theresa's infraspinatus and teres minor, which surprised her a great deal. Her roommate treated the muscles several times and showed Theresa how to self-treat them against a wall.

The massage improved the pain amazingly. To keep herself in shape for playing, Theresa began working on her shoulder before and after every practice session and performance.

Clinical Treatment

In treating the teres minor, a therapist should use supported fingers, searching high along the lateral border of the scapula, about an inch above the crease of the armpit (Figure 5.47). Paired supported thumbs can also be used. This muscle is about the size and thickness of an index finger. When it's tight, it can bunch up into a knot that feels like a small prune. Teres minor trigger points respond very well to massage if you can zero in on them. If you're unsure of just exactly where the muscle is, picture it crossing the outer edge of the shoulder blade toward its attachment to the back of the head of the humerus. Treat it as usual, with several short strokes. Always ask for numbers to stay in touch with the client's level of pain.

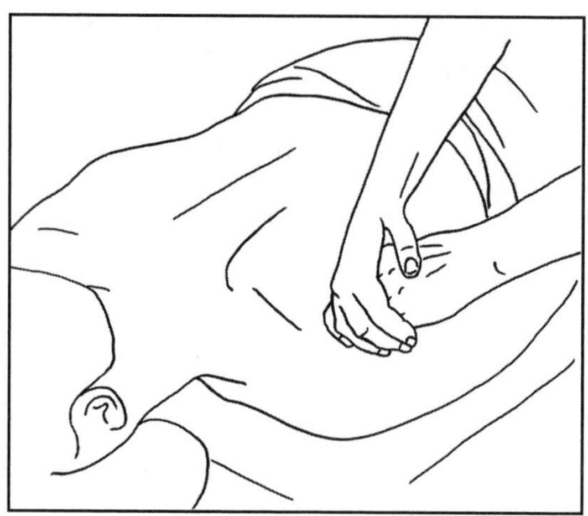

Figure 5.47 Teres minor massage right where the muscle crosses the outer edge of the shoulder blade

Chapter 6

Shoulder Treatment, Part B

Back Muscles Associated with the Shoulder

All the muscles in this chapter are located primarily or entirely on the back. This doesn't strictly apply to the deltoids, which might be more appropriately included with the arm muscles in the next chapter. But the deltoids are too important a factor in shoulder pain and dysfunction to be deferred to the next level. Along with the deltoids, the other muscles discussed here are the latissimus dorsi, teres major, trapezius, levator scapulae, rhomboids, serratus posterior superior, and iliocostalis thoracis.

The above-named muscles all have their specific individual functions, but one thing they have in common is the potential for directly or indirectly contributing to your shoulder trouble when afflicted with trigger points. Although this group has been placed in a position subordinate to the rotator cuff muscles, any muscle in this chapter can be the main cause of shoulder pain, depending on the circumstances. It would be a mistake to consider any of them insignificant.

Remember to review the information on anatomy and kinesiology in chapter 1 if you have difficulty locating any of these muscles or understanding how they should normally operate.

Latissimus Dorsi

"Latissimus dorsi" means "wide back muscle," and, indeed, it covers most of the mid and lower back (Figure 6.1). It attaches all along the spine from the mid to low back and across the top of the hip bone. Parts of the muscle attach to four or five of the lower ribs and to the inferior angle of the shoulder blade. The upper end of the muscle combines with the teres major at the back of the armpit, and their common tendon wraps around to attach high on the front of the humerus. The primary action of both muscles is to bring the arm down and in toward the chest. With the help of the posterior deltoid, they also extend the arm backward.

Stuart, *a thirty-seven-year-old anesthesiologist, injured his right shoulder working out on the gymnastic rings. As a physician, he was concerned that he might have torn his rotator cuff or separated the acromioclavicular joint. An orthopedist friend ordered an MRI but found no tissue injury. "You've just strained your muscles," his colleague said. "I'd stay off the rings for a while, but don't stop using your arm. What you don't need is a frozen shoulder."*

Over the next few weeks, Stuart made a point of using his arm. Nevertheless, to his great annoyance his shoulder pain only got worse, and he gradually lost range of motion until he could hardly move his arm at all. Reluctantly, he signed up for physical therapy, which he didn't like because of the pain. "Sure it hurts," the therapist told him, "but you gotta do it." It took several months, but he got his range of motion back and the pain gradually went away. Years later, however, the shoulder still hurt when he made certain movements. He also had a chronic deep ache in his mid back on the same side.

Using a book on myofascial pain that a patient had given him, Stuart discovered extremely painful trigger points in his latissimus dorsi and teres major muscles. It struck him that they were some of the muscles that would really get a workout on the rings. Had those trigger points just been lying there all this time? Using techniques from the book, Stuart was able to rid himself of his residual shoulder and mid back pain in less than a week.

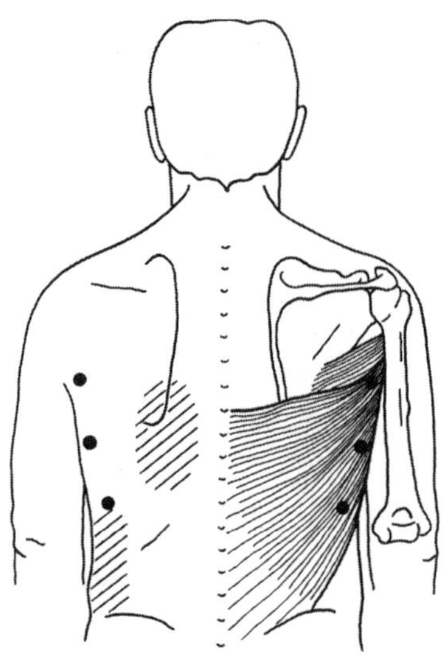

Figure 6.1 Latissimus dorsi trigger points and referred pain pattern

Symptoms

Although the latissimus dorsi is a muscle of the mid and lower back, it's included with the shoulder muscles because its trigger points can cause constant aching pain at the lower end of the shoulder blade (Figure 6.1). When a physician doesn't understand myofascial pain, this referred pain is apt to lead to a diagnosis of intrathoracic disease of undetermined origin and an order for a CAT scan, bronchoscopy, or angiogram (Simons, Travell, and Simons 1999, 572).

Pain can spread up over the shoulder blade and down over the triceps. When latissimus dorsi trigger points are unusually active, pain may extend to the inner side of the arm all the way down to the ulnar side of the hand and the fourth and fifth fingers (not shown). The lower trigger points sometimes cause pain in the front of the shoulder and low on the side of the abdomen (Figures 6.1 and 6.2). The pain in the front of the shoulder may be wrongly diagnosed as bicipital tendinitis (Simons, Travell, and Simons 1999, 580).

Trigger points in either the latissimus dorsi or the teres major can inhibit the full stretch that's necessary to reach up and forward or lift your arm all the way up. They can also increase your pain when you push down on the arms of a chair to get to your feet.

Latissimus dorsi trigger points cause only minimal restriction to movement of the arm, but they can contribute to frozen shoulder by fostering satellite trigger points in the

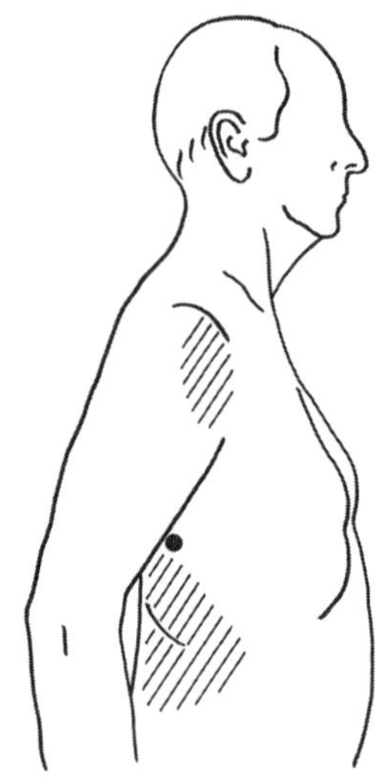

Figure 6.2 Latissimus dorsi trigger point and referred pain

subscapularis. Satellite trigger points may also develop in the lower trapezius, iliocostalis thoracis, and triceps. Latissimus dorsi trigger points themselves can be satellites of trigger points in the serratus posterior superior. Clearly, the latissimus dorsi is a muscle that should not be ignored.

Causes

When you consider the importance of the latissimus dorsi and teres major for strongly pulling the arm downward, it's easy to imagine the kinds of strains and overuse that can affect them. For the causes of trouble, look at activities such as skiing, gymnastics, tennis, swimming, rowing, chopping wood, pitching, or throwing a ball. Go easy with any exercise that involves pulling yourself up (chinning) or pushing down with your arms (workouts on the gymnastics horse). Walking with crutches can also overwork the latissimus dorsi. Wearing a tight bra restricts circulation in these muscles, which promotes trigger points (Simons, Travell, and Simons 1999, 578).

Be cautious with any work that makes you overstretch or repeatedly strain these muscles by reaching up and forward or overhead. In the workplace, an operation that requires you to repeatedly pull a lever downward is very likely to overwork the latissimus dorsi and teres major muscles. Travell and Simons tell of a woman who did just this by playing slot machines for six hours straight. Based on her referred pain, her doctor speculated that she surely must have gallbladder trouble, until she revealed that her gallbladder had already been removed (Simons, Travell, and Simons 1999, 574).

Self-Treatment

Pinching the wad of muscle behind the armpit with the fingers and thumb is very effective for locating latissimus dorsi and teres major trigger points, but massaging them that way (Figure 6.3) can quickly tire the hand. Luckily, these trigger points can be massaged with almost no effort with the Thera Cane or Backnobber or with a lacrosse ball against the wall (Figure 6.4). Use just six to twelve strokes on each trigger point that you find. For the latissimus dorsi, also explore the edge of your back from your lowest ribs to the back of your armpit. You may encounter an extremely tender area on the ribs under your arm just in front of the edge of the latissimus dorsi. This is a serratus anterior trigger point, which can make horrible pain in the side.

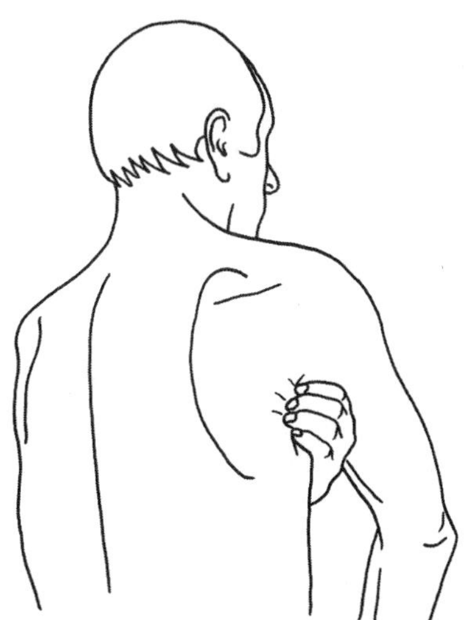

Figure 6.3 Latissimus dorsi and teres major massage between the fingers and thumb

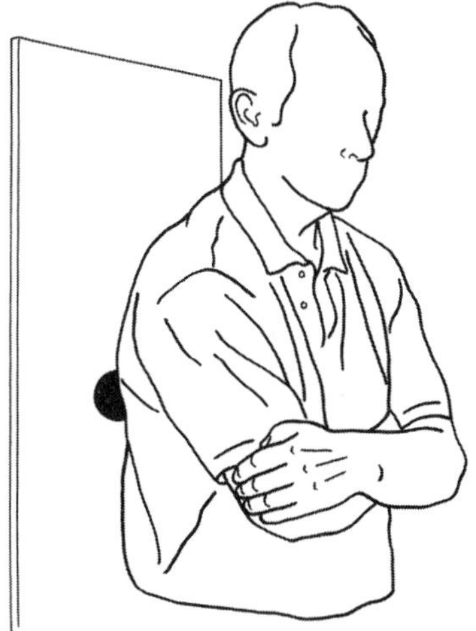

Figure 6.4 Latissimus dorsi massage with a lacrosse ball against the wall

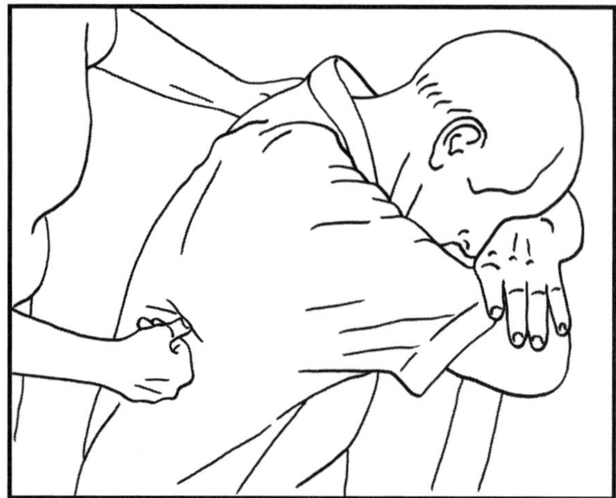

Figure 6.5 Partner massage of the latissimus dorsi with a supported thumb

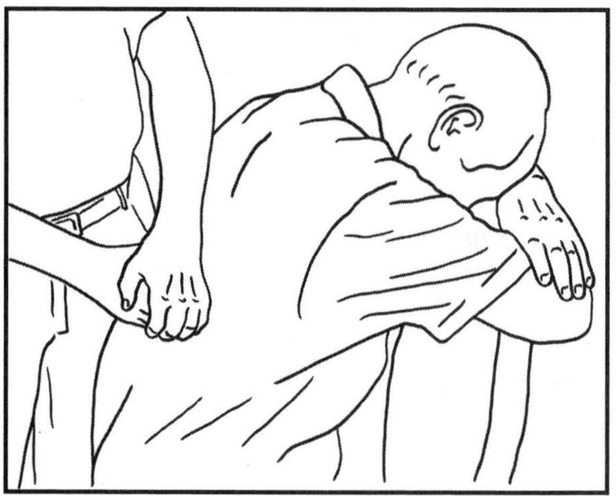

Figure 6.6 Partner massage of the latissimus dorsi with supported fingers

Partner Treatment

Working on someone else's latissimus dorsi can be a problem if the person is ticklish. Fortunately, most people should be able to take care of this area themselves with a ball against the wall. If you're called on to help an invalid or an elderly person, try using a supported thumb in the broad part of the muscle (Figure 6.5). Supported fingers are also very effective if you work from the opposite side (Figure 6.6). For trigger points in the web of muscle behind the armpit, you may be able to avoid the tickle response by using a loose fist while standing at the person's side.

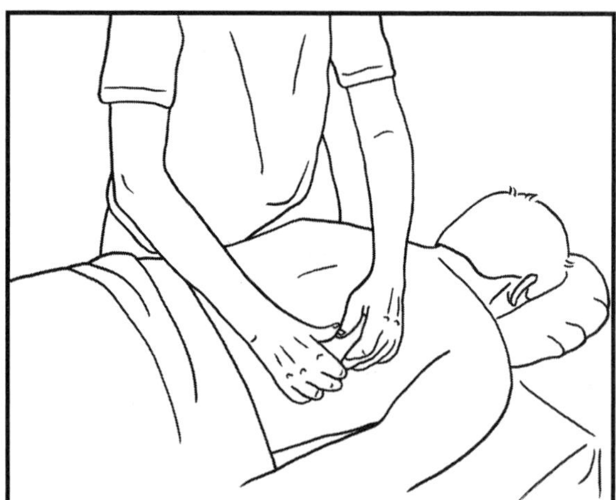

Figure 6.7 Latissimus dorsi massage by kneading between the fingers and thumbs of both hands

Clinical Treatment

Be aware that the mid back pain from latissimus dorsi trigger points can mislead you into massaging the mid back instead of the trigger points, which are more toward the border of the muscle. The latissimus dorsi can be treated by kneading with the fingers and thumbs of both hands (Figure 6.7). You can also use supported fingers. To make the most efficient use of your hands, focus on finding and treating specific trigger points instead of broadly massaging the entire area. Since the latissimus dorsi and teres major work together, they are usually involved together in causing myofascial pain. You will want to treat them both at the same time.

Teres Major

The teres major attaches to the back of the shoulder blade, near its inferior angle (Figure 6.8). At its upper end, it joins the latissimus dorsi, and together they then circle around to attach high on the front of the humerus. The teres major works with the latissimus dorsi to pull the arm down, back, and toward the body. The two muscles form the thick, muscular back wall of the armpit. Practice trying to find each muscle separately, feeling for a kind of trough between them. The teres major is the deeper of the two, right next to the edge of the shoulder blade.

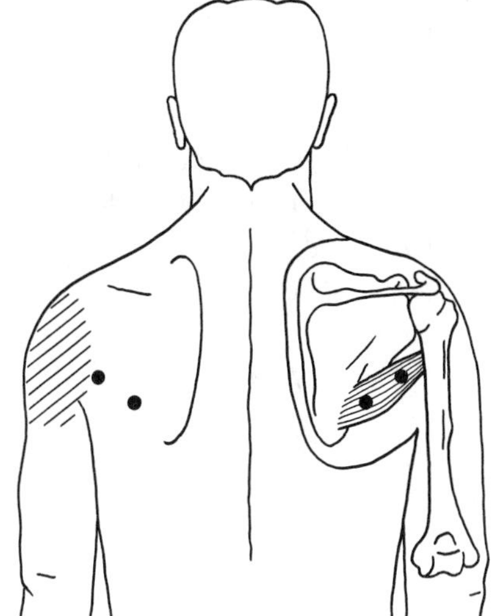

Figure 6.8 Teres major trigger points and referred pain

Symptoms

Trigger points in the teres major refer a deep ache to the posterior deltoid area, sometimes spreading down over the triceps. They can produce sharp pain in the back of the shoulder when you rest your elbows on a table or desk or when you reach up and forward to get something from a shelf. Reaching across your back or pulling down on something can also increase your pain. Pain referral is accentuated when you swing your arms while walking or running. Reaching high while serving in tennis can bring a sharp pain behind the shoulder (Simons, Travell, and Simons 1999, 589).

Teres major trigger points tend to create satellites in the posterior deltoid, teres minor, and subscapularis muscles. Tightness in the teres major pulls the shoulder blade away from the spine and places extra strain on the rhomboids. Don't let anybody tell you that your pain is caused by bursitis or tendinitis until you've taken a shot at treating teres major trigger points. Once you are able to locate the teres major, it's remarkably easy to treat, whether you do it yourself or have someone else do it.

Causes

Teres major trigger points develop when you overload or overwork the muscle in any of its normal actions. Pulling down and back against resistance is very taxing. An example would be having to wrestle the steering wheel of a large truck or motor home with deficient power steering. But strains can also occur during much more subtle activities. Stringed instrument players are especially vulnerable to repetitive strain injuries to their teres major and latissimus dorsi muscles.

> Holly, *a twenty-six-year-old graduate student in violin, was looking forward to a life in music. For several months, however, she'd regularly had to stop playing because of terrible pain in the back of her left shoulder that spread all the way across to her spine. She had tried ultrasound and other modes of physical therapy without benefit, so she began using prescription pain medications to get her through concerts. She also tried three different massage therapists but experienced negligible improvement in her problem.*
>
> *Trigger points were found in her scalenes, in all four rotator cuff muscles, and in the teres major and latissimus dorsi muscles. She had trigger points on both sides, but they were worse on the left side, where the pain was causing so much trouble. The therapist*

thought the problem probably began with excessive muscle tension. "I've always known I was too tense," Holly said, "but I didn't think it could do anything like this."

It appeared that Holly was keeping her left arm in extreme lateral rotation and locking all her shoulder muscles on the left side to get her hand in the correct position for fingering. Three treatments made her pain free. Six weeks later, she reported that she'd had no pain except for one time when she had played for two hours straight. She and her teacher were working on her technique to get her to relax while playing.

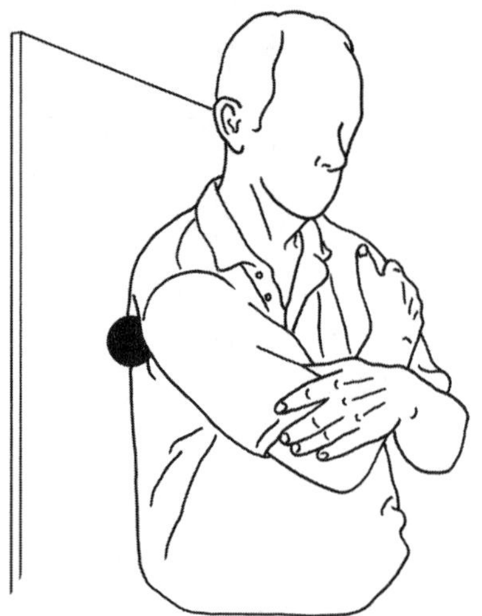

Figure 6.9 Teres major and latissimus dorsi massage with a ball against the wall

Self-Treatment

For treatment of teres major trigger points using a ball against the wall, the ball should be placed at the back of the armpit (Figure 6.9). You'll be massaging the muscle against the edge of your shoulder blade. There may be trigger points in both the teres major and the latissimus dorsi at this spot. Keep your arm up out of the way to improve access, as shown. You can also knead this wad of muscle with your hand, but concentrate on working efficiently to avoid straining your fingers.

Partner Treatment

To work on someone else's teres major, you'll have to risk tickling them while using the pincer grip (Figure 6.10). Don't try to massage the entire muscle, which can be quite thick and dense. Focus on finding trigger points and remember that just a few strokes comprise a treatment.

Clinical Treatment

To differentiate between the latissimus dorsi and teres major, feel for the narrow trough between them. The teres major is the deeper muscle. You really have to grasp a handful of muscle to get to it (Figure 6.11). You can also use supported fingers to press the teres major

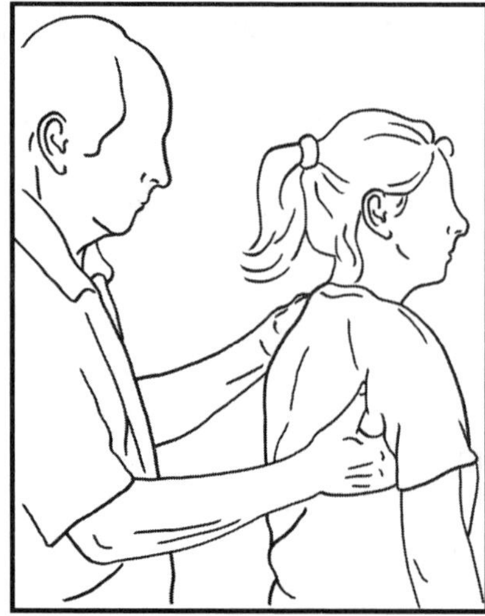

Figure 6.10 Partner massage of the teres major with a pincer grip

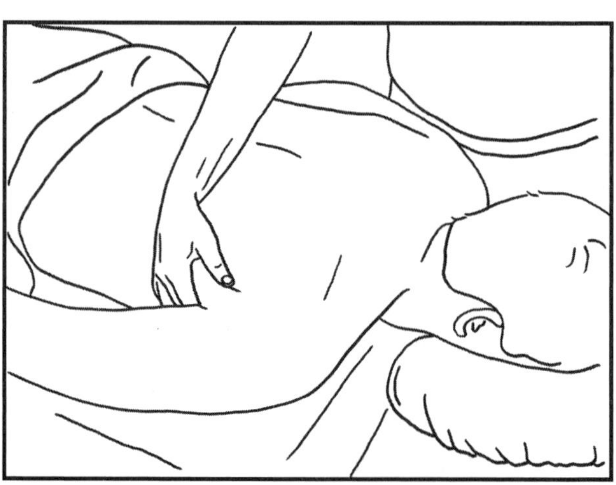

Figure 6.11 Latissimus dorsi and teres major massage between the fingers and thumb

against the bone halfway down the scapula's lateral border. You can do this by reaching across with your palms down or by working from the same side with your palms up.

Deltoid

If flattened out, the deltoid muscle would resemble the Greek letter delta, which has a triangular shape. On the body, the deltoid muscle completely surrounds the shoulder like a cap. Although the deltoid is technically a single muscle, it has three fairly distinct parts, the anterior, posterior, and middle deltoid, on the front, back, and outer side of the shoulder. Because of this, the deltoid muscle is often spoken of as "the deltoids."

The deltoid muscle attaches to the collarbone, the spine of the shoulder blade, and the acromion, the bony point of the shoulder. Its lower attachment is to the deltoid tuberosity, a slight lump about halfway down the outer side of the humerus. In conjunction with the supraspinatus muscle, the function of the deltoid is to raise the arm in any direction—to the front, back, or side. The anterior deltoid flexes the arm, raising it to the front. The posterior deltoid extends the arm, raising it to the rear. The middle deltoid, assisted by the anterior and posterior parts, abducts the arm, raising it to the side. The middle deltoid usually has the most strength and endurance.

Without some counterforce, the supraspinatus and middle deltoid would pull your shoulder joint apart when you raise your arm. Several other muscles prevent this, including the subscapularis, infraspinatus, teres minor, and anterior and posterior deltoids. Weakness caused by trigger points in any of these muscles can allow the supraspinatus and middle deltoid to pull the head of the humerus up against the acromion, painfully compressing the subacromial bursa and supraspinatus tendon. This is believed to be the cause of impingement syndrome (Simons, Travell, and Simons 1999, 623-632).

Sarah, *age twenty-eight, complained of an annoying pain in the front and outer side of her right shoulder that was affecting her work. She was a medical transcriptionist and sat at a computer all day. "I get a shot of pain every time I reach for the mouse," she said. "Sometimes I can barely lift my arm. I've been rubbing my shoulder so much now that I'm starting to get pain in my hand." She said she had tried several over-the-counter pain medications but nothing helped very much.*

By rubbing her shoulder, Sarah was intuitively self-treating trigger points in her deltoid muscle. Most of her work was wasted, however, because the deltoid trigger points were being maintained and perpetuated by trigger points in her infraspinatus. Extremely active and painful trigger points in both muscles were found and treated. Sarah said afterward that her shoulder felt much better.

Sarah was putting terrible strain on her deltoid and infraspinatus muscles in repeatedly reaching for her computer mouse beyond the right end of her keyboard. She used the mouse almost constantly, causing the muscles to be in nearly continuous contraction all day long without a chance to rest and recover. She avoided a recurrence of the problem by moving the mouse to the other side and learning to use it with her left hand.

Symptoms

Pain from deltoid trigger points is unusual in that it isn't referred to distant places—it's felt in the vicinity of the trigger point (Figures 6.12, 6.13, 6.14, and 6.15). Pain originating in the deltoid is felt mainly when you move your arm and less often when the arm is at rest.

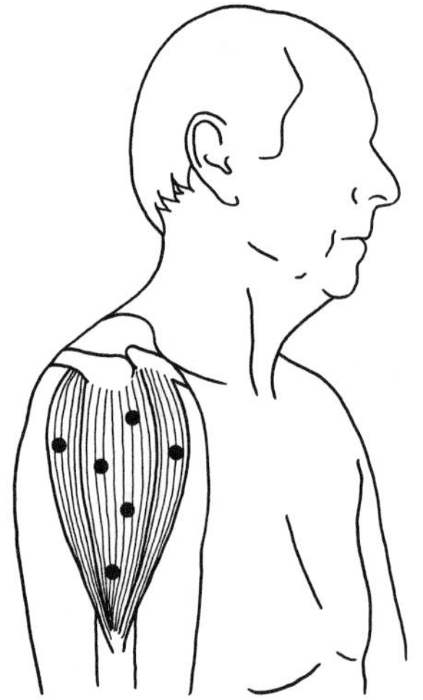

Figure 6.12 Deltoid trigger points

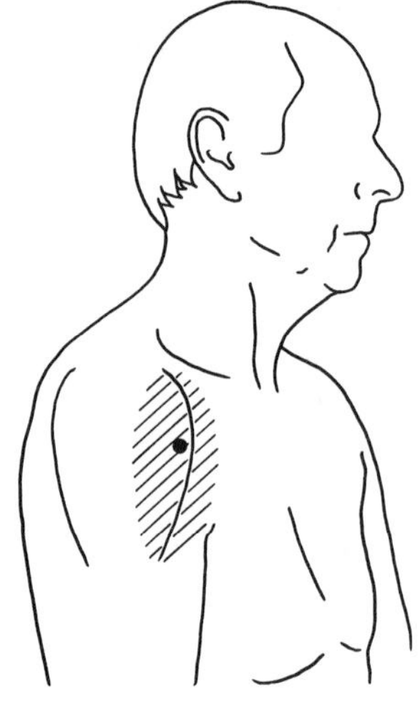

Figure 6.13 Anterior deltoid trigger point and pain pattern

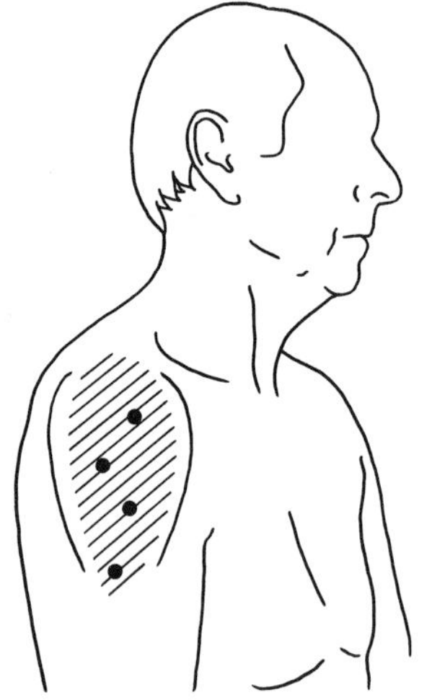

Figure 6.14 Middle deltoid trigger points and pain pattern

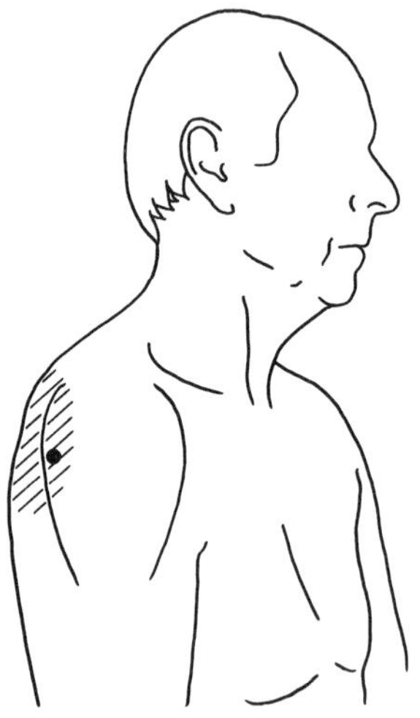

Figure 6.15 Posterior deltoid trigger point and pain pattern

Pain referred to the deltoids from elsewhere, on the other hand, is felt continuously or in relation to activity in other muscles. A continuous dull ache in the shoulder is more likely coming from the rotator muscles than from the deltoids. Trigger points arise quite frequently in the deltoids, but if you massage only the deltoids and ignore the rotators you won't solve your shoulder problem (Simons, Travell, and Simons, 623-624, 628-629).

Trigger points in any part of the deltoid weaken the shoulder and impair its efforts to raise the arm. This can seriously degrade your performance in sports or on the job. Look for trigger points in the anterior deltoid when it hurts to comb your hair or bring your hand to your face. Look for trigger points in the posterior deltoid when it hurts to put your hand in your back pocket. Trigger points in the anterior and middle deltoid contribute to difficulty in scratching your back.

When practitioners are unaware of myofascial causes, pain caused by trigger points in the deltoid muscles is apt to be blamed on arthritis, bursitis, impingement syndrome, cervical nerve entrapment, or rotator cuff tendinitis. These conditions can occur, but trigger points are the more probable cause (Simons, Travell, and Simons 1999, 628-631; Reynolds 1981, 111-114).

Causes

Deltoid trigger points rarely exist by themselves, and they're rarely the primary cause of shoulder pain. They're frequently created as satellites of trigger points in the scalenes, pectoralis major, or rotator cuff muscles, all of which send pain to the deltoid area—the front, back, and side of the shoulder. However, the deltoid can also suffer overuse and strain independently.

The deltoid muscle is frequently overloaded in athletic activities that require forceful flexion of the shoulder, particularly swimming, skiing, weight lifting, and ball throwing. In the workplace, the deltoid is overused by having to hold heavy hand tools up to do a job, or by repeatedly reaching up, out, or back, hour after hour. Picking up and carrying a baby or small child is a very common way to abuse the deltoid and other shoulder muscles (Simons, Travell, and Simons 1999, 628-629; Jonsson and Hagberg 1974, 26-32).

To reduce repetitive strain to the deltoids, try to work in ways that will help keep your elbows at your sides. Typing taxes the deltoids when the keyboard is too high. Good ergonomics dictates keeping the elbows tucked in and the keyboard level with them. Support the elbows whenever possible and avoid sitting in chairs that don't have arms. In sports, muscle problems come from playing too long and too hard and from not giving due attention to the condition of your muscles. Any athlete, amateur or professional, should learn to self-treat trigger points and do it as a daily discipline.

Keep in mind that the deltoid muscles must work hard to keep the arm from being pulled from its socket when you carry or lift heavy weights. They're also likely to suffer during any accident or fall that wrenches, jams, or pulls on the arms. An impact injury to the shoulder from an auto or sports collision can be expected to set up trigger points in the deltoids. Other impact traumas occur with repeated recoil from a rifle or shotgun or when the deltoid is struck hard during a fall or by a tennis ball or baseball (Simons, Travell, and Simons 1999, 628-629).

Self-Treatment

Note that trigger points will be found only at the midpoint of the muscle in the anterior and posterior deltoids. Because of the bipennate arrangement of the middle deltoid's muscles fibers, its trigger points can occur anywhere from the point of the shoulder to the muscle's attachment in the middle of the upper arm (Figure 6.12). Most deltoid trigger points will be found in the middle deltoid because it's the largest part of the muscle and works the hardest.

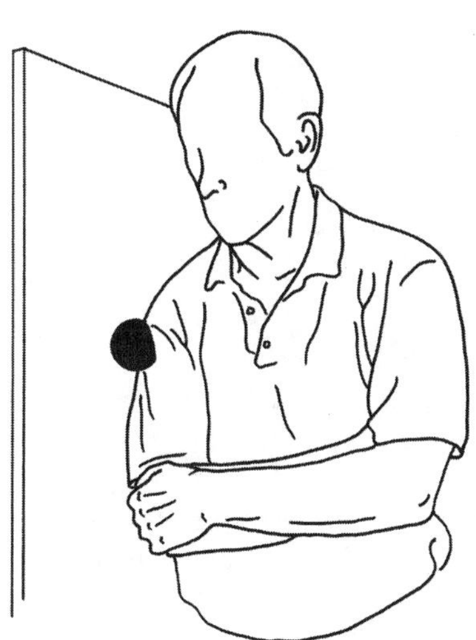

Figure 6.16 Deltoid massage with a ball against the wall

The middle deltoid's complex structure is difficult to illustrate, and it isn't well represented in Figure 6.12. It's actually made up of more than a dozen smaller overlapping heads that individually look like Figure 2.19 (see letter C). This fiber arrangement makes the middle deltoid an intrinsically much more powerful muscle than the anterior and posterior deltoids with their simpler fiber pattern.

Trigger points are easy to find in the deltoid, but don't try to massage this muscle extensively with your hand. Use a tennis or lacrosse ball against the wall instead. Turning at an angle to the wall, to the front or to the back, will allow you to roll the ball selectively over any of the three parts of the muscle. Lean in and roll the ball from top to bottom and back again, checking every inch of the muscle's area (Figure 6.16). When you find a tender spot, treat it with six to twelve short strokes and then move on to the next. Remember that the object is not to kill the trigger point. Just flush it a few times to stimulate healing, then leave it alone for a few hours to let the body do its work.

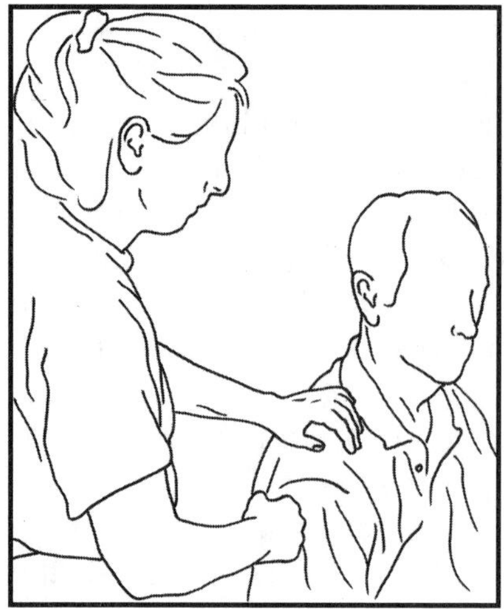

Figure 6.17 Partner massage of the middle deltoid with a loose fist

Partner Treatment

Treating the deltoid on someone else is not difficult if you assume a position that allows you to apply sufficient pressure. The best strategy is to have the person seated and treat the shoulder from a standing position using a loose fist (Figure 6.17). The person can help by leaning toward you to counter the pressure as you work. Move around to the front, side, and back, searching for trigger points in each of the three heads of the deltoid. Usually one trigger point will be worse than the others, and that's the one to focus on. Unless the person is disabled, you should encourage self-treatment with a ball against the wall. The deltoid may be the easiest of all the shoulder muscles to self-treat in this manner.

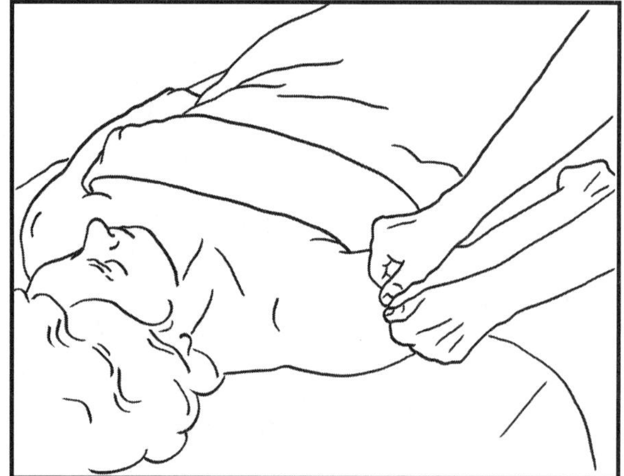

Figure 6.18 Clinical massage of the deltoids with paired supported thumbs

Clinical Treatment

With the client on a massage table, the deltoid muscles can seem to be in an awkward position for professional massage. The solution is to treat the deltoid as three separate muscles. You can use supported fingers on the anterior and posterior deltoids with the client lying faceup or facedown, respectively. You'll want to use paired supported thumbs on the middle deltoid (Figure 6.18). You can also use a loose fist, locking your elbow against your hip to take the strain off your own shoulder.

Trapezius

The trapezius covers the upper back and the back of the neck and is made up of three parts that function differently because of varying orientation of their muscles fibers. The upper trapezius raises the shoulder and helps turn the head, the middle trapezius pulls the shoulders back, and the lower trapezius aids in positioning and stabilizing the shoulder blade for various movements of the arm.

Alison, *age thirty, bought a set of free weights so that she could increase her upper body and arm strength. The day after her first workout session, she awakened with the worst headache she'd ever had. The pain was strongest in her right temple and in the back of her neck at the base of her skull. Associated with the headache was a terrible ache behind her right eye. She was also dizzy and nauseous, and she'd been vomiting in the night. To top it off, her shoulders were so sore she could hardly lift her arms.*

Trigger points were found in Alison's sternocleidomastoid and trapezius muscles and the muscles in the back of her neck. Squeezing a trigger point in her right upper

trapezius accentuated the pain in her temple and behind her eye. Several sessions of self-applied massage over the course of a single day got rid of all her symptoms. It took a couple more days to get rid of her shoulder pain and to get all the movement back in her arms. Her therapist told her it was perfectly all right to continue with her workouts as long as she also kept up with treating her trigger points.

Symptoms

Of all the muscles in the body, the trapezius is the one most commonly afflicted with trigger points. Although its trigger points often contribute to shoulder pain, they aren't usually involved in limiting movement of the arm. You may be surprised to learn that trapezius trigger points play a role in most headaches, and sometimes they can be the sole cause.

The first trapezius trigger point, trapezius #1, is located in the very topmost fibers of the roll of muscle on top of the shoulder, but don't look for it in the thickest part of the muscle. You can find it only by pinching a tiny roll of skin in the angle of the neck, right where the shoulder and neck come together. This is where the trapezius starts up the back of the neck. The taut band that contains the trigger point will feel like a knitting needle between your fingers.

Trapezius #1 is the primary cause of a temple headache, but it may also send pain to the masseter muscle at the angle of the jaw, down the side of the neck behind the ear, and deep behind the eye (Figures 6.19 and 6.20). Its effects are most often identified as a tension headache. Researchers have found it to be the most common trigger point. Almost everyone has trapezius #1 trigger points at one time or another (Simons, Travell, and Simons 1999, 278-287).

The trapezius trigger point #1 is also a frequent cause of dizziness that's indistinguishable from that caused by a trigger point in the clavicular branch of the sternocleidomastoid. Moreover, it's capable of inducing trigger points in muscles in the temple and jaw, making it an indirect cause of temporomandibular joint (TMJ) dysfunction, jaw pain, earache, and pain in the lower molars (Simons, Travell, and Simons 1999, 279).

The trapezius trigger point #2 is actually a pair of trigger points an inch or two apart, very deep in the roll of muscle on top of the shoulder. It's important to know that they are a major cause of pain at the base of the skull, which may be felt either as a headache or as neck pain (Figure 6.21). This referred pain frequently induces satellite trigger points in the muscles of the back of the neck. When neck massage feels good but doesn't get rid of the pain, the problem is probably in the trapezius muscles, not the muscles of the back of the neck.

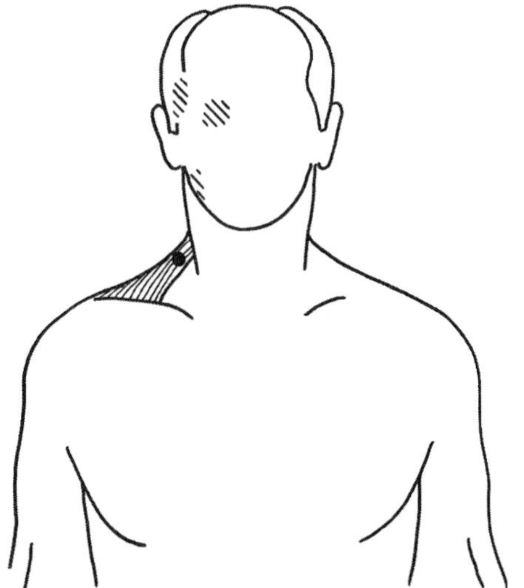

Figure 6.19 Trapezius #1 trigger point and referred pain pattern, front view

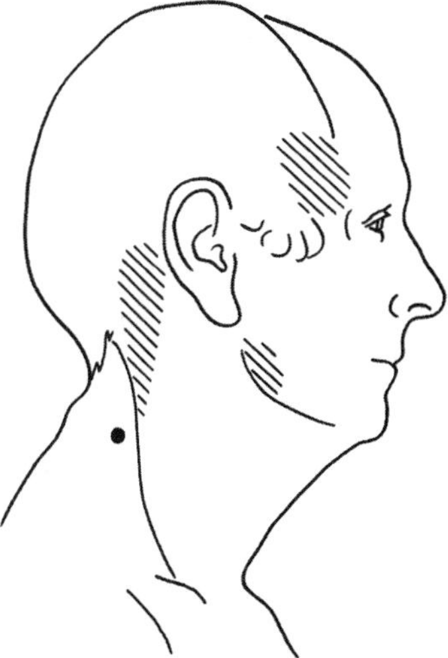

Figure 6.20 Trapezius #1 trigger point and referred pain pattern, side view

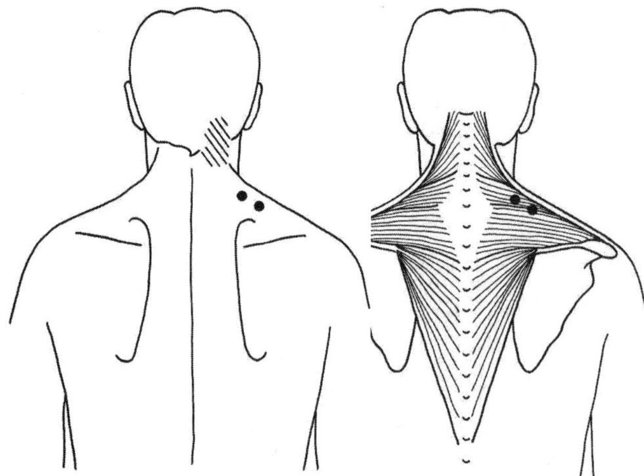

Figure 6.21 Trapezius #2 trigger points and referred pain pattern

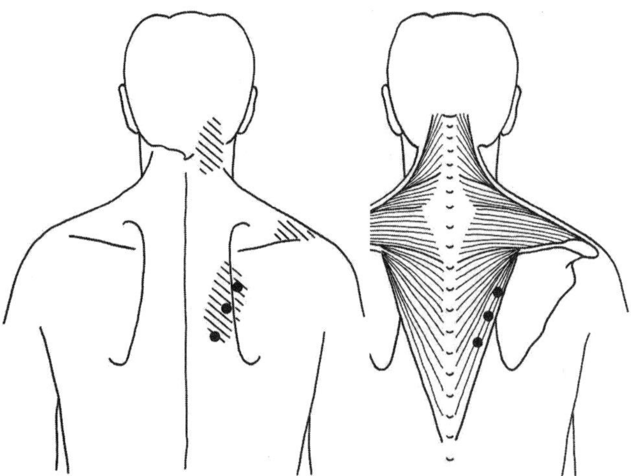

Figure 6.22 Trapezius #3 trigger points and referred pain pattern

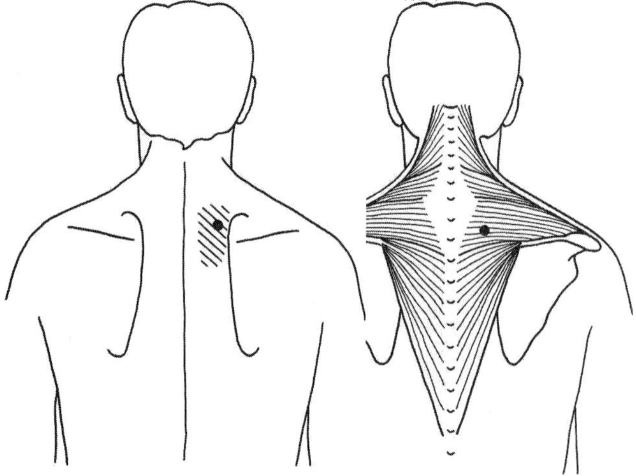

Figure 6.23 Trapezius #4 trigger point and referred pain pattern

The trapezius #3 is actually a set of trigger points found along a diagonal line in the border of the lower trapezius, which crosses the inner edge of the shoulder blade about halfway up (Figure 6.22). These extremely common but easily missed trigger points refer pain to the base of the skull like trapezius #2 and can also send pain to the upper trapezius itself.

Satellite trigger points produced on top of the shoulders and in the back of the neck can cause several kinds of headache. This cascade or domino effect of myofascial trigger points is one reason why headaches can be so hard to understand and treat effectively. Trapezius #3 extends its mischief by creating satellite trigger points in the supraspinatus and iliocostalis muscles, which can make it a significant indirect source of shoulder pain.

Trapezius #3 is also responsible for an oppressive ache or burning pain in the mid back that can come after a long spell at the computer without elbow support. Backaches at this site are very familiar to piano players, who also hold their arms out in front of them unsupported for long periods of time. Although trapezius #3 is a long way from the neck, it's one of the many causes of a stiff neck. When trigger points weaken the lower trapezius muscles, they may contribute to "winging" of the shoulder blades (Simons, Travell, and Simons 1999, 280).

Trapezius trigger point #4 occurs next to the inner border of the shoulder blade in the broad middle part of the trapezius (Figure 6.23). It causes a burning kind of pain nearby, alongside the spine. Superficial trigger points in this area can cause goose bumps on the back of the upper arm and, amazingly, sometimes on the thighs (Simons, Travell, and Simons 1999, 281-282).

The symptoms generated by trapezius trigger points are widely misinterpreted, producing a whole catalog of misdiagnoses and misdirected treatments. Travell and Simons give us a long list: cervical radiculopathy (nerve root compression), spinal stenosis, subacromial bursitis, chronic intractable benign pain, occipital neuralgia, scapulocostal syndrome, and atypical facial neuralgia. Headaches caused by trapezius trigger points may be labeled as cervogenic, vascular, cluster, or migraine when their true cause isn't understood. Although there can be true medical causes of headaches, an examination for trigger points should be near the top of any doctor's list. Trigger point massage is far safer and more effective for headaches, upper back pain, and shoulder pain than most of the remedies currently employed (Simons, Travell, and Simons 1999, 291-293).

Causes

The trapezius covers most of the upper half of the back, extending upward to cover the central part of the back of the neck. This uppermost part of the trapezius is what gives the back of the neck its shape. The muscle attaches to the base of the skull, the spine, the collarbones, and the shoulder blades. The trapezius supports the weight of the shoulders and must contract strongly to rotate the shoulder blade every time you raise your arm. Another primary function is to hold the shoulder blade solidly in place as a base for the finer operations of the arm and hand.

The uppermost part of the trapezius helps support the weight of the head and neck when you bend your head forward or to the side. Poor posture, such as slumping while seated or habitually carrying your head forward, places an unnecessary burden on your trapezius muscles. Pectoral muscles shortened by trigger points, indicated by a round-shouldered posture, exert a constant pull on the shoulders that the trapezius muscles must constantly counteract.

Another common cause of trapezius trigger points is emotional tension that keeps your shoulders up. Any work or physical activity that keeps the shoulders raised can also create trigger points in the trapezius. Trigger points are produced in all parts of the trapezius when you work with your arms held out in front of your body for extended periods of time. You subject your trapezius muscles to constant strain when you sit without elbow support, so it's wise to use a chair with arms when working at the computer or any other desk job.

Heavy-breasted women may be especially vulnerable to any of the trapezius symptoms. The strain of supporting heavy breasts can make trapezius trigger points a constant problem, an excellent reason for getting very good at self-treating them. Carrying a heavy backpack or a heavy purse hanging from a shoulder strap can be the simple explanation for that chronic "migraine" or stiff neck. It might be time to question the importance of all that stuff you're packing around from place to place all day long (Simons, Travell, and Simons 1999, 287).

Travell and Simons suggest that you not hold your telephone handset to your ear with your shoulder. If your hands must remain free, use a speakerphone or a headset. If your trapezius is chronically in trouble, take the weight off it by keeping your hands in your pockets when you're on your feet and even when walking (Simons, Travell, and Simons 1999, 301).

Tom, *age sixty-six, had been the manager of a service station. When he retired, he decided to learn to play the piano, something he'd wanted to do all his life.*

Unfortunately, he began to have a dull aching in his left shoulder, mid back, and at the base of his skull the moment he sat down to play. The problem was having to hold his arms out in front of him while he played—he just wasn't used to it. He became very discouraged because the pain came on so quickly, and he was annoyed at himself for not taking up the piano sooner, when he was still strong and had the physical stamina for it.

Luckily, another one of Tom's retirement hobbies was studying about trigger points, and he eventually found a trigger point in his lower trapezius that was evidently the cause of all the trouble. Self-applied massage with a tennis ball against the wall immediately eased the dull aching in his back, at the base of his skull, and out near the point of his shoulder. Tom made it part of his routine to massage the spot before he played and then again afterward. Several weeks later, he noticed that he wasn't getting his piano-playing pains anymore.

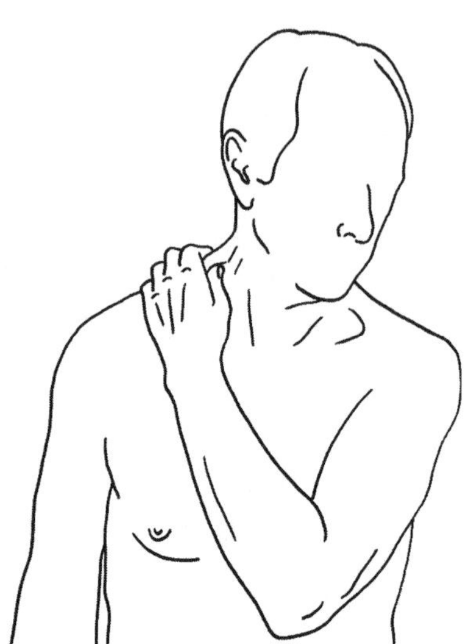

Figure 6.24 Massage of trapezius #1 with a pincer grip

Self-Treatment

There are four primary locations for trigger points on each side of the trapezius muscle. Trapezius #1 is in the upper trapezius, right under the skin in the angle of the neck. You need to take only a shallow pinch to get hold of it (Figure 6.24). Feel for a firm strand or cord as small as a pencil lead or the tube of a ballpoint refill. In larger people, it can be as thick as a knitting needle. Search for the tender spot in this tiny cable and massage it by rolling it between your thumb and first two fingers.

A good strong squeeze of trapezius #1 will very often reproduce or accentuate a temple headache, which confirms it as the cause. If your upper shoulders are very tight or thick with muscle or fat, you may have difficulty grasping the small roll of skin inhabited by this trigger point. To make this strand of muscle easier to get hold of, loosen the trapezius by putting your hand in your pocket. If massage with fingers and thumb is too tiring for your hand, try pressing trapezius #1 against a ball on a wall with a supported thumb (Figure 6.25). Virtually everyone has this trigger point and it causes an incredible amount of grief, so it's important to master it.

Massage trapezius #2 with the Thera Cane (Figure 6.26) or the Backnobber. This is one of the best uses for the Backnobber. Its smaller knob is very effective for digging deep into the upper trapezius, which is usually a strong, thick muscle, even on a small person. Notice that maximum pressure and control is obtained when the opposite hand is in the crook of the cane. Use the weight of your arm to stroke forward across the muscle fibers and take the pressure off between strokes. If you rub back and forth with constant pressure, you don't give the blood a chance to flow in and out of the tissue. Remember that there are two trigger points in

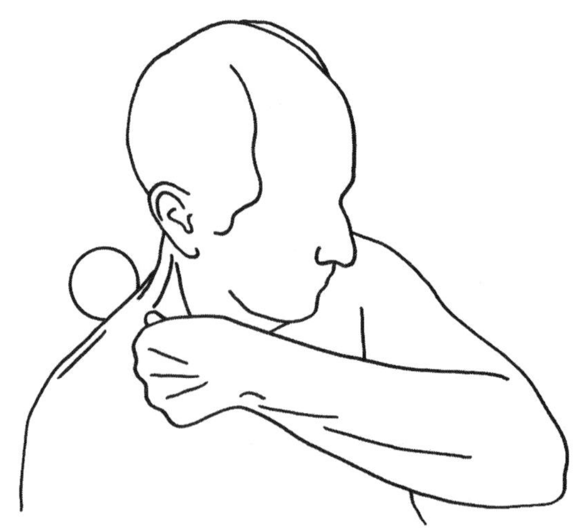

Figure 6.25 Massage of trapezius #1 with a supported thumb against a ball against the wall

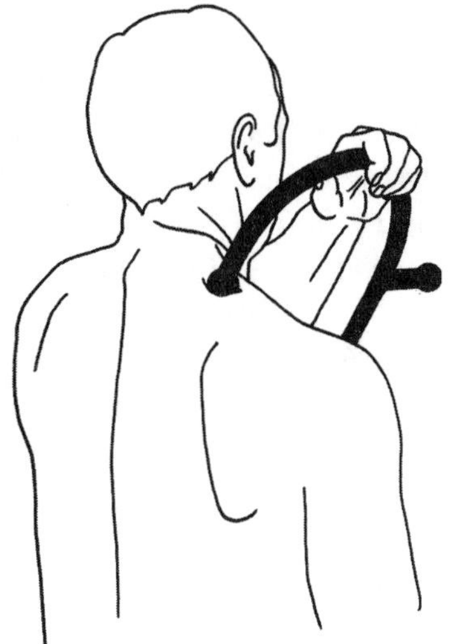

Figure 6.26 Massage of trapezius #2 with the Thera Cane

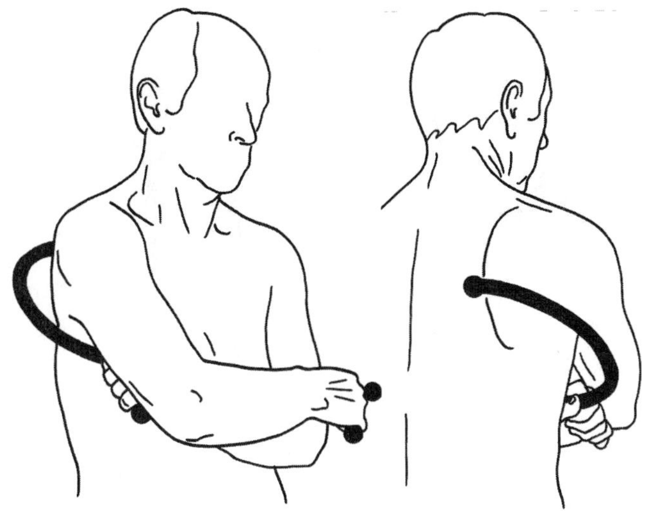

Figure 6.27 Massage of trapezius #3 with the Thera Cane

this part of the upper trapezius. The one further out toward the tip of the shoulder is in a thin part of the muscle and can be truly vicious.

Trapezius #3 can also be worked with the Thera Cane (Figure 6.27). Note that crossing your arms will give you greater leverage and control. You can better relax the muscles you're working on in this position, too. In Figure 6.27, the right hand is the one applying the pressure and the knob is stroking downward over the trigger point. Search three or four inches along the diagonal lower border of the muscle. You'll probably find more than one tender spot.

Employing a ball against the wall is especially effective for trapezius #3 (Figures 6.28 and 6.29). Stroking upward along the edge of the shoulder blade, you'll feel a kind of "speed bump" as the ball goes over the diagonally oriented border of the muscle. There's likely to be more than one trigger point at this site, one on each side of the edge of the shoulder blade and possibly one nearer to the spine. Use a tennis ball if the trigger points are especially tender. A lacrosse ball is better if you have to penetrate a lot of tissue. You can see right away that this technique works very well on any part of the back and buttocks.

Massage trapezius #4 by reaching over the shoulder to the opposite side with the Thera Cane or Backnobber (Figure 6.30). Again, the

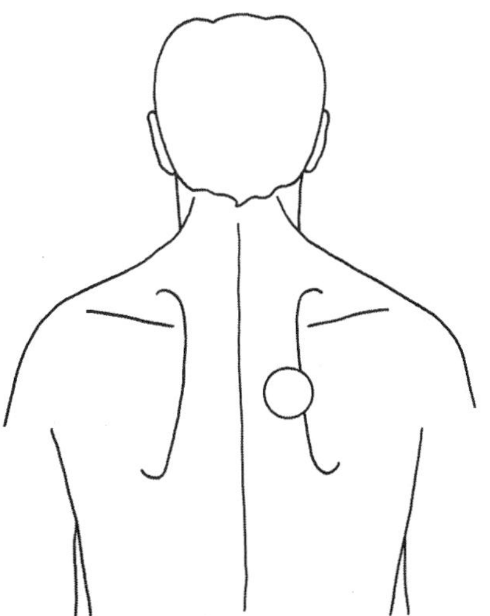

Figure 6.28 Massage of trapezius #3 with a ball against the wall

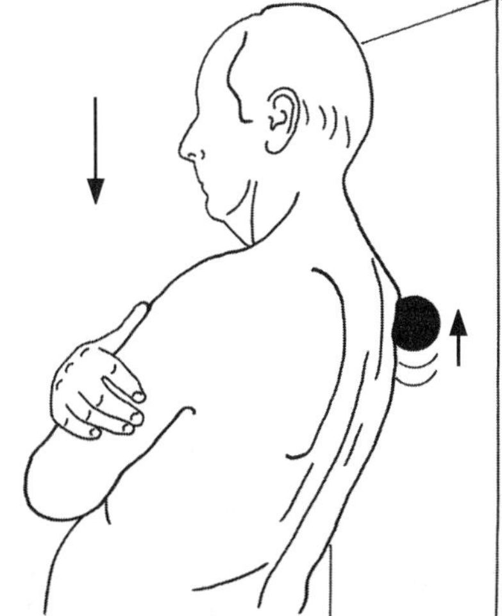

Figure 6.29 Massage of trapezius #3 with a ball against the wall

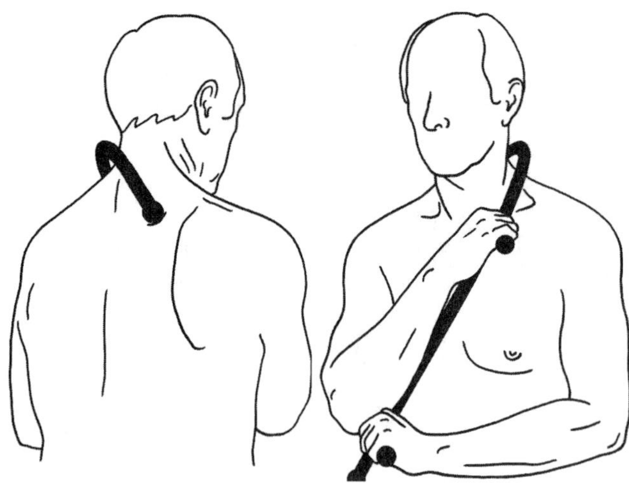

Figure 6.30 Massage of trapezius #4 with the Thera Cane over the opposite shoulder

arms are crossed for leverage, comfort, and control. The upper hand guides the tool and the lower hand applies pressure in a downward direction. For clarity, the Thera Cane is shown being applied to bare skin in the illustrations, but always wear a shirt so there's an intervening layer of cloth.

Trigger points should be massaged three to six times a day for best results, but limit the session to six to twelve strokes per trigger point. Don't try to kill them; let your body's natural processes do the healing.

Partner Treatment

When working on someone else's upper trapezius you can knead the muscle, but pair your hands to make the job less fatiguing. You can approach the trapezius either from behind or from in front (Figures 6.31 and 6.32). If you have the person sit while you stand, you can use supported fingers and take advantage of your weight for applying pressure.

Everyone has trouble in the upper trapezius and a friendly rub is always appreciated. Unfortunately, the upper trapezius is one of the most difficult muscles to treat, whether you do it yourself or have someone else do it. It helps to know that upper trapezius trigger points tend to be located closer to the front of the muscle. So concentrate your efforts in the front of the muscle rather than the back of it. If you work from behind, as in Figure 6.31, your fingers will be digging in. If you work from in front, as in Figure 6.32, focus on pressing with your thumbs. As always, use short, repeated moving strokes, not static pressure.

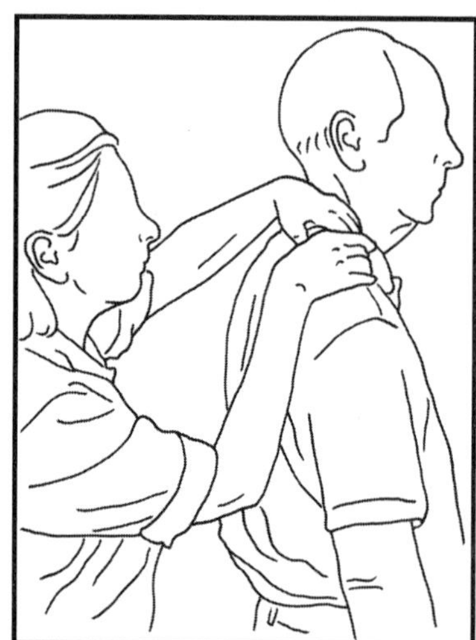

Figure 6.31 Partner massage of the upper trapezius from behind

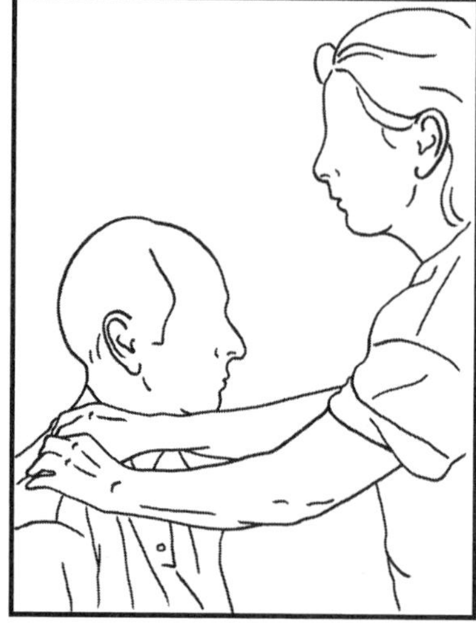

Figure 6.32 Partner massage of the upper trapezius from in front

Clinical Treatment

Treat your client's trapezius #1 with one hand, kneading between your thumb and two fingers (Figure 6.33). Work trapezius #2 with the fingers and thumbs of both hands (Figure 6.34). Focus your efforts on the front side of the muscle. If you use supported fingers, also an

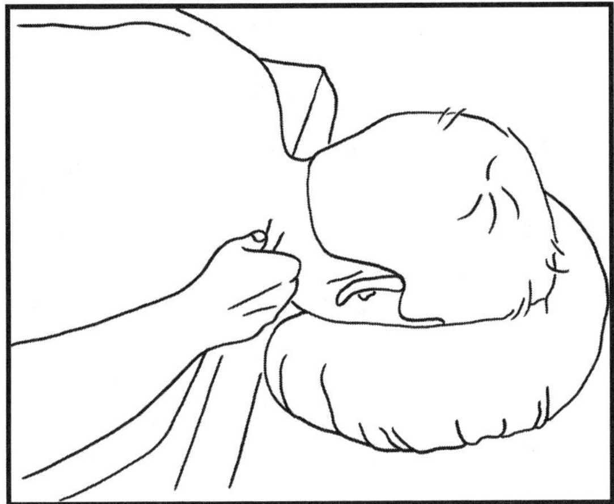

Figure 6.33 Trapezius #1 kneaded between the fingers and thumb

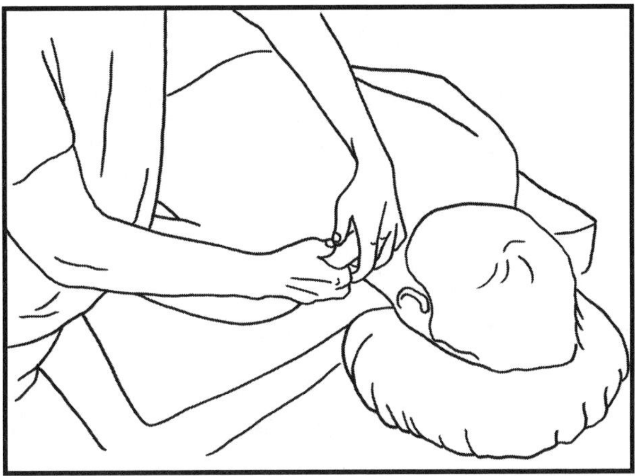

Figure 6.34 Trapezius #2 massage with paired hands, stroking with the thumbs toward the outer shoulder

excellent method here, stroke toward the outer shoulder. You may have noticed that many of your clients have an apparent "speed bump" in their upper trapezius that you feel when working with supported fingers. This is the underlying levator scapulae, whose fibers run at approximately a 90 degree angle to those in the trapezius. When you feel that bump, it's a sign that the levator scapulae needs work too.

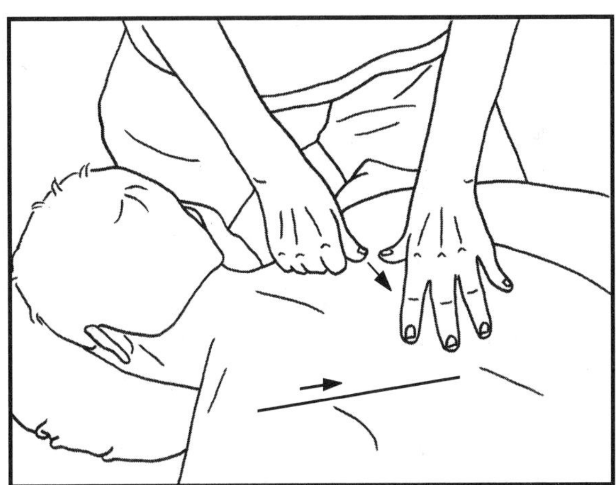

Figure 6.35 Trapezius #3 massage with a supported thumb. The other thumb keeps the muscle's lower border from moving.

Trapezius #3 can be treated with extraordinary precision using a supported thumb as shown in Figure 6.35, where the right thumb is stroking with the fibers along the diagonal lower border of the muscle. Make short strokes away from yourself in the direction of the arrow. The left thumb is held stationary in a position that keeps the edge of the muscle from squirting out from under your right thumb. The diagonal line and arrow on the left side of the body indicates the border of the lower trapezius on that side.

For treating trapezius #4, use supported fingers. This is the area that massage therapists usually call the rhomboids. Four different muscles actually overlap here. The middle trapezius is on top, then the rhomboids, then the iliocostalis thoracis, and finally the serratus posterior superior on the bottom, lying on the rib cage. The levator scapulae is only an inch or two away.

As you know, this wide place between the shoulder blade and spine always needs a lot of work. You can improve your effectiveness in this area if you learn the exact location of each muscle and relate it to specific kinds of pain. Broadly applied massage often falls short in solving pain problems because it never zeroes in on specific trigger points. You'll become better at solving problems if you proceed analytically and learn precisely where everything is.

Levator Scapulae

The levator scapulae muscle lifts the shoulder blade, a task perfectly reflected in its name. "Levator" is from the same Latin root as "elevator." *Scapula* is Latin for "shoulder blade." Don't be thrown by the word ending "ae" in scapulae. In common usage, "levator scapulae" is usually pronounced as though it were spelled "levator scapula." Levator scapulae trigger points occur nearly as often as those in the trapezius. They're the primary cause of the kind of neck stiffness that keeps you from turning your head. In fact, Travell and Simons call the levator scapulae the "stiff neck muscle."

Tony, *age thirty-three, had typical levator scapulae trouble. He'd had constant pain and stiffness in the right side of his neck ever since a fender bender three months earlier. He couldn't turn his head to the right at all. His insurance was paying for physical therapy, but the stretching and traction seemed to be making his pain worse. Electrostimulation helped, but the relief didn't last.*

Massage to Tony's levator scapulae muscles cut through his pain at once and gave him his first lasting relief. He was shown various ways to do the massage himself, which he was encouraged to do several times a day. Within a week, his pain was gone. In three weeks, he could turn his head again with full range of motion.

Symptoms

Trigger points in the levator scapulae cause pain and stiffness in the angle of the neck (Figure 6.36). When sufficiently active, they also refer a lesser degree of pain along the inner edge of the shoulder blade and to the back of the shoulder (not shown). The pain sent to the posterior shoulder can foster satellite trigger points in the deltoid muscle. The main area of pain in the angle of the neck promotes satellites in the trapezius and middle scalene. In this way, levator scapulae trigger points can be the ultimate source of all the symptoms produced by those two muscles, including headaches and shoulder pain.

Levator scapulae trigger points are what keep you from turning your head to look behind you when you're backing up in your car. You may not be able to turn your head at all toward the side that has the trigger point (Simons, Travell, and Simons 1999, 491-492). Pain usually is present only when you try to turn your head, though you can have a constant dull aching in your neck without movement if the trigger points are bad enough. Levator scapulae trigger points are not responsible for the condition known as torticollis, or wryneck, where your head continuously pulls over to one side. Wryneck is caused by sternocleidomastoid trigger points.

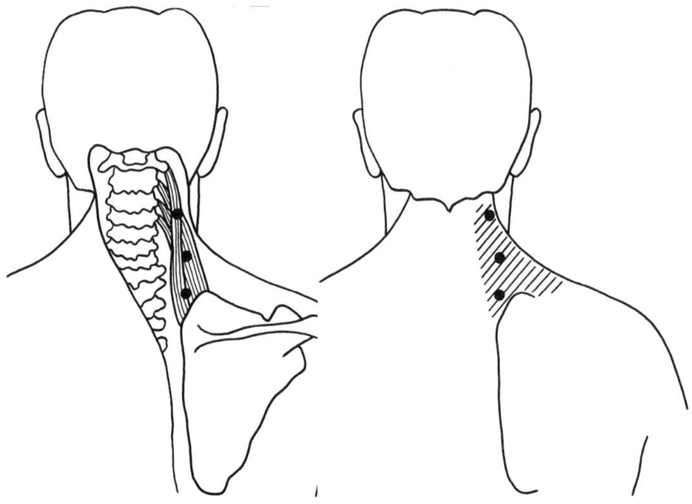

Figure 6.36 Levator scapulae trigger points and referred pain pattern

Pain in the upper back, the neck, and between the shoulder blades is commonly given the medical label scapulocostal syndrome. Physicians unfamiliar with myofascial trigger points have a multitude of explanations and treatments for the condition, including steroid injections and braces to correct your posture. Poor posture does favor development of trouble with your levator scapulae muscles, but trigger points are usually the true cause of the problem and trigger point therapy will take the pain away (Simons, Travell, and Simons 1999, 495, 498; Cailliet 1991, 253-257).

Since there are a number of small bursas around the superior angle of the shoulder blade, levator scapulae trigger points can be misdiagnosed as scapulothoracic bursitis. A favored medical approach is to perform a scapulothoracic bursectomy, which is to cut out the presumably offensive bursa and part of the shoulder blade (Lehtinen et al. 2004, 99-105). It's true that a bursa can sometimes become irritated and swollen, but the trouble can usually be traced to trigger points in nearby muscles. The right approach is to treat the trigger points and let the bursa heal on its own, which it will do when the myofascial origin of its irritation is relieved.

Causes

The lower end of the levator scapulae muscle attaches to the superior angle of the shoulder blade. Its upper end attaches to the transverse processes of the four uppermost neck vertebrae. This arrangement allows the levator scapulae to help raise the shoulder blade and thereby raise the shoulder. This is the function, of course, that gets the muscle into trouble, usually from simple overuse. When stress and bad posture habits keep your shoulders up, you can be sure that the levator scapulae muscles are being strained unnecessarily.

Because of the attachments to the cervical vertebrae, the levator scapulae on each side is also able to help turn your head to that same side. When trigger points disable parts of the muscle, it's reluctant to contract and perform this function. The muscle also resists lengthening, which can keep you from turning your head in the other direction, too (Simons, Travell, and Simons 1999, 494).

Many things can make trouble for a levator scapulae, including sleeping on your side without support for your head, typing while looking at copy out to one side, and holding the phone clamped between your head and shoulder. Backpacks and purses suspended from shoulder straps are as bad for levator scapulae muscles as they are for the trapezius. Both muscles have to stay strongly contracted to counter the downward pull. You'll notice that a woman who carries her purse on a shoulder strap has to keep her shoulder hiked up to keep the purse from sliding off.

Levator scapulae muscles are also stressed by overexercise, emotional tension, and armrests that are too high or too low. In addition, the levator scapulae is one of many muscles strained by whiplash. Trigger points set up by an auto accident or a fall can persist undetected for years and be the unknown source of chronic pain and disability (Simons, Travell, and Simons 1999, 494-495).

As a pair, the levators serve as a checkrein for the head when it hangs forward. They are consequently severely abused if you habitually carry your head forward. Levator scapulae and trapezius muscles can be strained beyond endurance by habitually reading material that's flat on a desk or table, since all the muscles of your neck and upper back have to remain contracted the entire time your head is hanging forward in that position. Prop your book up when you read so you can keep your head up; you can purchase several styles of bookstands at any college bookstore or online to help with this.

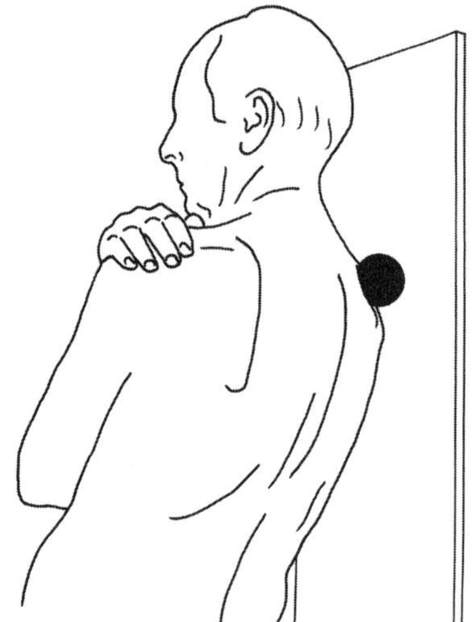

Figure 6.37 Massage of levator scapulae #1 with a ball against the wall

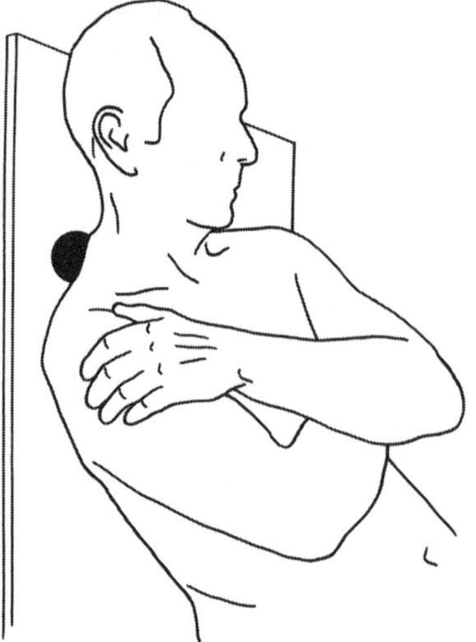

Figure 6.38 Massage of levator scapulae #2 with a ball against the wall

Self-Treatment

There are three trigger points to address in treating the levator scapulae. Levator scapulae trigger point #1 is very easy to find; it's just above where the muscle attaches to the superior angle of the shoulder blade. Unfortunately, this is an attachment trigger point, so it isn't the one that needs the most attention. It feels good to work this spot and helps to some degree, but it won't get rid of your neck pain and stiffness.

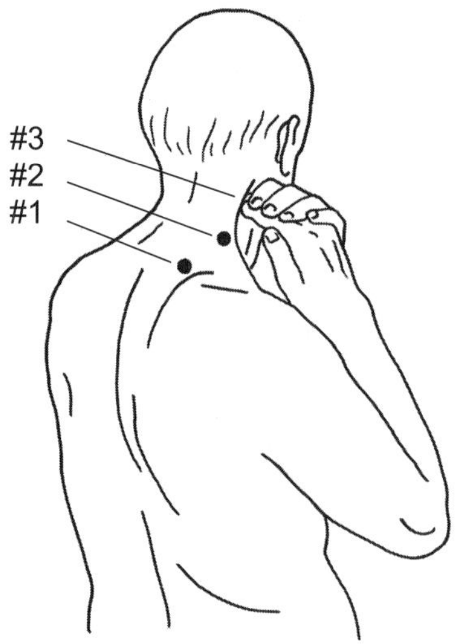

Figure 6.39 Massage of levator scapulae #3 with supported fingers

Levator scapulae #2 is a central trigger point, and it's the one to go after. It's buried under the thick upper trapezius, so you'll need to apply strong pressure to get to it. Use a ball against the wall for the lower two trigger points (Figures 6.37 and 6.38). A Thera Cane or Backnobber also works well when you use the technique shown for the middle trapezius (see Figure 6.30).

Don't neglect levator scapulae #3, high on the side of the neck just behind the top of the sternocleidomastoid muscle. Work it with a supported thumb or supported fingers (Figure 6.39). To confirm the location of the muscle by isolated contraction, hold your fingers in place as you repeatedly raise and lower your shoulder.

Sometimes the tissue in the upper back feels gritty or gravelly as you massage it. Called *palpable crepitus*, it's believed to be calcified nodules associated with the tendons. These deposits are evidence of muscle strain. Massage helps the body dissolve them and carry them away (Simons, Travell, and Simons 1999, 496).

Partner Treatment

The two lower levator scapulae trigger points can be massaged effectively with supported fingers (Figure 6.40). Have the person raise and lower their shoulder to better locate the superior angle of the shoulder blade. You may also be able to feel the levator scapulae itself as it repeatedly contracts beneath the upper trapezius. Be aware that the fibers of the two muscles run at a right angle to one another. Levator scapulae #3, on the side of the neck, can be gently massaged with a supported thumb or a pair of fingers. When you do this, support the opposite side of the neck with your other hand.

Clinical Treatment

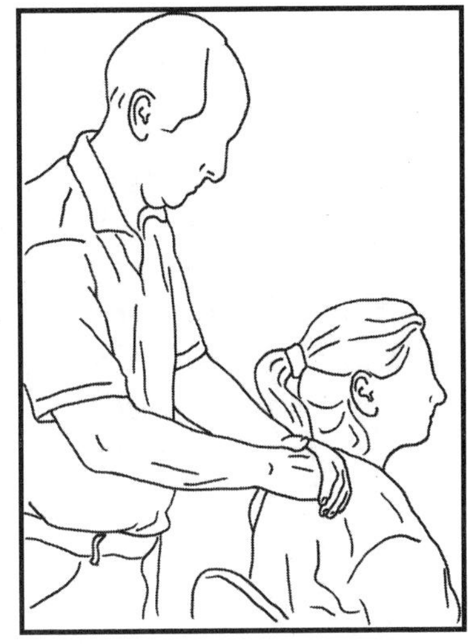

Figure 6.40 Partner massage of the levator scapulae with supported fingers

With a client whose upper trapezius is loose enough, you can push its front edge back and dig under it to massage levator scapulae #1 (Figure 6.41). Otherwise, you can use supported fingers and push down through the trapezius. Visualize the levator scapulae crossing beneath the trapezius at 90 degrees. If you stroke the levator scapulae across its fibers, you'll feel the taut muscle very clearly as a "speed bump."

You'll find levator scapulae #2 right where the muscle begins to come out from under the trapezius in its travel up the neck. Use a supported thumb to press it against the transverse processes of the vertebrae as you execute repeated strokes (Figure 6.42). Trigger point #3, on the side of the neck, can be treated with a pair of fingers.

If you search an area the diameter of a baseball encompassing the levator scapulae's two lower trigger points, you may find additional tender spots. These are likely to be satellite trigger points in the splenius cervicis and iliocostalis cervicis. They contribute to neck pain and stiffness and will need work as part of the treatment.

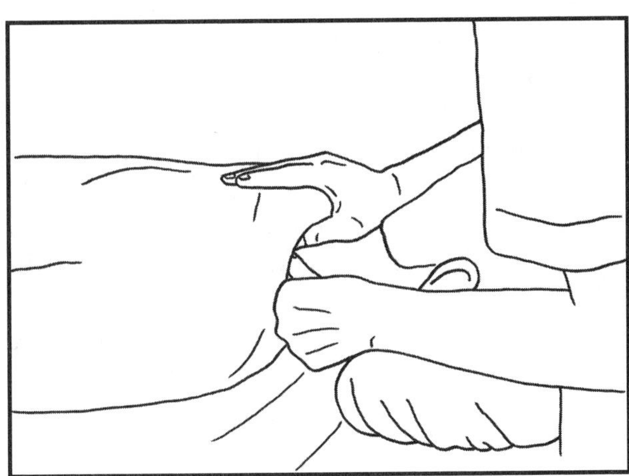

Figure 6.41 Massage of levator scapulae #1 with access under the front edge of the upper trapezius

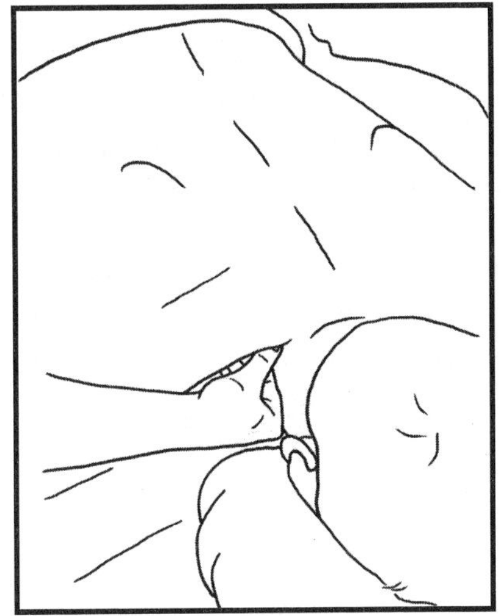

Figure 6.42 Massage of levator scapulae #2 with a supported thumb

Rhomboids

The rhomboid muscles attach to several vertebrae of the upper back and to the inner edge of the shoulder blade. The rhomboid minor is higher and somewhat separate from the rhomboid major, but the two are indistinguishable by touch. The function of the rhomboids is to move the shoulder blade toward the spine, to help raise the shoulder blade, and to hold the shoulder blade still when needed, as a solid support for the operations of the arm and hand.

Patti, *age twenty-nine, came to the weekend clinic at a large massage school with tightness and pain in her upper back and neck. She woke up with the problem the day after waxing her truck. The therapist noted that Patti carried her shoulders rolled forward and that her shoulder blades were "winging" through the back of her shirt. "I have pain most of the time between my shoulder blades," she said. "But this is about as bad as it's ever been."*

Extremely tender trigger points were found in Patti's trapezius, levator scapulae, rhomboids, pectoral muscles, and the muscles of the back of her neck. The initial treatment reduced her pain considerably and brightened her up as well. The therapist then showed her how to work on her upper back herself with a tennis ball against the wall. He said that if she came back to the clinic, she was to tell the student assigned to her that her pectoral muscles should be worked on again. They were part of the problem with the chronic pain in her back because they caused the rhomboid muscles between her shoulder blades to work harder. In the unaccustomed waxing of her truck, Patti had severely overworked both sets of muscles.

Symptoms

Trigger points in the rhomboids refer pain along the inner edge of the shoulder blade (Figure 6.43). It's an aching kind of pain that becomes even more noticeable when you're sitting still. A significant amount of pain at this site may also be coming from the serratus posterior superior muscle and iliocostalis thoracis, which lie beneath the rhomboids, and from the middle trapezius, which lies over them. There are likely to be trigger points in all four layers. Other muscles that send pain to the area between the shoulder blades include the scalenes, infraspinatus, latissimus dorsi, serratus anterior, and levator scapulae.

It's important to check for trigger points in your scalenes before going to the trouble of treating any of these other muscles. Surprisingly, the scalenes are among the most common sources of pain in the upper back. Without first taking care of the scalenes, massage applied to the rhomboids or to any of the other muscles listed here can fail to bring lasting relief, even though it may feel great. The constant aching caused by rhomboid trigger points may provoke an erroneous and useless diagnosis of scapulocostal syndrome, which is only another way of saying that you have chronic pain in your upper back. Sadly, many physicians still consider this pain to be a condition with an unknown cause (Simons, Travell, and Simons 1999, 618).

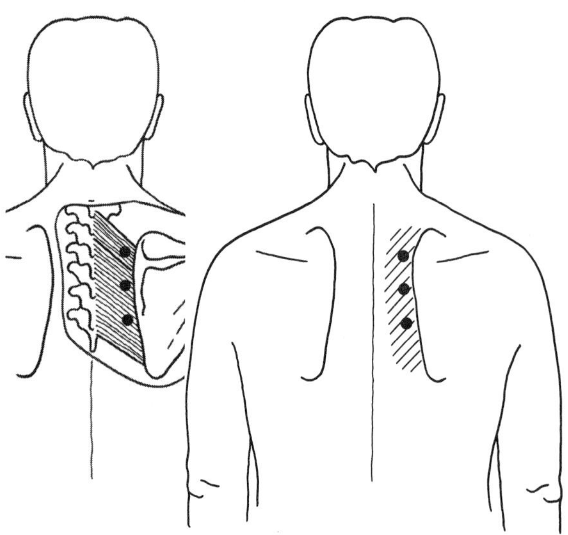

Figure 6.43 Rhomboid trigger points and referred pain pattern

A symptom that may help verify rhomboid involvement in upper back pain is *crepitation*, the sound of snapping or crunching in the rhomboids during shoulder movement due to calcium deposits in the tendons caused by constant strain. This strain is traceable to the shortening and stiffening effects of trigger points in the muscles (Simons, Travell, and Simons 1999, 616). Massage can help the body remove these deposits.

Shortening of the rhomboids limits movement of the arm when reaching forward or raising the arm overhead. Pain may increase when you stretch down to pick something up off the floor (Simons, Travell, and Simons 1999, 614). Any such limitation to your range of motion affects the functioning of the entire shoulder complex and predisposes you to the development of a frozen shoulder.

Causes

To avoid overuse of the rhomboids, it's wise to moderate any activity that requires continuously or repeatedly raising your shoulders or pulling with your arms. Keeping the shoulders pulled back in an unnatural military posture requires that the rhomboids remain continuously contracted. Throwing a ball or rowing a boat can exhaust the rhomboids. Habitual tension that keeps the shoulders up stimulates formation of trigger points in many muscles, including the rhomboids.

One cause of trouble in the rhomboids that might never occur to you is tight pectoral muscles. When trigger points keep the pectoral muscles shortened, they pull the shoulder blade forward. The rhomboids must then tighten in response to keep the shoulder blade in place. The rhomboids are easily overstretched when they're contracting to counter the pull of the pectoral muscles. This is an exhausting kind of muscle work called *eccentric contraction*, and it's guaranteed to set up trigger points (Simons, Travell, and Simons 1999, 613, 616).

The pull of tight pectorals causes your shoulder blades to stick out in back and gives you a round-shouldered, flat-chested posture. It's very difficult to correct your posture or give relief to the rhomboids without first deactivating trigger points in the pectoral muscles. Attempts to stretch the rhomboids for the purpose of therapy when they're already being held in a lengthened state by the pectoral muscles can strain them even further, irritating their trigger points and making the pain worse. Wait to stretch until the trigger points are gone (Simons, Travell, and Simons 1999, 618; Kendal, McCreary, and Provance 1993, 282-283).

Self-Treatment

Rhomboid massage can be applied easily and efficiently with the Thera Cane or Backnobber, although a tennis ball against the wall is a friendlier tool (Figure 6.44). Use a lacrosse ball for greater pressure and even more control. Long-term, chronic knots in the rhomboids will give the ball a bumpy ride. Carry a ball with you or keep one at work and look for opportunities during the day to be alone for a few minutes with your ball and your rhomboids.

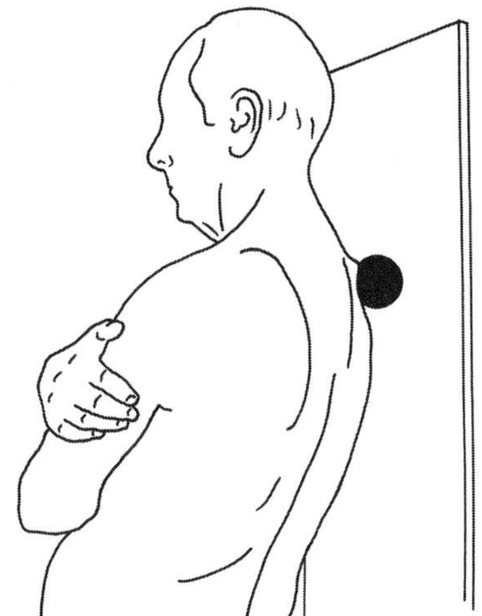

Figure 6.44 Rhomboid massage with a ball against the wall

Partner Treatment

Treating someone else's rhomboid trigger points is easier with the person seated and you standing behind (Figure 6.45). A supported thumb may be an adequate tool in this area, but you can get more pressure with supported fingers, as illustrated. Everyone likes to have this region rubbed, and it usually feels like just the right thing to do for the pain that's so

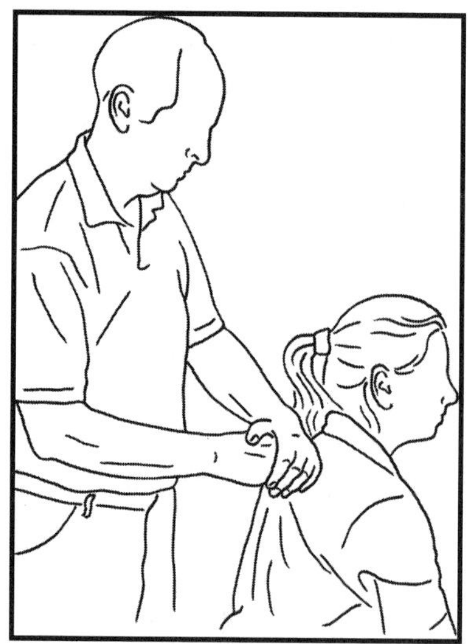

Figure 6.45 Partner massage of the rhomboids with supported fingers

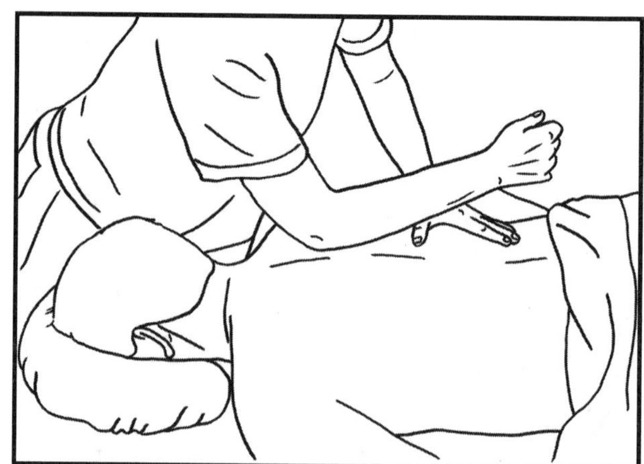

Figure 6.46 Rhomboid massage with the elbow, the thumb of the opposite hand serving as a guide

common here. Just don't forget that this is a favorite place for the scalenes to send pain. If you ignore the scalenes, you may not solve the problem.

Clinical Treatment

Some massage therapists like to treat the rhomboid area with the client lying faceup. The advantage is in using the client's weight to apply pressure, but it can be quite a strain for the fingers. If you want make it less of a trial for your hands and fingers, have the client lie facedown and use an elbow (Figure 6.46). This allows you to use your own weight for the pressure, and you don't have to use your hands at all. If your elbow feels too pointy and aggressive, use your forearm. The ulna bone of the forearm is plenty aggressive for a thin client. Using supported fingers in this area also works well and doesn't overtax your fingers.

Serratus Posterior Superior

Although the serratus posterior superior muscles attach to the spine like the rhomboids and run in the same direction, they don't attach to the shoulder blade. Instead, they go underneath the shoulder blade to attach to several upper ribs (Figure 6.47). The serratus posterior superior muscles function to raise the ribs during inhalation to help fill the lungs.

Elaine, *age forty-four, was troubled by a constant oppressive ache in her upper back that felt like it was deep under one shoulder blade. It was worrisome and her doctor had ordered an X-ray to check for lung disease. Fortunately, he found none. She remarked that her job was particularly stressful. She was a school administrator and traveled all day between schools. "It's not problems at the schools that wear me out, it's the traffic. I never get a chance to relax. I find myself holding my breath at stoplights."*

Not surprisingly, all the muscles in Elaine's upper back were extremely tight. She groaned from relief during treatment. It was interesting to the therapist that massage to Elaine's serratus posterior superior made her little finger tingle, a classic sign of that mus-

cle's involvement in the problem. Two more treatments got rid of the ache under her shoulder blade and the therapist showed her how to self-treat to keep it from coming back.

Symptoms

The referred pain pattern of the serratus posterior superior is very broad (Figure 6.48), and it overlaps the patterns of several other muscles. A deep ache under the shoulder blade is the most characteristic symptom. Pain may also be felt in the back of the shoulder, the point of the elbow, and the pinky side of the wrist and hand. Pain in the little finger is, in fact, a signature of serratus posterior superior trigger points. The referral pattern in the hand is sometimes experienced as numbness. Occasionally, pain may occur over the entire triceps, down the ulnar side of the forearm, and even into the pectoral area (not shown). The referred pain deep under the shoulder blade has the potential to create satellite trigger points in the subscapularis muscle, which can be the place where a frozen shoulder begins. Serratus posterior superior trigger points can themselves be satellites caused by the scalenes, again indicting the unappreciated scalenes as the possible distant origin of frozen shoulder (Simons, Travell, and Simons 1999, 900-905).

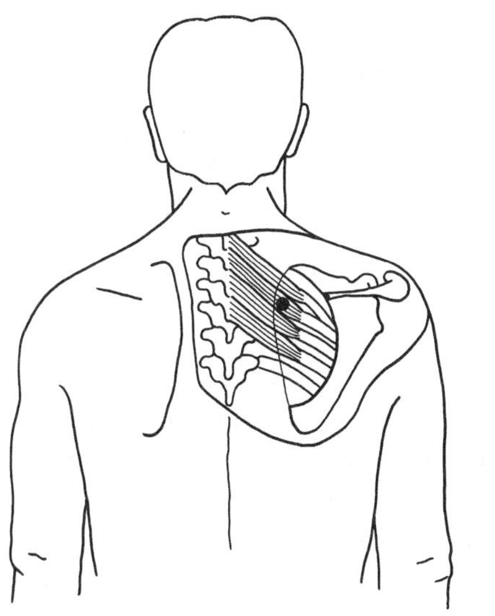

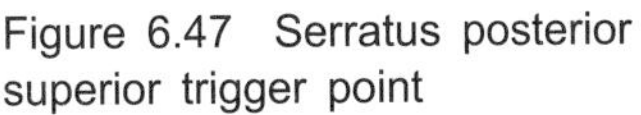

Figure 6.47 Serratus posterior superior trigger point

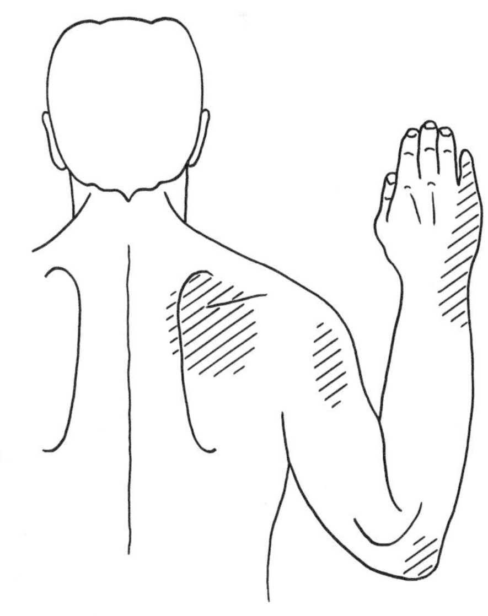

Figure 6.48 Serratus posterior superior referred pain pattern

Serratus posterior superior trigger points were among the first discovered by Janet Travell. One of her earliest studies found them to be present in 98 percent of her patients who experienced shoulder pain (Travell, Rinzler, and Herman 1942, 417-422). Even though these trigger points and their effects have been known about for over sixty years, doctors still misdiagnose them. One confusing factor is the numbness they can refer to the hand and fingers, which closely mimics cervical nerve root compression caused by a herniated disk in the neck. This numbness can also be misconstrued as peripheral neuropathy, a disease of the sensory nerves. The elbow pain can be wrongly labeled olecranon bursitis (Simons, Travell, and Simons 1999, 905).

The serratus posterior superior muscles are very often cited as the cause of scapulocostal syndrome, which is pain affecting mainly the posterior shoulder area (Simons, Travell, and Simons 1999, 905; Ormandy 1994, 105-108). Some surgeons believe that a serratotomy (severing the serratus posterior superior) is the perfect solution to the problem (Fouri 1991, 721-724). But you can probably keep your muscles intact and whole if you learn to treat your own trigger points.

Causes

Strenuous breathing during heavy exertion has the potential to create trigger points in the serratus posterior superior. Nervous hyperventilation or habitually breathing with your chest instead of your diaphragm can also overwork them. Especially taxing for them is the struggle for breath incident to respiratory illnesses such as asthma, bronchitis, pneumonia, emphysema, bronchitis, and smoker's cough (Simons, Travell, and Simons 1999, 902).

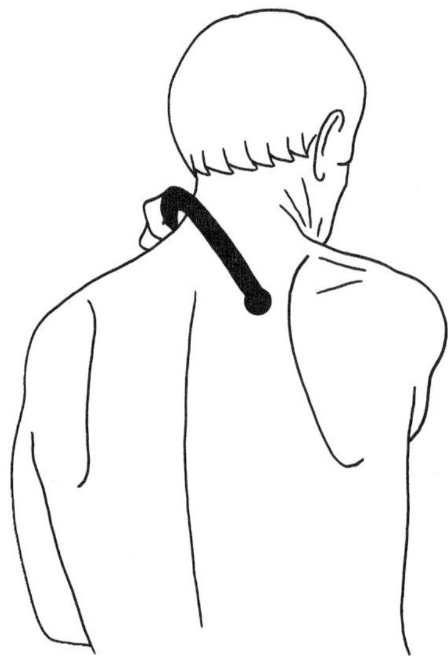

Figure 6.49 Serratus posterior superior and rhomboid massage with a Thera Cane or Backnobber

Self-Treatment

Because the serratus posterior superior is largely hidden by the shoulder blade, its trigger points are inaccessible with your arm at your side. (The big bite taken out of the shoulder blade in Figure 6.47 illustrates this.) Luckily, the shoulder blade can be moved out of the way by simply placing the hand on the opposite shoulder while applying massage. Work with the Thera Cane or Backnobber over the opposite shoulder with the hand in the bow (Figure 6.49). A ball on the wall works well, provided the arm is held across the body to move the shoulder blade aside. Use the same technique as you would for the rhomboids (see Figure 6.44).

Partner Treatment

Self-treatment with the ball is straightforward enough if you get the shoulder blade out of the way and get the ball in the right place. If disability stands in the way of self-care, however, you may want to corner some noble soul to do it for you. Treatment of the serratus posterior superior by a partner is just the same as with the rhomboids and levator scapulae. In Figure 6.50, only one hand is shown working on the trigger point. This is to show exactly where to place your fingers relative to the superior angle of the shoulder blade. You need to be a little above the rhomboid trigger points and a little below levator scapulae #1. For the actual therapy, use supported fingers.

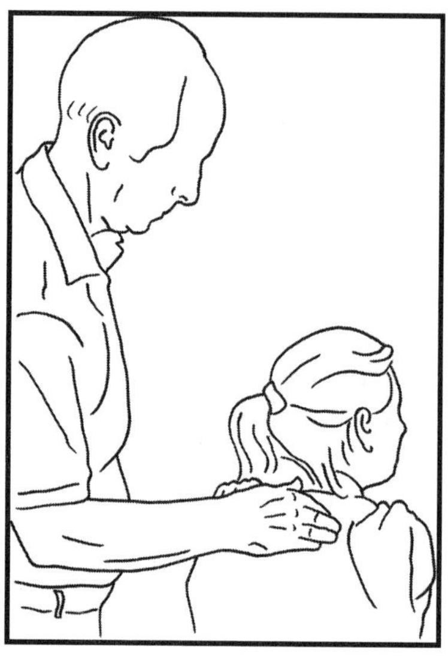

Figure 6.50 Partner massage of the serratus posterior superior

Clinical Treatment

Treat the client with the same technique that you use for the rhomboids, but be sure to use the blade of the ulna, not the point of the elbow (Figure 6.51). The muscle will bear very little pressure because it's thin and lies right on the ribs, making its trigger points excruciatingly tender. Note that the client's arm is hanging off the table to move the shoulder blade aside.

Take special care not to overtreat. Give it six to twelve easy strokes and then leave it for the natural healing processes to take over. You aren't required to force a release. The worst mistake you can make with a trigger point is to compulsively try to erase it. You may get away with this with some clients, but with others you risk having them swear off trigger point massage forever, and maybe swearing off you, too.

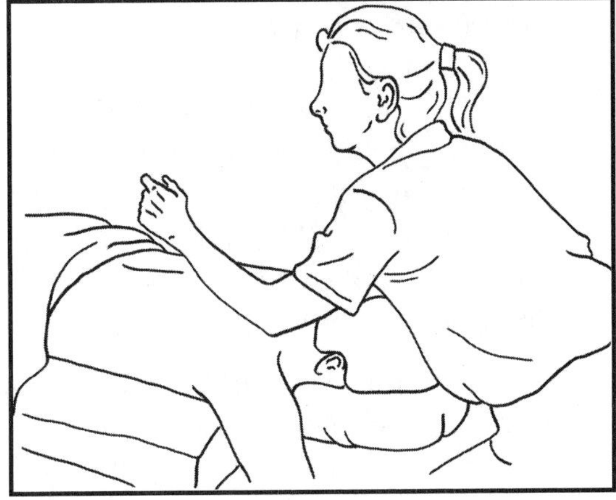

Figure 6.51 Serratus posterior superior massage with the blade of the ulna

Iliocostalis Thoracis

There are three long back muscles side by side between the shoulder blades and the spine. As a group, they're known as the *erector spinae*. The *spinalis* (spin-AH-liss) lies right along the spine. The *longissimus thoracis* (long-ISS-ih-mus thor-RA-cis) is an inch or so further out. The *iliocostalis thoracis* (ILL-ee-oh-kuh-STAHL-iss thor-RA-cis) is the furthest from the spine, although the distance may be no more than two inches. It lies right along the inner edge of the shoulder blade, and sometimes under it, when the arm is parallel with the body (Figure 6.52).

These three long muscles can have trigger points anywhere along their length, causing back pain in various places, but only the iliocostalis thoracis has any involvement with shoulder pain. The iliocostalis thoracis trigger point that can cause shoulder pain is located an inch or so below the bottom edge of the lower trapezius, next to the inferior angle of the shoulder blade (Figure 6.52). Sometimes this trigger point will be found just below the inferior angle, or it may be hidden underneath it. The exact placement of the iliocostalis varies a little from person to person. To search for the trigger point, move your shoulder blade out of the way by placing your hand on the opposite shoulder.

Symptoms

In addition to pain, trigger points in the long back muscles cause tightening over their entire length. This can make them bulge out in a hard contraction, giving the impression that one whole side of the back is in trouble, when a single trigger point somewhere is actually the prime instigator. Although this is commonly called a "back spasm," it's not a true spasm that will respond to treatment with heat and stretching. A contraction that's being maintained by trigger points won't give up until you locate the trigger points and deactivate them (Simons, Travell, and Simons 1999, 921, 926). Rick's story is an illustration of how misleading trigger point symptoms can be.

> Rick, *age thirty-four, was a muscular power-company lineman who suffered pain and tightness over the entire length of his back, from his tailbone to the base of his skull. He was conscious of his aching back and shoulders even when sleeping. His insurance had paid for CAT scans, MRIs, X-rays, and many visits to two different chiropractors, but he'd experienced no improvement and received no definitive diagnosis. Exploratory surgery was being held open as an option. In the meantime, he'd been instructed to exercise and stretch.*

"I keep doing the stretching," he said, "but it never does any good. My back's so stiff I feel like an old man."

Rick's back muscles were like wooden posts, and constantly guarding against pain was making his stiffness worse. Trigger points were found in several places along his erector spinae on both sides, and trigger point massage gave him great relief. A month of working on himself with a tennis ball against the wall erased most of his pain. This enabled the muscles to stop guarding, and he soon felt loose enough to profit from the stretching exercises that had been prescribed.

A trigger point in the iliocostalis thoracis causes a diffuse kind of pain that can be felt all along the inner edge of the shoulder blade, although it tends to concentrate at the inferior angle. It can occasionally send pain to the front of the body in the area of the upper abdominal and lower pectoral muscles (Figure 6.53). The arrhythmia trigger point is located near the center of this region and may be activated as a satellite of the trigger point in the iliocostalis thoracis.

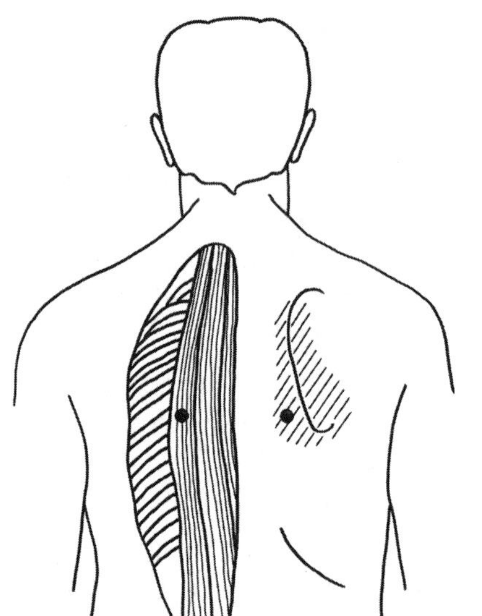

Figure 6.52 Iliocostalis thoracis trigger point and referred pain pattern

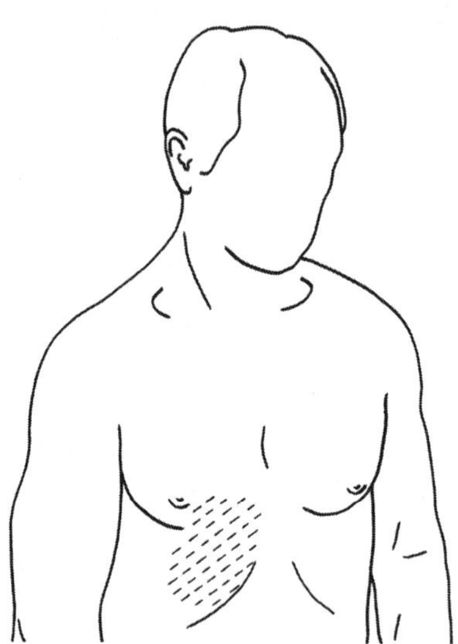

Figure 6.53 Iliocostalis thoracis anterior pain pattern. The dotted lines indicate occasional pain.

Referred pain from iliocostalis trigger points can be mistaken for the pain of angina, pleurisy, appendicitis, or other visceral diseases. Even when you have one of these more serious conditions, remember that myofascial pain from trigger points is likely to be contributing to your discomfort (Simons, Travell, and Simons 1999, 924-925).

Causes

Picking up something that's too heavy for you is a major cause of trigger points in your long back muscles, especially if you lift suddenly or your body isn't straight and centered. The back muscles are particularly vulnerable when you do anything strenuous while bending or twisting to one side. Lifting while twisted puts the full load on just one half of the back, in effect doubling the strain. In all aspects of your work and play, stay balanced on both feet and squarely face the object you're dealing with.

Whiplash is another common cause of trigger points in the long back muscles. They can also be created by prolonged immobility or staying in a strained position too long. Repetitive motion on the job is sure to make trouble. Repetitive tasks never give your muscles a chance to rest and catch up.

Self-Treatment

The best approach for massage of the iliocostalis thoracis is simply to back up to a wall with a tennis ball (Figure 6.54). Use a lacrosse ball or high-bounce ball if you need deeper penetration. If you put the ball in a long tube sock, you'll have a handle for better control of positioning. Several other muscles that contribute to shoulder problems can be treated at the same time in this way, including the levator scapulae, rhomboids, serratus posterior superior, and lower trapezius. Treat these muscles sequentially, beginning with the levator scapulae above the shoulder blade and working your way down the inner edge of the shoulder blade to the iliocostalis thoracis at the inner edge of the inferior angle.

Simply seek out the exquisitely tender spots and roll the ball repeatedly over them. Use short, slow strokes, parallel with the muscle fibers. Minimize bending of your knees by rocking your pelvis forward and back to roll the ball. The Thera Cane is also a great tool for the back.

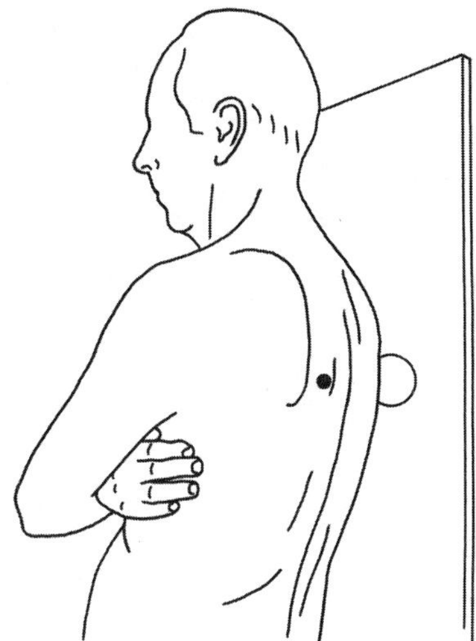

Figure 6.54 Iliocostalis thoracis self-treatment with a ball against the wall. The black dot is the corresponding trigger point of the opposite side.

Partner Treatment

It's best to treat the iliocostalis thoracis trigger point with the person standing (Figure 6.55). Seated, the person would tend to lean forward, and this tightens the back muscles. This area in the mid back is a little awkward to work on, so you'll want to concentrate your efforts and make them efficient. Use either a supported thumb or the knuckles of a loose fist. Move the skin and clothing with each stroke, and keep the strokes very short and specific to the trigger point. As always, six to twelve strokes are an optimal amount of treatment.

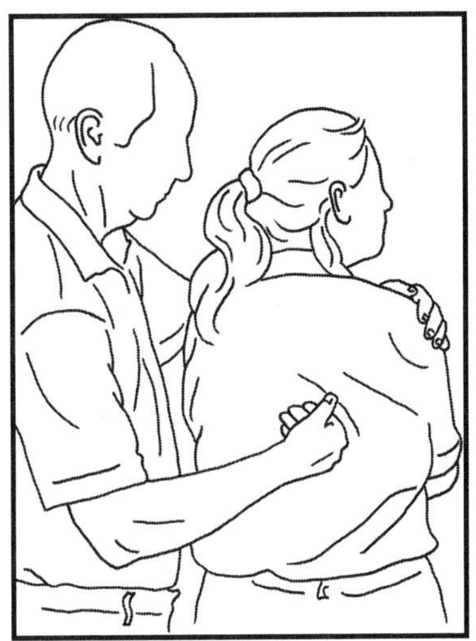

Figure 6.55 Iliocostalis thoracis partner treatment with a supported thumb

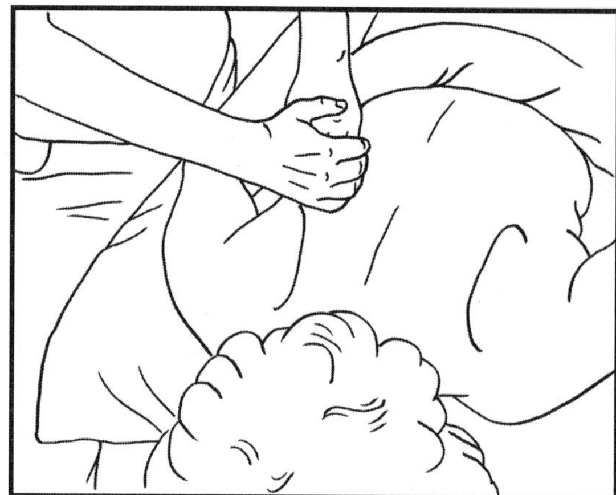

Figure 6.56 Iliocostalis thoracis clinical massage with supported fingers

Clinical Treatment

Supported fingers are an ideal tool for treating the iliocostalis thoracis (Figure 6.56). You can also use paired supported thumbs (see Figure 4.22), keeping the thumbs touching to lock the hands together, then leaning in to make the stroke and letting your body weight do the work. You should view your hands as an integrated tool and use body motion to make the stroke rather than stroking with the action of the thumb joints. Many therapists overuse their thumbs and have a chronic aching in their thumb muscles. To give your thumbs a total rest, use supported fingers. To rest your hands altogether, use your elbow. To find a trigger point that may be hiding under the inferior angle, move the shoulder blade a little to the side by having the client's arm hang over the side of the table.

Chapter 7

Shoulder Treatment, Part C

This chapter has to do with two categories of muscles, those of the upper arm and those of the chest and pectoral area. Both groups have the potential for contributing to shoulder pain. When you have a frozen shoulder or an arm severely limited in its range of motion, most of the muscles discussed in this chapter can be expected to harbor trigger points.

At first glance, certain muscles in these groups might seem to be of very little consequence. For instance, you might think that the diaphragm is too far from the shoulder to be of any concern. To the contrary, diaphragm trigger points can send part of their pain to the top of the shoulder, encouraging development of satellite trigger points in the upper trapezius. As for the upper arm muscles, all of them either send pain to the shoulder or directly affect its operation. In fact, one of their major roles is to help keep the shoulder joint together.

At issue with the upper arm, chest, and pectoral muscles is their propensity for sponsoring trigger points in the rotator cuff muscles, which are directly responsible for most of the pain and stiffness in your shoulder. It would be a mistake to slight any muscle in this book, no matter how insignificant it might seem. The functions of the muscles in the shoulder area are so interwoven that a small or remote muscle can have far-reaching effects on many others. The small scalene muscles of the neck, discussed in chapter 5, are a notable example of this kind of thing. They're famous for stirring up trouble in many other places, including the shoulder, arm, hand, upper back, and pectoral area.

Pectoral Muscles

Trigger points in the pectoral muscles can be a critical factor in the development of a frozen shoulder. To begin with, they usually send their pain to the front of the shoulder. In addition, tightness in a pectoral muscle resulting from trigger points can undermine the function of other muscles of the shoulder complex, making more trigger points almost inevitable. If one muscle in the shoulder area gets a trigger point that remains untreated, it's only a matter of time before they all get them. It's almost as if there were a trigger point virus. The shoulder muscles eventually all call in sick, and you end up with some of the worst pain you've ever known and unable to move your arm. And it can all start with a pectoral trigger point (Simons, Travell, and Simons 1999, 833).

An even bigger issue with pectoral trigger points is their ability to mimic the pain of a heart attack. The left shoulder and arm pain so typical of a heart attack occurs in exactly the same areas as the pain referred from trigger points in pectoral muscles (Lange 1931, 118-135). Severe (or mild) chest pain that lingers long after a heart incident may be coming from these pectoral trigger points (Simons, Travell, and Simons 1999, 819-821; Edeiken and Wolferth 1936, 201-210).

Amazingly, cardiac disease can also be the instigating factor in a frozen shoulder because heart pain can create satellite trigger points in the chest and shoulder muscles. As you'll recall, Janet Travell began her career as a cardiologist. One of the things that led to her interest in trigger points was the surprising number of frozen shoulders among her heart patients.

Pectoralis Major

The pectoralis major muscles are the muscular part of the breasts in both men and women. "Pectoralis" comes from *pectus*, the Latin word for "breast." "Major" means it's the largest of the pectoral muscles.

> Doug, *age forty-nine, had pain in the front of his right shoulder and collarbone. It had been chronic for at least ten years. "It hurts to raise my arm. I have to use my left arm to raise my right arm at work." He was suspicious of the whiplash he'd suffered in a rear-end collision thirty years earlier, but he believed his present problem more likely stemmed from the high demands of his work in an automotive assembly plant.*
>
> *Doug's collarbone was very sensitive to tapping, and trigger points were found in many areas, including his scalenes, sternocleidomastoids, trapezius, and rotator cuff muscles. Trigger points in his pectoralis minor and the upper part of his pectoralis major were extremely tender. The first treatment, with a focus on the pectoral muscles, significantly moderated the pain in his collarbone and the front of his shoulder. Self-treatment over a period of four weeks made his job much more tolerable.*

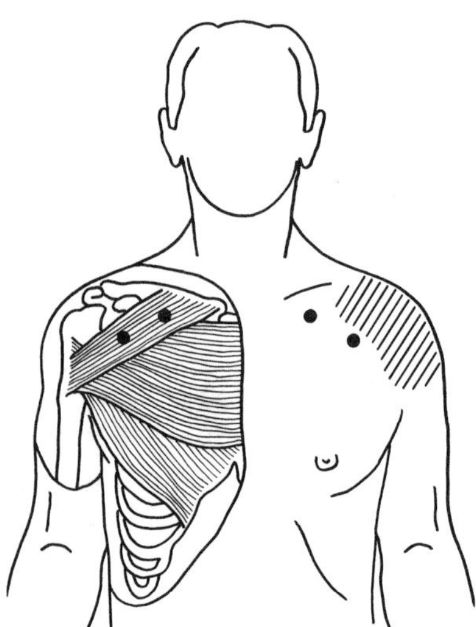

Figure 7.1 Pectoralis major, clavicular section: trigger points and referred pain pattern

Symptoms

Pain from pectoralis major trigger points is felt in the chest and the front of the shoulder. Especially active trigger points also send pain to the inner arm, the inner elbow, the pinky side of the hand, and the fourth and fifth fingers. The exact location of the pain depends on the location of the trigger point in the three sections of this complex muscle. The clavicular section is the highest and attaches to the collarbone. The sternal section lies in the middle and attaches to the breastbone. The costal section is the lowest and attaches to the ribs. The three sections combine to attach to the front of the humerus.

Trigger points will be found in four areas of the pectoralis major. You can locate them by relating them to their different patterns of pain. Trigger points in the clavicular section send pain to the front of the shoulder (Figure 7.1). This upper part of the muscle assists the anterior deltoid in raising the arm to the front. Clavicular trigger points are apt to create satellites in the front part of the deltoid (Simons, Travell, and Simons 1999, 826-827).

Trigger points in the sternal section refer pain to the inner arm and the inner elbow. They can also cause an intermittent, frightening pain and sense of constriction in the central part of the chest that is easily confused with angina pectoris, the pain created by heart disease (Figure 7.2). These two origins of chest pain can be distinguished somewhat by the fact that trigger point pain tends to occur when you move your arm. True angina can be present at rest and isn't necessarily associated with arm movement. A disturbing reality about trigger points in the pectoral muscles is that they can actually induce a reduction in the diameter of the coronary arteries thus reducing the oxygen available to the heart muscle (Simons, Travell, and Simons 1999, 838). False heart pain can also come from trigger points in the scalenes, the upper part of the rectus abdominis, and muscles of the upper back (Simons, Travell, and Simons 1999, 832).

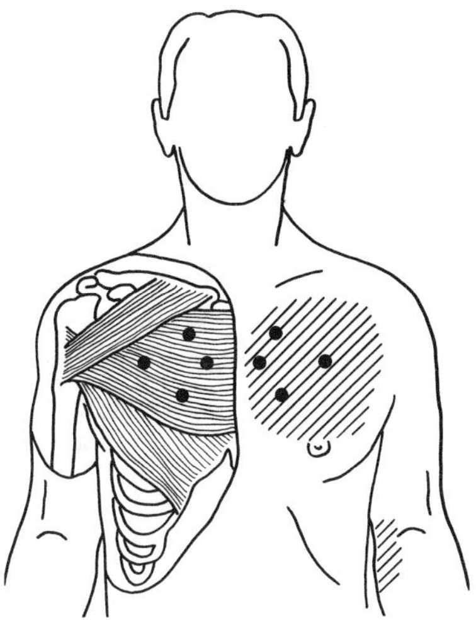
Figure 7.2 Pectoralis major, sternal section: trigger points and referred pain pattern

Trigger points in the thick lateral border of the costal section cause hypersensitivity in the nipple along with tenderness and pain in the breast itself (Figure 7.3). This breast tenderness can make a woman's bra exceedingly uncomfortable, and a man with the same problem can find his shirt to be very irritating. Tension in the pectoralis major from costal trigger points can actually interfere with lymph drainage, creating edema of the breast along with a degree of enlargement and a sense of congestion. Given the current focus on breast cancer, symptoms from these fundamentally harmless trigger points can be responsible for a great deal of unnecessary alarm if you and your health care providers are not aware of them (Simons, Travell, and Simons 1999, 819-831; Long 1956, 102-106).

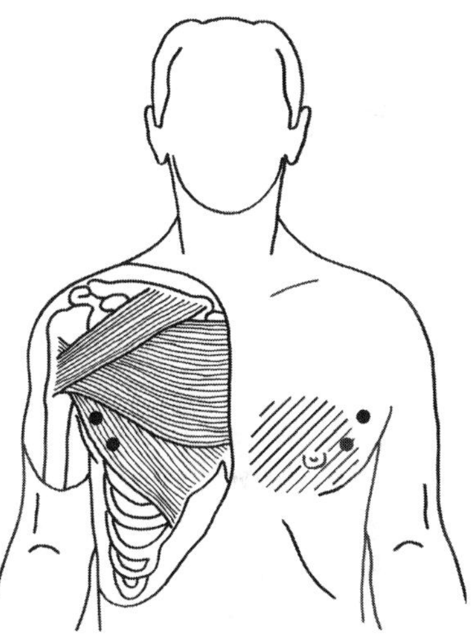
Figure 7.3 Pectoralis major, costal section: trigger points and referred pain pattern

A trigger point in the lower border of the pectoralis major between the fifth and sixth ribs can cause an irregular heartbeat (Figure 7.4). This is called an *ectopic* heartbeat, meaning that the activation of the irregular heartbeat originates outside the sinoatrial node, the nerve center in the heart that normally controls heart rate (Thomas 1997, 637). The pectoralis major trigger point's involvement in disturbing the heart's rhythm is a somatovisceral effect, wherein muscles affect the function of internal organs. In this case, the effects are manifested in a fast heartbeat, a sense of spasming, or premature contractions. You might think a trigger point affecting the heart would be on the left side, nearer to the heart, but this arrhythmia trigger point occurs only on the right (Simons, Travell, and Simons 1999, 832).

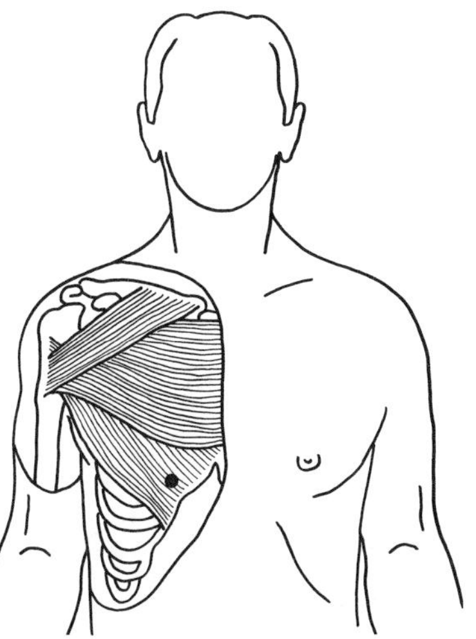
Figure 7.4 Pectoralis major, arrhythmia trigger point

An irregular heartbeat can be a particularly worrisome thing that suddenly takes your attention away from everything else, leaving you in a state of breathless apprehension. But all this heightened awareness and concern are completely unwarranted when trigger points are the cause. Trigger point massage immediately restores normal heart rhythm when trigger points are disturbing it (Simons, Travell, and Simons 1999, 832).

Tightness from trigger points in the pectoral muscles makes it hard to reach back at shoulder level and keeps the shoulder pulled forward, which puts the back muscles under constant strain and can be a hidden cause of back pain. Pectoral tightness also produces a round-shouldered posture that causes the head and neck to be kept projected forward, sponsoring trigger points in the sternocleidomastoid and scalene muscles. It's easy to understand how the overload imposed on shoulder and upper back muscles by a shortened pectoralis major can lead to the development of trigger points throughout the region, progressively limiting movement of the arm and ending in a frozen shoulder (Simons, Travell, and Simons 1999, 827-828, 833).

> Anna, *age seventy-three, didn't realize she was a victim of pectoral trigger points. She strapped on a TENS unit (transcutaneous electrical nerve stimulator) every day for her chronic mid back pain. Unable to wear the unit at night, she regularly had to take a narcotic painkiller to enable her to sleep. Trigger points had shortened her pectoral muscles to such an extent that she couldn't pull her shoulders back to stand up straight, so she was developing a dowager's hump. After her first trigger point massage, she was able to go to sleep without taking her pain medication for the first time in years. Though she's never eager to massage her own pectoral muscles, which are still very tender, her back always feels better when she does.*

The round-shouldered posture fostered by pectoral trigger points can have many other indirect effects, including excessive pressure on spinal disks, compression of nerves, jaw problems, restricted breathing, chronic fatigue, and neck pain (Simons, Travell, and Simons 1999, 809). Unfortunately, attempts to force a correction of your posture generally fail unless you first find and deactivate the specific trigger points that are keeping the pectoral muscles tight. Efforts to stretch these sensitive muscles without releasing their trigger points can make your symptoms worse. After the trigger points are gone, stretching and working on your posture are quite appropriate and beneficial.

When your muscles are limber, pain free, and responsive, you can achieve the most healthful posture simply by raising the crown of your head and standing tall. In the absence of pectoral trigger points, your shoulders will find their own good place. Never aim at keeping your shoulders pulled back in a soldierly stance, which is neither normal nor healthy (Simons, Travell, and Simons 1999, 809-810, 833).

All of these diverse symptoms deriving from myofascial trigger points in the pectoralis major muscle lead to a very long list of mistaken diagnoses:

- Acid reflux
- Bicipital tendinitis
- Bronchitis
- Cervical nerve root impingement
- Chest wall syndrome
- Colitis
- Costochondritis
- Hiatal hernia
- Intercostal neuritis
- Intestinal gas

- Lateral epicondylitis
- Lung cancer
- Medial epicondylitis
- Mediastinal emphysema
- Pleurisy
- Precordial catch syndrome
- Rib-tip syndrome
- Slipping rib syndrome
- Subacromial bursitis
- Supraspinatus tendinitis
- Tietze's syndrome

Causes

In vigorous sports activities and many kinds of work, the pectoralis major can be overused when the arm is thrust forward, upward, or across the body with excessive force or too many repetitions. The woman in the previous chapter who overused her trapezius muscles while waxing her truck also overused her pectorals. The unaccustomed use of hedge clippers is another example of the kind of forceful arm motion that can get your pectoral muscles into trouble.

Be alert for anything that fosters a round-shouldered posture, particularly when muscular effort is involved. Chronic nervous tension or anxiety can keep your shoulders rounded and tight. Carrying a backpack can create trigger points in muscles of the chest, abdomen, upper back, and neck. Tune in to any muscle tension you feel when you've got the backpack on. Having to walk with your head and body thrust forward to balance the weight of a backpack should give you a clue to the strain it imposes. Part of your trigger point therapy should be figuring out how to lighten your load or finding another way to carry it (Simons, Travell, and Simons 1999, 847-953).

Self-Treatment

A ball against the wall is an awkward tool for treating the pectoral region, especially for women, because breasts of even medium size get in the way. Supported fingers or supported knuckles, however, do an excellent job (Figure 7.5). Note that the man on the left is using the flats of his fingers, which tires the fingers quickly since so much more force is

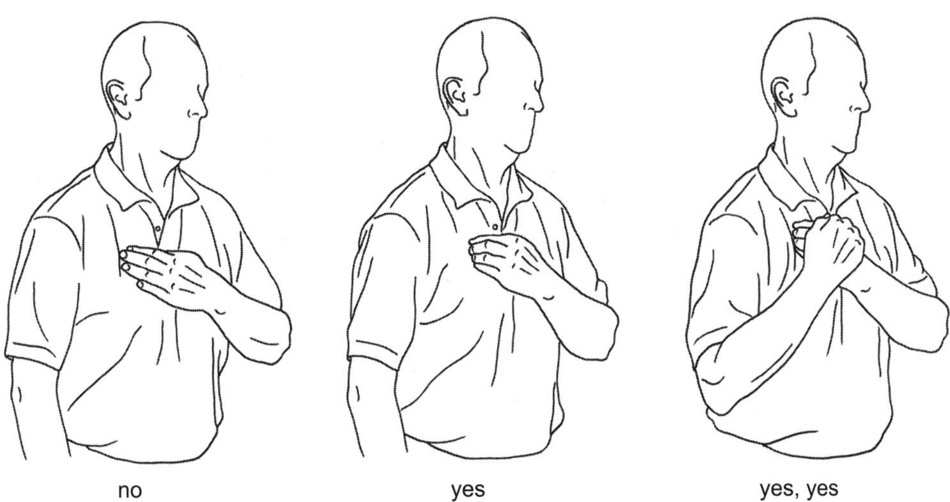

Figure 7.5 Pectoralis major massage with supported fingers

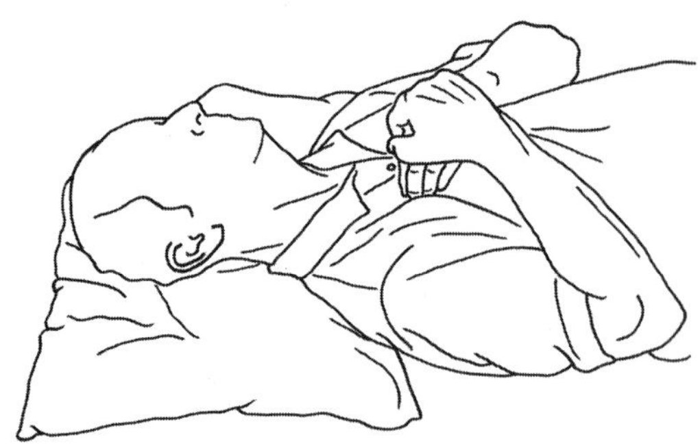

Figure 7.6 Massage of the pectoralis major with supported fingers, lying down

needed to penetrate. The man in the middle is using the tips of his fingers to dig deeply into the muscle. The man on the right is doing the right thing to save his fingers by exerting most of the pressure with his other hand. These supported fingers are the best tool because they penetrate easily with minimal effort. If you're handicapped by long fingernails, you may be tempted to press with the flats of your fingers. You'll find that your fingers tire very quickly when used in that way. Try supported knuckles, a Thera Cane, or a Knobble instead.

Men will find all parts of the pectoralis major directly accessible through the skin. For women, the upper half is similarly accessible, but the lower half must be approached through breast tissue or by moving the breast aside. Don't let large breasts be an impediment to massage. Lying on your back (Figure 7.6) will let gravity move both breasts aside, allowing better access to areas of the pectoral muscles that the breasts cover when you're sitting or standing. For massage of trigger points in the outer border of the pectoralis major, knead them between your fingers and thumb (Figure 7.7).

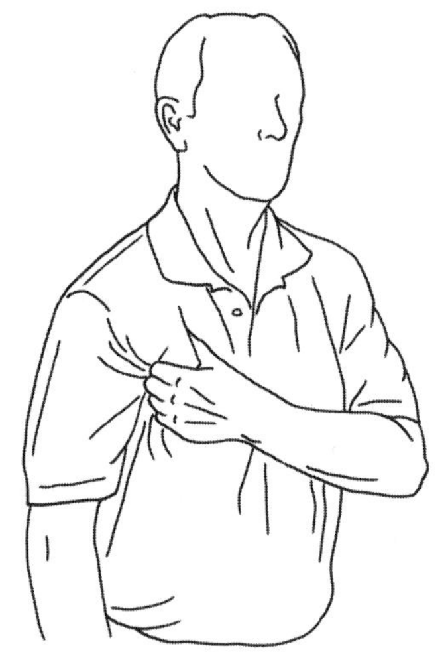

Figure 7.7 Massage of the lateral border of the pectoralis major

The trigger point for heart arrhythmia is found between the ribs, a couple of inches to the right of the *xiphoid process*, the lower tip of the breastbone. Massaging this trigger point is sharply painful, but the heart rhythm will straighten out right away if the trigger point is to blame. This trigger point can be difficult to resolve if emphysema engages you in a constant battle to exhale (Simons, Travell, and Simons 1999, 838).

You may find a large number of trigger points in the pectoral area, and they can be some of the most painful that you'll encounter anywhere. Pain in or around the breasts can be a serious cause of concern for women, because it naturally arouses fears of breast cancer. Great efforts are being made to get women to do regular self-examinations so they can familiarize themselves with the natural state of breast tissue and learn to recognize changes that may represent potential tumor growth. However, physicians and others who monitor women's health believe that most women don't do self-examinations, either because they're terrified at the thought of what they might find or because they don't clearly understand what they're looking for (Hackett 2000).

This is unfortunate, because breast self-examination is an ideal time to learn to distinguish between normal and abnormal lumps in breast tissue and the sometimes lumplike trigger points in the underlying muscles. Very often, pain in the breast area is nothing more serious than pain from trigger points in the chest muscles. A breast self-exam, if done thoroughly and with attention to possible trigger points, should allay fear, not increase it. Working with a doctor or nurse who understands both myofascial pain and the anatomy of the breast can be enormously helpful (Hackett 2000).

Partner Treatment

The pectoral area is such a personal space that most people prefer self-treatment or professional massage. If you need to help a friend or family member with their pectoralis major, work with the fingertips of one hand with the person sitting or standing. An alternative would be to have the person lie down and use supported fingers as you would for clinical treatment. Use the thumb and fingers to knead the lateral border of the muscle as shown for self-treatment (Figure 7.7). The pectoral area is a sensitive place even under the best of circumstances, so proceed delicately.

Clinical Treatment

Surprisingly, many professional massage therapists never treat the front of the body. This may have more to do with personal squeamishness than consideration for the client. Therapists who regularly address these places rarely encounter a client who declines the work. People with myofascial trigger points benefit greatly from treatment of their pectoral and abdominal muscles.

Supported fingers are the best way to treat all of the broad area of the chest. Work from the head of the table as shown (Figure 7.8). Expect to find many tiny trigger points, especially in the sternal section of the pectoralis major. Work through the sheet for the lower half of the chest. Use very short, repeated strokes as usual, moving the sheet and the skin with each stroke. When treating the majority of women, most of the breast will fall to the side and out of the way. Although this makes it easier to treat most of the muscle, it makes it harder to treat the lateral border, as the breast will be lying right on it. Simply have the client pull her breast toward the center with her opposite hand. You can then knead the lateral border between the fingers and thumb of one hand (Figure 7.9).

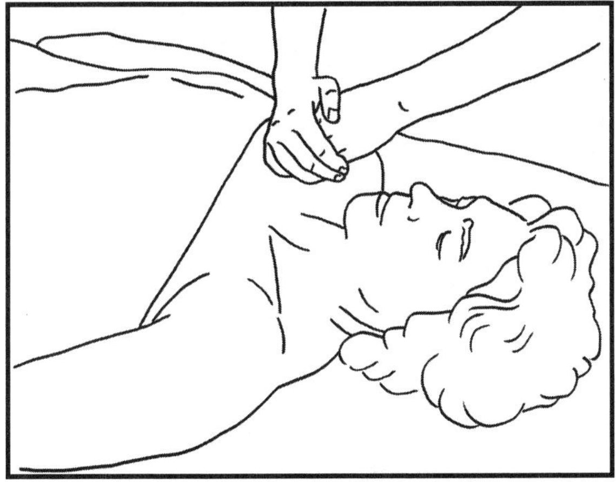

Figure 7.8 Pectoral massage with supported fingers. You can also treat through the sheet.

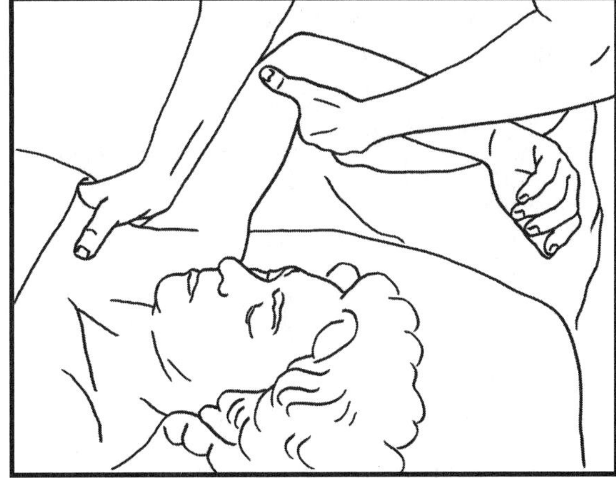

Figure 7.9 Massage of the outer border of the pectoralis major between fingers and thumb

Subclavius

The subclavius muscles lie just under the collarbones. They attach to the middle of the collarbones and to the ends of the first ribs near where they join the breastbone. The specific function of the subclavius muscles hasn't been established, but it's likely that they help keep

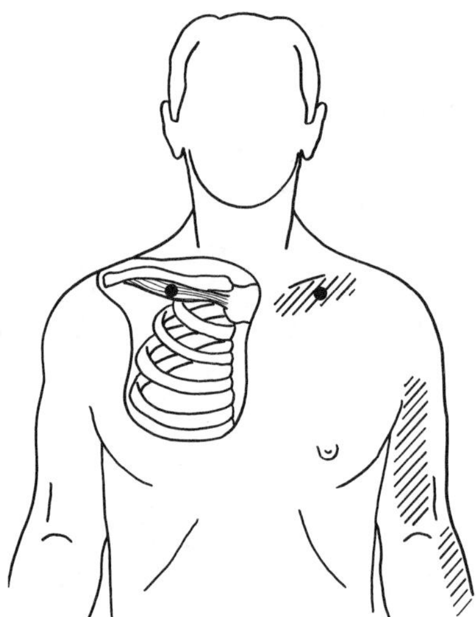

Figure 7.10 Subclavius trigger points and referred pain pattern

the sternoclavicular joint from pulling apart. They're sure to be overworked by the same actions that overwork the pectoral muscles.

Considering their small size, the subclavius muscles have a disproportionately widespread referred pain pattern (Figure 7.10). Subclavius trigger points cause pain just below the collarbone. They also send pain to the biceps and the *radial* side (thumb side) of the forearm. Sometimes they cause pain in the radial side of the hand, the thumb, and the index and middle fingers (not shown). When trigger points shorten a subclavius muscle, it can keep tension on the collarbone, pulling it down and squeezing the subclavian artery and vein against the first rib, which restricts circulation in the arm and hand. The edema from this compression is apt to be misdiagnosed as vascular thoracic outlet syndrome (Simons, Travell, and Simons 1999, 821, 828, 830).

You won't be able to feel the subclavius directly, because it's covered by the clavicular section of the pectoralis major. But search for the exquisite tenderness of its trigger point deep under the middle of the collarbone. Supported fingers work well for massage here, as shown in Figures 7.5 and 7.8. Focus the pressure on the middle finger and work deeply, trying to get up behind the collarbone.

Pectoralis Minor

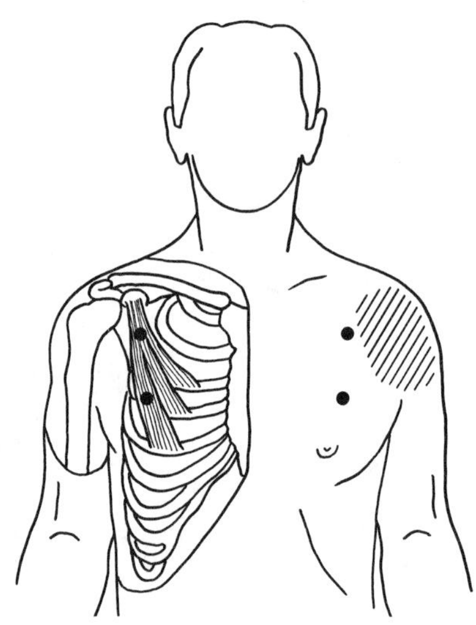

Figure 7.11 Pectoralis minor trigger points and referred pain pattern

The pectoralis minor muscle lies completely hidden under the pectoralis major and has a different orientation and very different attachments. Though generally a smaller muscle, it can still be very strong and thick. The pectoralis minor attaches at its upper end to the coracoid process, the odd little projection of the shoulder blade that sticks through to the front of the shoulder (Figure 7.11). With your arm at rest in your lap, you can feel the coracoid process as a hard roundness, something like a marble under the skin, just below your collarbone, next to the ball of your shoulder (the head of the humerus).

The other end of the muscle divides into three or more sections, which attach to individual ribs in the center of the breast area. The action of the pectoralis minor is to pull down on the coracoid process to fix the shoulder blade in place for various operations of the arm. A secondary function is to pull up on the ribs to help expand the chest during forced breathing, such as in vigorous sports activity. Trigger points in the pectoralis minor cause symptoms similar to those of pectoralis major trigger points, but a troubled pectoralis minor can have peculiar effects all its own, as illustrated by Aaron's case.

Aaron, *a fifty-two-year-old executive with an automobile company, had recurrent pain in the front of his left shoulder ever since he messed it up in a volleyball game ten years ear-*

lier. He also had numb fingers in his left hand most of the time. "I've tried everything, including a lot of physical therapy, but it just doesn't go away." In an effort to strengthen his shoulder, Aaron had been doing water aerobics in the pool at the YMCA, but so far, this had just made the pain worse.

Active trigger points were found in Aaron's scalene and pectoralis minor muscles. All were far more tender on the left side than the right. Pressure on his left pectoralis minor accentuated the pain in the front of his shoulder and the numbness in his hand. He could hardly believe the problem and its solution were so simple. After a single professional massage and instruction in self-applied trigger point massage, Aaron got rid of his chronic, long-term pain and numbness in less than three weeks.

Symptoms

The referred pain pattern for the pectoralis minor is nearly the same as for the clavicular section of the pectoralis major, being felt primarily in the front of the shoulder (Figure 7.11). Pain sometimes spills over to the entire breast area and the inner arm, inner elbow, ulnar (pinky) side of the hand, and third, fourth, and fifth fingers (not shown). As with trigger point symptoms in other muscles of the pectoral region, this distribution of pain can be mistaken for signs of heart disease. Other misdiagnoses can include thoracic outlet syndrome, cervical nerve root impingement, supraspinatus tendinitis, bicipital tendinitis, and medial epicondylitis (Simons, Travell, and Simons 1999, 844-852).

Tightness from trigger points often causes the pectoralis minor muscle to compress the neurovascular bundle, which consists of the nerves and major artery that supply the arm and hand (Figure 7.12). Blood flow to the arm and hand can be restricted in this manner by the pectoralis minor, even to the point of making the pulse at the wrist undetectable. Swelling in the hand and fingers, however, is not a symptom of pectoralis minor trigger points. Swollen hands are usually caused by tight scalenes compressing the axillary vein, which runs under the scalenes but not under the pectoralis minor (Simons, Travell, and Simons 1999, 847-851; Rubin 1981, 107-110).

Numbness in the forearm, hand, or fingers caused by a taut pectoralis minor squeezing the brachial nerves may be misdiagnosed as carpal tunnel syndrome or peripheral neuropathy. As you may recall, the scalenes provoke similar numbness and a similar misinterpretation. Pain from the scalenes is often sent to the chest in the exact location of the pectoralis minor and can be one reason for development of pectoral trigger points (Simons, Travell, and Simons 1999, 844-851).

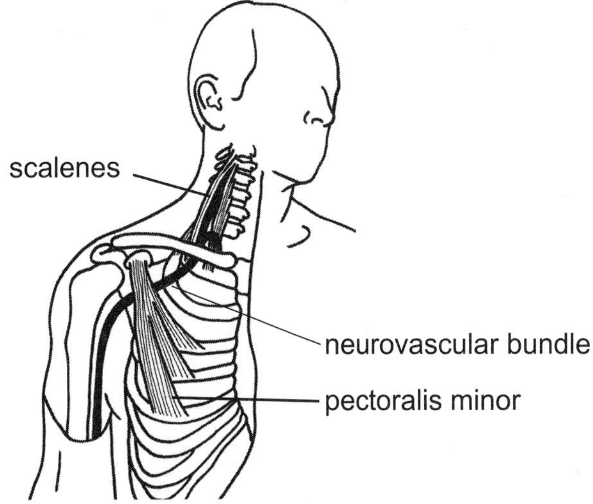

Figure 7.12 Neurovascular bundle (dark line), consisting of the nerves, artery, and vein that serve the arm and hand

The round-shouldered posture imposed by shortened pectoralis minor muscles can cause an ache in the mid back from the strain on the lower trapezius muscles. Excess tension in the pectoralis minor pulls the shoulder blade forward and causes it to stick out in back. This "winging" of the shoulder blade is made worse when the lower trapezius is weakened by its own trigger points and can't resist the pull of the pectoralis minor. This tightness in the pectoralis minor also restricts movement of the shoulder blade. As a consequence, it may be difficult to your raise arm above your head or reach for something behind you. Attempts at therapeutic stretching of the pectoralis minor are not advisable because of the stress placed on its vulnerable attachments (Simons, Travell, and Simons 1999, 852; Lewit 1991, 198-199).

Causes

Hyperventilation or a tendency to breathe shallowly, into the chest rather than the abdomen, can seriously overtax the pectoralis minor, as can a chronic cough. Whiplash injuries can overstretch the pectoralis minor muscles and set up trigger points. Pressure from the straps of a backpack or a heavy purse can cause them by cutting off circulation. Repetitive forceful, downward motions of the arms in sports or in the workplace can promote trigger points. A slumped, round-shouldered posture with the head forward can also set up trigger points in the pectoralis minor and make them very persistent.

If you have recurrent trouble with your pectoralis minor muscles, start watching for situations that tend to cause or perpetuate their trigger points. Under stress, you may be unconsciously holding your breath, hyperventilating, or breathing very shallowly. A hunched posture can be keeping your chest muscles shortened and tight. Heavy lifting will get you in trouble with the pectoralis minor, just as with the scalenes. Working for long periods with your arms out in front of you or up overhead will do the same.

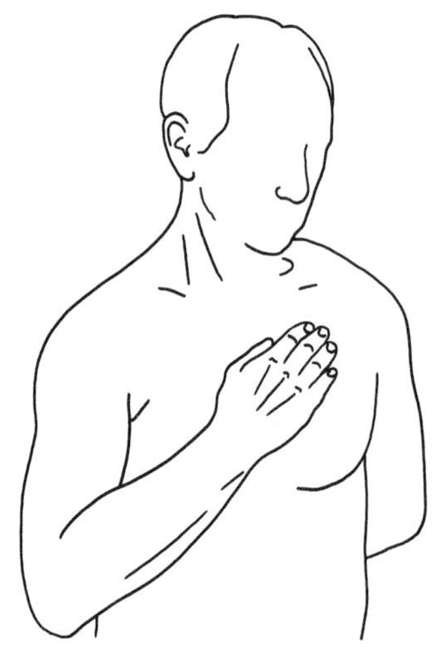

Figure 7.13 Locating the pectoralis minor. The hand behind the back is pushing against the wall.

Self-Treatment

You can locate the pectoralis minor by feeling it bulge up when it contracts. If you put your opposite hand on your chest as you would for the Pledge of Allegiance, your fingertips will be in the right position to feel the pectoralis minor contract (Figure 7.13). To make the pectoralis minor contract without contracting the pectoralis major, put your hand behind you and push back against a wall or the back of your chair.

There may be more than one trigger point in pectoralis minor muscles because of the varying length of muscle fibers in its different heads. Massage them with supported fingers, beginning at the coracoid process and pulling downward on a diagonal line across the chest with very slow, deep, short strokes. The "supporting" hand helps exert pressure (see Figure 7.5). For partner treatment and clinical treatment, use supported fingers for the pectoralis minor in the same way you'd use them for the pectoralis major.

Chest Muscles

There are only two chest muscles besides the pectorals whose trigger points can affect the shoulder. These are the serratus anterior and the diaphragm. Ironically, serratus anterior trigger points don't cause shoulder pain, although the muscle itself participates in many functions of the shoulder and arm and may need treatment in cases of serious shoulder dysfunction, such as frozen shoulder.

The diaphragm also has an odd role in that it neither sends pain directly to the shoulder, nor is it involved in operating the shoulder. But diaphragm trigger points may occasionally send pain to the upper trapezius, conceivably giving the diaphragm an indirect role in shoulder problems, especially in runners and other athletes who put extraordinary demands on the diaphragm in extended periods of forceful respiration. Interestingly, the diaphragm and the serratus anterior work together as part of your breathing apparatus. When one of them has trigger points, the other probably has trigger points too.

Serratus Anterior

Although the serratus anterior is located under the arm (Figure 7.14), it's actually a shoulder muscle. The muscle's attachments to your ribs and to the inner border of the shoulder blade gives it leverage for rotating the shoulder blade so that the socket of the shoulder joint faces more in an upward direction, allowing you to raise your arm. Without this ability to reposition the shoulder blade, you wouldn't be able to raise your arm above your head. The serratus anterior muscles also aid inhalation by assisting expansion of the ribs when you need more air than usual. Serratus anterior trigger points cause trouble for chest breathers like Judy, who habitually overwork them because of nervous tension.

Judy, *a twenty-seven-year-old social worker, got such a sharp pain in her sides when she was under stress that it was almost impossible to breathe. In her job, she was under stress every day. "When I've got that pain, I feel like I can only use about 10 percent of my lung capacity and I have to breathe quicker. I can't climb stairs, I can't move, I can't do anything! It's like I've got a metal band strapped around me. I can't take a deep breath at all, and if I laugh or cough or sneeze, it's just awful. I feel like I can't get enough air. I start getting dizzy. When it gets really bad, I get back spasms too."*

Extremely tender trigger points were found in Judy's serratus anterior muscles on both sides of her upper chest. She was shown how to do serratus anterior massage with her fingertips when she felt an episode coming on. Even when the attack is severe, she's usually able to get rid of the pain in her sides within a couple of hours. As a preventive measure, she's trying to learn to relax and breathe with her abdomen.

Symptoms

Pain from trigger points in the serratus anterior muscles is usually felt in the side and often in the mid back at the lower end of the shoulder blade (Figures 7.15 and 7.16). Note that the mid back pain pattern coincides with the trigger point in the iliocostalis thoracis and may be the factor perpetuating it. Sometimes pain spills over to the inner side of the arm and forearm and the pinky side of the hand (not shown). This pain pattern can suggest lung disease—or a heart attack if it's on the left side. Its true source can remain a mystery unless

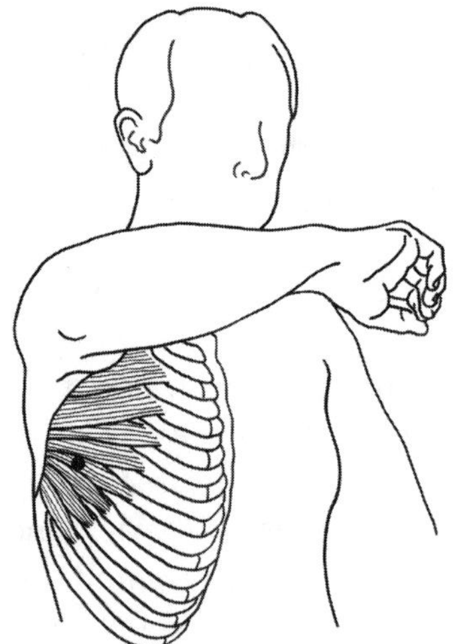
Figure 7.14 Serratus anterior primary trigger points may be in any of the muscle's branches.

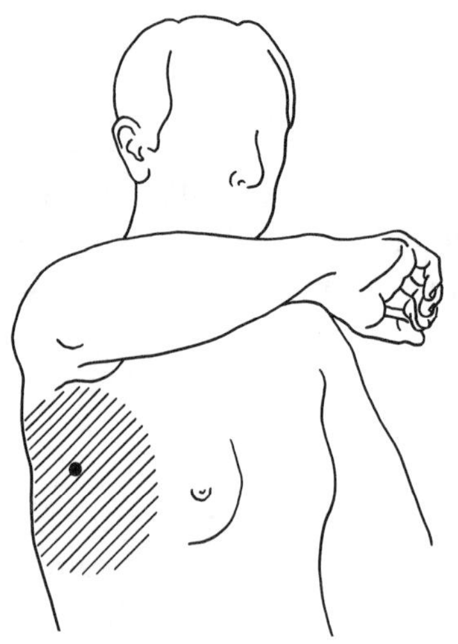
Figure 7.15 Serratus anterior referred pain pattern (side stitch)

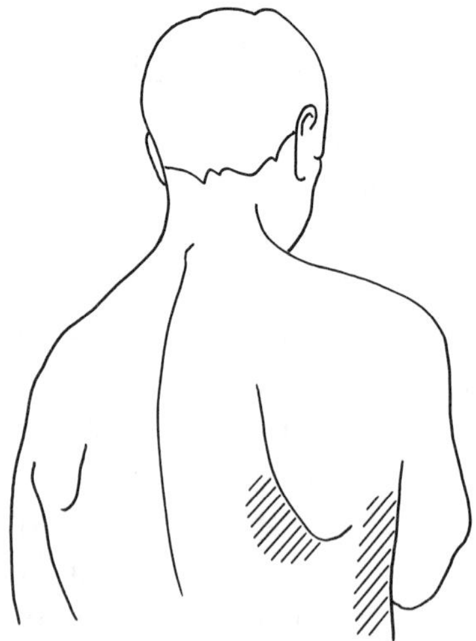
Figure 7.16 Serratus anterior referred pain pattern in the back

you're aware of what myofascial trigger points can do (Simons, Travell, and Simons 1999, 887-892).

With serratus anterior trigger points, you can't take a deep breath without pain, nor can you exhale completely. Diaphragmatic breathing hurts, so you're limited to shallow chest breathing. A troubled serratus anterior can be the main cause of the painful stitch in the side so familiar to runners. Side stitch can also come from trigger points in diaphragm, intercostal, or abdominal oblique muscles. Tightness in the serratus anterior makes it hard to reach back behind yourself or pull your shoulders back. The pull on your ribs can make your breasts feel abnormally sensitive (Simons, Travell, and Simons 1999, 887-894).

Emphysema isn't thought to promote trigger points in the serratus anterior, but when trigger points are present for other reasons, they can add significantly to the pain and difficulty in expelling air experienced by those with emphysema. When the serratus anterior is in trouble, additional stress is put on the scalenes, sternocleidomastoid, and serratus posterior superior, all of which aid in forced breathing. This can result in a growing cascade of symptoms, from headaches and jaw pain to dizziness and numb hands, making a long list of mistaken diagnoses possible (Simons, Travell, and Simons 1999, 892-894).

Serratus anterior trigger points don't directly limit the movement of the shoulder and arm. However, they do cause weakness in the muscle, which requires other muscles to work harder or in an unaccustomed manner. The pectoralis minor, trapezius, levator scapulae, and rotator muscles can all be affected, making the serratus anterior an unsuspected participant in shoulder trouble.

Causes

When you need extra breath quickly, as in any vigorous activity, the serratus anterior muscles assist respiration by pulling on the ribs to expand the chest. For this reason, athletic exertion can quickly overtax these muscles, especially when you're out of shape. It's usually amateur or weekend athletes who get a stitch in the side, not well-conditioned enthusiasts and professionals. Since the serratus anterior is so active in movements of the arm and shoulder, it's particularly vulnerable to unaccustomed participation in tennis, swimming, running, chin-ups, push-ups, weight lifting, and workouts on the pommel horse or the flying rings.

Respiratory illnesses that involve strenuous coughing can activate trigger points in the serratus anterior muscle, causing pain in your sides and back that can make you think you're progressing to pleurisy or pneumonia. Habitual tension and hyperventilation under emotional duress can activate latent trigger points in serratus anterior muscles. The pain they cause can make you fear the problem is worse than it really is, but the serratus anterior responds exceptionally well to self-treatment.

Self-Treatment

You can find the primary serratus anterior trigger point on the most prominent rib on your side. Search for it three or four inches straight down from your armpit at the level of your nipple—or where the nipple used to be, as one older woman remarked. Generally, this will be the site of greatest tenderness. When this trigger point is very active, you won't like touching it because it can really hurt. Luckily, it doesn't take much pressure to have a beneficial effect. Be aware, however, that trigger points can exist on any of the nine ribs this muscle attaches to. If you have trouble getting rid of the pain in your side, search the whole rib area under the arm, clear up into the armpit. Trigger points in the abdominal obliques that attach to your lowest ribs also cause pain in the side, as can trigger points in the diaphragm.

Part of the extreme discomfort experienced when you reach into your armpit to massage a subscapularis muscle probably comes from inadvertently applying pressure to nearby parts of the serratus anterior. The back half of the serratus lies between the subscapularis and the ribs. Picture your shoulder blade and ribs as the two slices of bread of a ham and cheese sandwich. Then visualize the subscapularis as the ham and the serratus anterior as the cheese. When your fingers are in the slot back of your armpit searching for the subscapularis, as in Figure 5.24, they're between the ham and the cheese. In this position, your nails contact the subscapularis and the flats of your fingers are on the serratus anterior.

The fingertips can be used for massage of serratus anterior muscles (Figure 7.17). To save your fingers, try using a tennis ball against the wall (Figure 7.18). Or just hold the ball in your hand and pull it slowly across the trigger point. Additional pressure can be applied by using your arm to clamp the ball and your hand against your side.

Simply being informed about the serratus anterior can keep you out of trouble. Stay alert for early symptoms, like the classic sharp stitch in your side when you take a deep breath or the sense that you can't get enough air. Early intervention with the serratus can stop trouble in its tracks. If you want to avoid trouble in the first place, remember that emotional stress promotes habitual muscle tension, which predisposes the

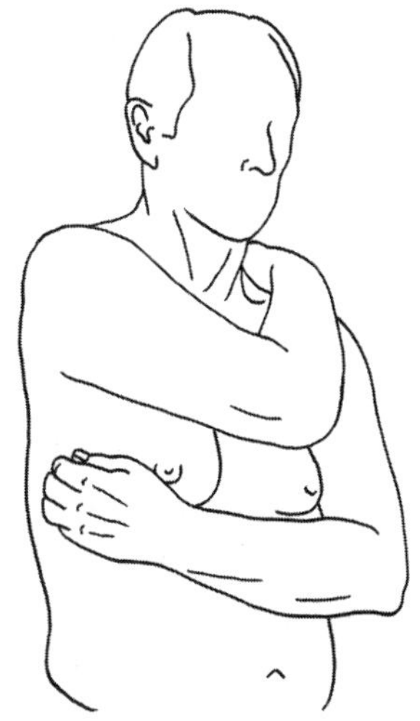

Figure 7.17 Serratus anterior massage using the fingertips

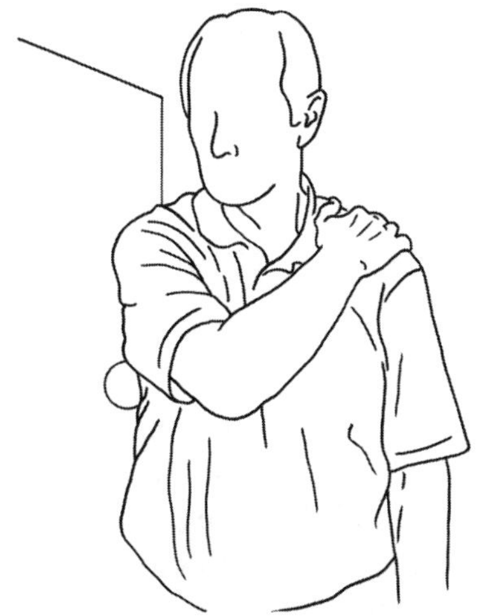

Figure 7.18 Serratus anterior massage with a ball against the wall

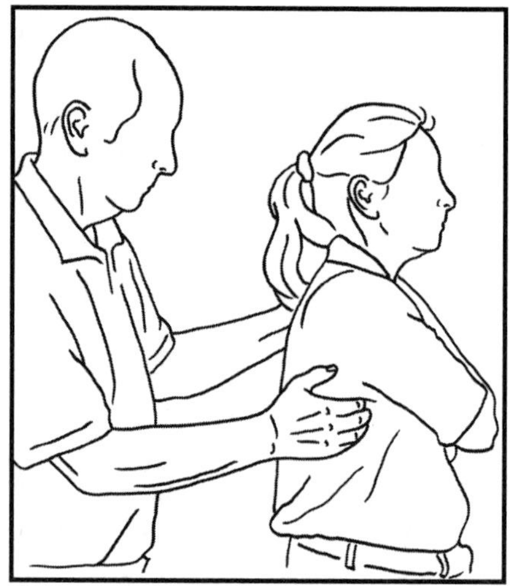

Figure 7.19 Serratus anterior partner massage with the fingertips

serratus anterior to trigger points. Learn to be aware of when you're holding your breath or breathing with your chest. It's also wise to avoid overdoing vigorous athletic activities, especially running, before you're in proper condition.

Partner Treatment

You may have some difficulty treating someone else's serratus anterior, because you'd have to use your fingertips (Figure 7.19), which would get the tickle response from almost everybody. If for this reason you can't treat the other person, you may be able to demonstrate how to self-treat.

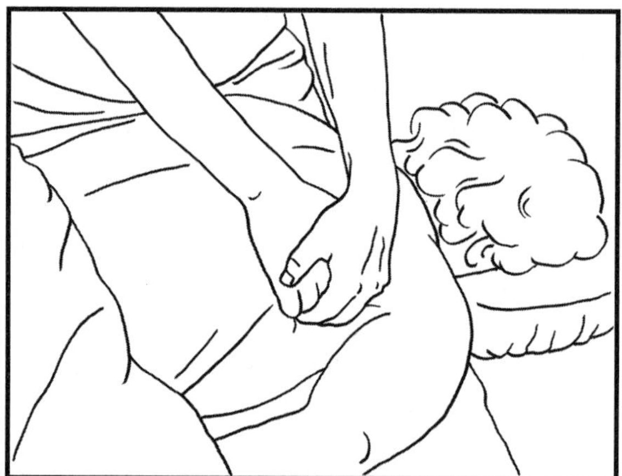

Figure 7.20 Serratus anterior massage with paired hands, three finger widths down from the armpit.

Clinical Treatment

The tickle response is much less likely to occur in the context of a full body massage with the client facedown. If you work cross-body as shown in Figure 7.20, you can simply hold your hands together and lean back a little to execute the stroke. It's also possible to approach the serratus anterior with the client faceup, using supported fingers (both palms up) on the side nearest you. When working on a woman, have her pull her breast out of the way.

A serratus anterior trigger point can be a horribly tender spot, so begin with great caution and watch the client's face for signs that you're being too aggressive. Keep asking for numbers on the pain scale. Don't ask, "Is this too much pressure?" A client who believes in "no pain, no gain" may not give you a truthful answer. Ask for a number; it's a much more exact measure, anyway. Remind the client to keep breathing and to concentrate on relaxing.

Diaphragm

The diaphragm is a thin muscle inside the body that separates the organs of the chest from those of the abdomen. It attaches to the inside of the lowest ribs all the way around. At rest, the diaphragm has a dome shape, bowing up into the lower chest. When you inhale, the diaphragm contracts and pulls down, flattening out and creating a vacuum in the chest that causes the lungs to inflate. To exhale, ordinarily all you do is relax the diaphragm. To inhale properly, the lower abdominal organs must move out of the way to make room for the diaphragm to come down.

A number of muscles can't be treated with massage because they are simply too deep inside the body to be accessible. The muscles lining the inside of the chest fall into this class.

Luckily, the muscles that make the most trouble are on the outside. The diaphragm muscle is on the borderline. Most of it is inaccessible, of course, but the edge of the diaphragm can be reached where it attaches to the ribs in front. It's precious little access to this important muscle, but it's enough to do a significant amount of good.

Symptoms

Trigger points in the diaphragm cause pain under the ribs in front near the muscle's attachments behind the bottom ribs (Figure 7.21). You can also have pain in your sides—the classic side stitch—a little lower than the pain from the serratus anterior (not shown). Pain from diaphragm trigger points typically occurs on exhalation, whereas with the serratus anterior it's worse on inhalation. Trigger points in either muscle give you a sense of shortness of breath.

Myofascial pain associated with the ribs is frequently mislabeled costochondritis, or inflammation of the ribs. Or you may be told you have a separated rib, gastroesophageal reflux, ulcers, or gallbladder trouble. Treatment for these conditions is unlikely to solve the problem when trigger points are the cause (Simons, Travell, and Simons 1999, 862-879).

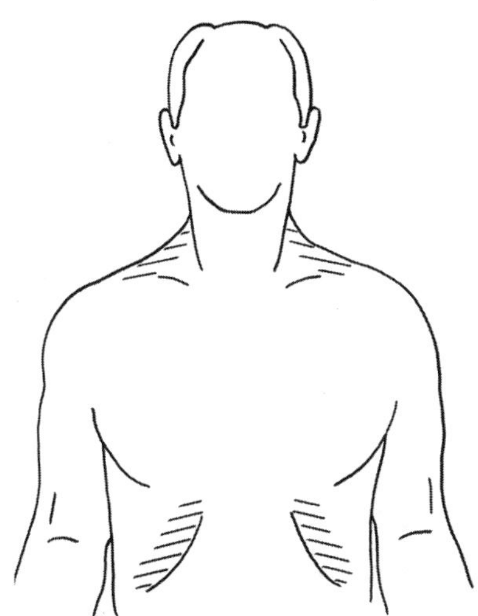

Figure 7.21 Diaphragm referred pain pattern. The trigger points are hidden behind the ribs.

Causes

Emotional distress, a chronic cough, chest breathing, and overexertion in athletics can all cause trigger points in the diaphragm, as can a slumped posture or any condition that makes you struggle to get your breath. If you strive to keep your stomach in at all times for the sake of your appearance, you unnecessarily hamper the mechanics of natural breathing. But you don't have to let it all hang out over your belt, either. Try to find a reasonable compromise.

Self-Treatment

To treat the diaphragm trigger points that are accessible, dig under your ribs in front with supported fingers and do as much deep stroking massage as you can manage, up to twelve strokes per trigger point (Figure 7.22). This area is easier to access if you exhale completely and pull your stomach in. This also stretches the diaphragm, which can be beneficial when done along with the massage. For the deepest

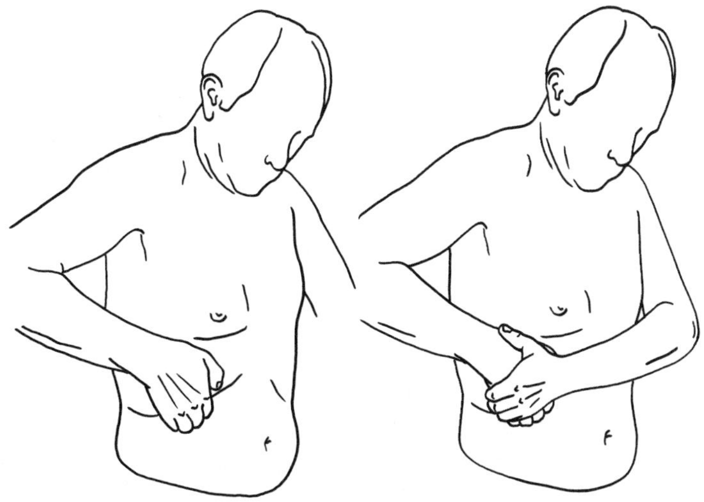

Figure 7.22 Diaphragm massage up under the ribs with supported fingers. For the deepest penetration, sit down and lean forward.

penetration, sit and lean forward or lie on your back with your knees up. Any work you do on the diaphragm's peripheral trigger points will benefit other trigger points in its unreachable central dome. Note that taking a deep breath can overcontract your diaphragm, so it's wise to avoid extreme athletic exertion until you've made some progress with the trigger points.

Partner Treatment

You probably won't be called on to treat someone else's diaphragm since access to it lies in a fairly personal space. However, you might want to demonstrate the self-treatment technique for someone who's having trouble getting the hang of it. If you have occasion to treat a friend or family member, make sure you commence cautiously and gently. There can be extremely tender trigger points in the abdominal muscles in this same area, and the diaphragm trigger points themselves can be horribly painful if you press too hard.

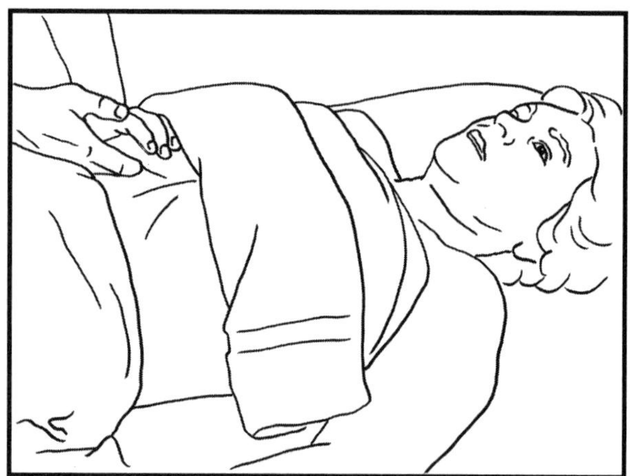

Figure 7.23 Diaphragm massage up under the lowest rib with supported fingers

Clinical Treatment

Treatment of the diaphragm will be integrated into your abdominal massage protocol, the only difference being the insertion of your fingers up under the ribs (Figure 7.23). To counter the sense of invasiveness, stroke very slowly and calmly. When the client allows abdominal massage, it implies a great deal of trust. This is where you must be at your best: calm, centered, and controlled. Work as though you were treating a baby or small child.

Upper Arm Muscles

Bodybuilders have an intense interest in their upper arm muscles and are likely to know the anatomical names of all four of them: the biceps, brachialis, triceps, and coracobrachialis. Everyone else is inclined to ignore this important group unless the muscles begin to hurt. When your upper arm muscles are out of condition, your job or recreational activities can put demands on them that easily exceed their strength and endurance. The upper arm muscles have to support the weight of whatever is in your hand, whether it's a baby, a bag of groceries, or a heavy tool. In athletics, sometimes the upper arm muscles are called on to support the weight of the entire body. Simply getting in and out of chairs or in and out of your car can sponsor trigger points in the upper arm muscles, especially if you're carrying a few extra pounds of body weight.

Trigger points in any of your four upper arm muscles can contribute to pain in the shoulder. The function of the shoulder can be affected too, because three of the four upper arm muscles cross the glenohumeral (ball-and-socket) joint to attach to the shoulder blade.

Biceps

The biceps has two heads, the short head attaching to the coracoid process, the long head attaching to the shoulder blade just above the socket (Figure 7.24). This attachment to the shoulder blade lets the biceps help raise the arm. The two heads come together to attach to the radius bone of the forearm, which allows the muscle to bend the elbow and help turn the hand over with the palm side up.

Another extremely important function of the biceps is to participate in keeping the arm firmly in its socket. Many muscles work to maintain this joint, but without the biceps it would be impossible to carry any weight at all without pulling the joint apart. Biceps trigger points weaken the muscle, making other muscles work harder than usual in order to compensate.

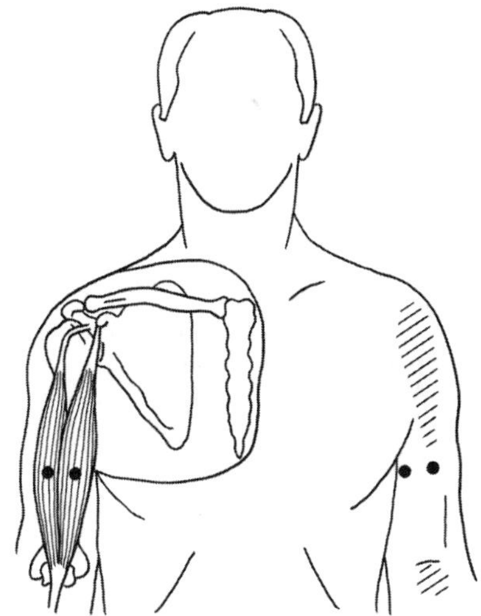

Figure 7.24 Biceps trigger points and referred pain pattern

Symptoms

Trigger points in the biceps cause pain or aching in the front of the shoulder and just below the crease of the elbow (Figure 7.24). They can cause pain in the biceps itself when the muscle contracts. You may also experience weakness in the arm and difficulty in completely straightening your arm with your palm facing down. A vague ache may occur in the upper trapezius area behind the shoulder (not shown). Pain referred to the shoulder from the biceps may be mistaken for subdeltoid bursitis, bicipital bursitis, bicipital tendinitis, or arthritis.

You may get a sharp catch in your shoulder when raising your arm, which some will mistakenly diagnose as impingement syndrome. The biceps tendon in the front of your shoulder can become extremely tender, which may be labeled tenosynovitis, but it's usually only a secondary effect of trigger points in the long head of the biceps. Treating the site of the pain in the shoulder won't help if biceps trigger points are causing the problem (Simons, Travell, and Simons 1999, 648, 654).

Causes

Referred pain from the infraspinatus, scalene, or subclavius muscles can create trigger points in the biceps. Other common causes of biceps trigger points are overexertion in sports, lifting heavy weights at arm's length with the palm up, and exercises that strongly flex the elbow, such as chin-ups. Repetitive strain in the workplace—repetitively turning a screwdriver, for example—can also exhaust the biceps (Simons, Travell, and Simons 1999, 652).

Be mindful of any activity that necessitates maintaining a contracted biceps. Playing the violin, for instance, requires keeping the left biceps in continuous contraction to keep the hand in the correct position on the fingerboard. Violinists' right biceps muscles often develop trigger points from the continual contracting and lengthening during bowing.

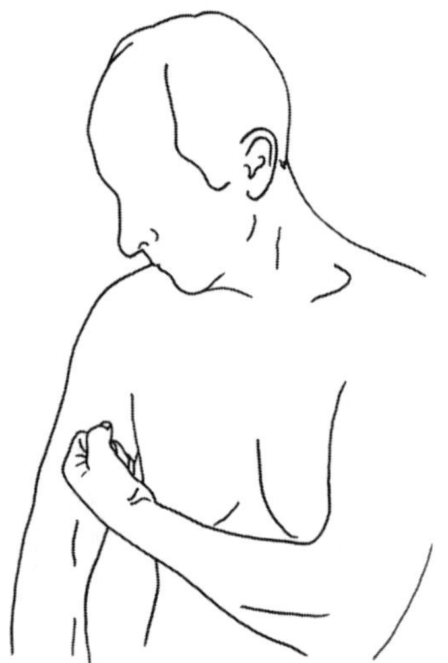

Figure 7.25 Biceps massage with the knuckles of a loose fist

Self-Treatment

Trigger points may be found in either head of the biceps at the midpoint of the muscle. Massage the muscle with a supported thumb or rake it deeply with the knuckles of a loose fist (Figure 7.25). It's a waste of time and energy to get caught up in massaging the tender referral area on the front of the shoulder.

Partner Treatment

As with self-treatment, use a loose fist for treating someone else's biceps. Support the person's arm with your other hand, as shown in Figure 7.26. Remember that there may be a trigger point in each head of the muscle, located approximately side by side about halfway down the front of the arm. There's no need to massage the whole length of the muscle.

Clinical Treatment

Treat the client's biceps with the same loose fist technique that you would use in treating yourself or informally treating a friend or relative (Figure 7.26). To really zero in on a specific trigger point, use supported thumbs (Figure 7.27). It's important to find out how the client spends the day, because specific activities cause specific kinds of pain.

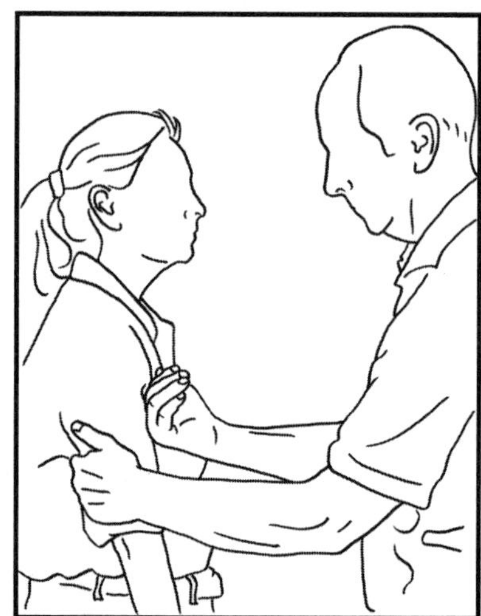

Figure 7.26 Biceps partner massage with the knuckles of a loose fist

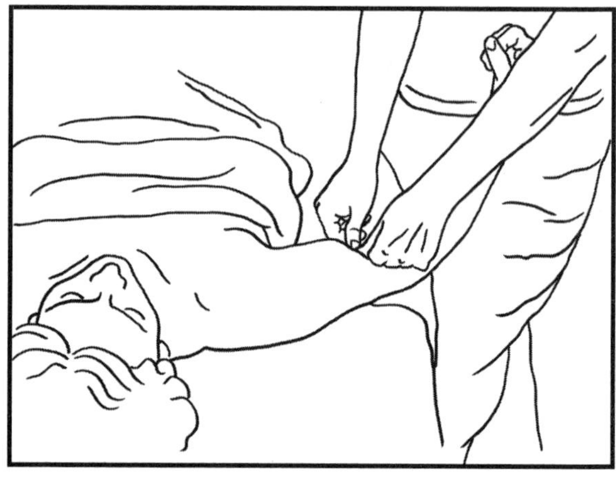

Figure 7.27 Biceps clinical massage with supported thumbs

Emma, *age twenty, majored in the oboe and minored in the cello. Both instruments contributed to her chronic pain. Playing the cello gave her pain in her right biceps and made her shoulder pop when she was bowing. Playing the oboe gave her a constant ache at the base of her right thumb that grew worse when she was holding the oboe. Playing either instrument made the front of her shoulder ache.*

Trigger points were found in many muscles, all on the right side, where Emma was having all her trouble. Her scalenes, sternocleidomastoid, forearm muscles, and all four rotators were involved, but the muscles in her upper arm were the worst of all because they were the ones most severely overused in her intense practice schedule.

Emma was highly motivated to learn how to self-treat her problems since her health insurance wouldn't pay for professional massage (even though it had paid for many sessions of chiropractic and physical therapy, which had done less for her than a single trigger point massage). Within three weeks of beginning to treat her own biceps and brachialis muscles, the pain in her right arm and shoulder had become negligible. Even the shoulder popping had stopped.

Brachialis

The brachialis muscle is the workhorse of the elbow, doing much of the work normally credited to the biceps, such as bending your elbow to lift something. The brachialis lies under the biceps, covering the front of the lower half of the humerus (Figure 7.28). Its upper end attaches to a bony mound on the outer surface of the humerus about halfway down, just below the attachment of the deltoid muscles. The other end of the brachialis attaches to the ulna, one of the two bones of the forearm.

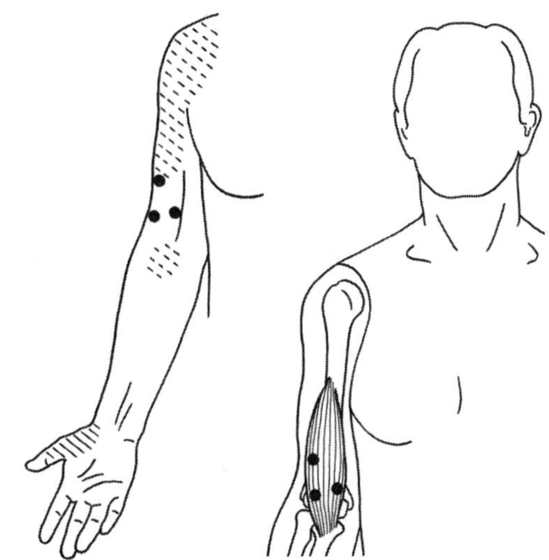

Figure 7.28 Brachialis trigger points and referred pain pattern. The dotted lines indicate occasional or vague pain.

Symptoms

Brachialis trigger points make it difficult to straighten the elbow, but the pain they create is felt primarily at the base of the thumb (Figure 7.28). They can also create less intense pain in the front of the shoulder and just below the crease in the elbow. There may be an oppressive ache or tightness on the outside of the upper arm near the elbow. Compression of the radial nerve, which passes through the brachialis, can make the thumb and the back of the forearm tingle or feel numb (Simons, Travell, and Simons 1999, 660-663).

Many muscles are capable of referring pain to the base of the thumb, but the brachialis and scalene muscles are always the prime suspects. It's natural to massage the thumb when it hurts, but remember that it isn't going to solve the problem if the pain is being sent from somewhere else.

Causes

Many kinds of activity overwork the brachialis. A frequent cause is keeping the elbow bent while under a load—carrying heavy bags of groceries, carrying a baby around, picking up growing children, or carrying a purse hanging on the forearm. Brachialis muscles are also stressed by holding up heavy tools for long hours and by any repetitive action of the elbow. You can foster trigger points in your brachialis muscles by doing too many chin-ups or by any other strained bending of the elbow in exercise or sports. Working all day at a computer keyboard with your arms held out in front of you requires continuous contraction of the brachialis muscles of both arms. For this reason, computer users nearly always have brachialis trigger points.

You may not be aware of the connection between your symptoms and an activity that overworks one or both of your brachialis muscles. This often happens to musicians who have to hold their instrument up in front of them for long periods of time. Oboe players, for example, often suffer from chronic pain and numbness in the thumb of their right hand, which has to continuously support the weight of the instrument. Though the thumb itself may seem to be in trouble because that's where the pain is felt, the real problem is in the brachialis muscle, which has to stay contracted the entire time the oboe is being held. Oboists and other musicians with this problem should put the instrument down at every opportunity and let the arm hang at their side, allowing the brachialis to lengthen and relax. Frequent self-applied trigger point massage, however, is the best remedy. While appropriate rest is a vital part of any therapy for trigger points, trigger point massage attacks the problem directly.

Self-Treatment

Brachialis trigger points are found under the outer edge of the biceps, just above the crease of the elbow (Figure 7.28). Push the biceps aside to access the brachialis and massage it against the bone with a supported thumb (Figure 7.29). Note that the arm getting the massage is braced against a table. You can also brace your arm against your thigh. The trigger point that causes nerve entrapment lurks in a slippery sort of lump in the muscle, about the size and shape of an almond, a short way above the elbow on the outside of the arm. This lump tends to squirt out from under a supported thumb, but it's less elusive when worked with a ball against the wall. Occasionally, trigger points occur under the inner edge of the biceps, the side closest to the body.

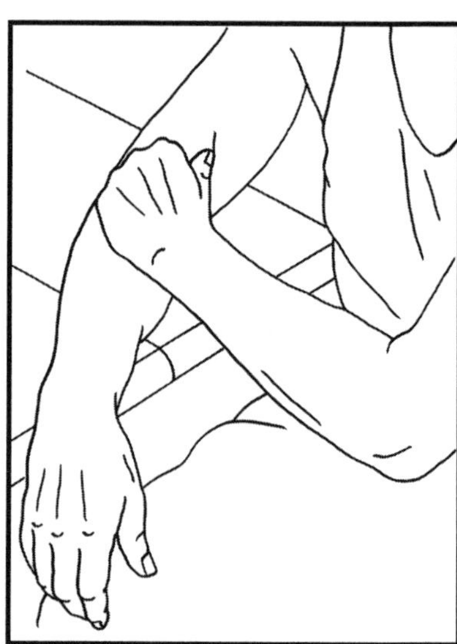

Figure 7.29 Brachialis massage with a supported thumb, pushing in under the biceps with the thumb

Partner Treatment

You need to use a supported thumb to get to the brachialis muscle, which is completely covered by the biceps (Figure 7.30). Support the person's arm with your other hand. Obviously, you'll want to check the brachialis any time you're treating the biceps, and vice versa. Use a supported thumb to work on both muscles.

Clinical Treatment

Treat the client's brachialis muscle with a supported thumb for ease in getting under the biceps (Figure 7.31). Slacken the biceps and brachialis by keeping the elbow slightly flexed. Begin just above the crease in the elbow for the trigger point causing thumb pain. Work your way about halfway up the arm, still trying to work underneath the biceps. Search for the "almond" if thumb numbness is an issue.

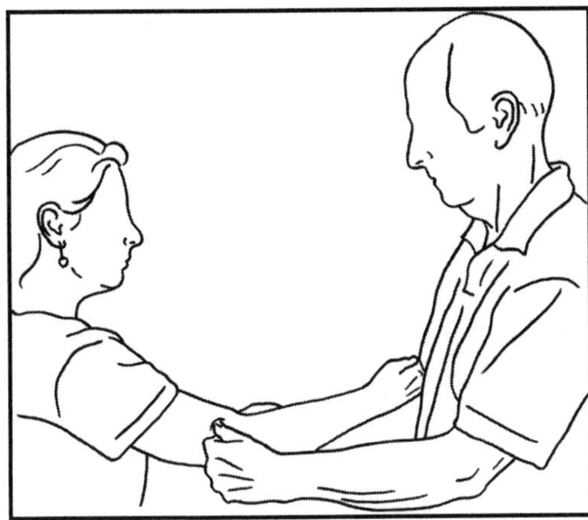

Figure 7.30 Brachialis partner massage with a supported thumb, supporting the arm with the opposite hand

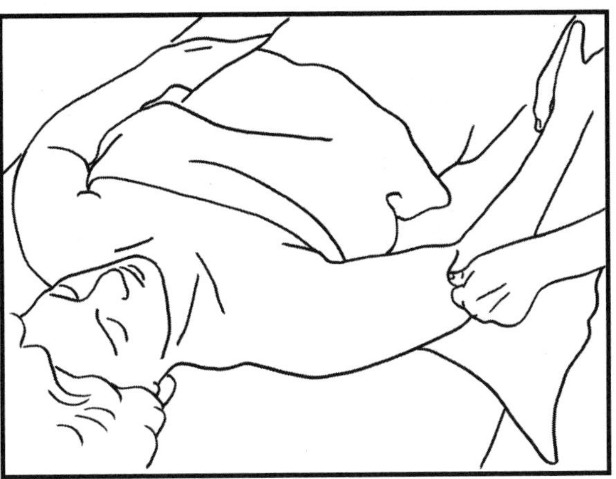

Figure 7.31 Brachialis clinical massage with a supported thumb pushing the biceps aside

Triceps

The triceps is a long, broad muscle with three branches or heads. The attachment of the long head of the triceps to the shoulder blade helps keep the arm in its socket. The lateral and medial heads attach to the humerus. The medial head lies right on the bone under the other two heads and is sometimes called the "deep" head. All three heads come together to cross the elbow joint and attach to the ulna, one of the two bones of the forearm. This gives the triceps great leverage for straightening the elbow. Triceps trigger points occur at five different sites and evoke five different pain patterns.

Symptoms

Triceps trigger point #1 sends pain to the back of the shoulder, the outer elbow, and sometimes to the back of the forearm (Figure 7.32). When bad enough, it can cause an ache in the upper trapezius, the base of the neck, and the triceps itself (not shown). Although this is the most common triceps trigger point, its location in the inner half of the triceps (closest to the body) makes it easy to overlook (Simons, Travell, and Simons 1999, 667-668).

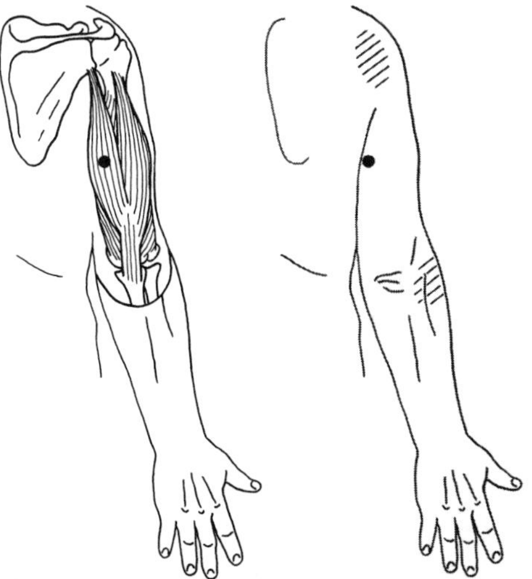

Figure 7.32 Triceps #1 and referred pain pattern in the back of the shoulder and in the outer elbow

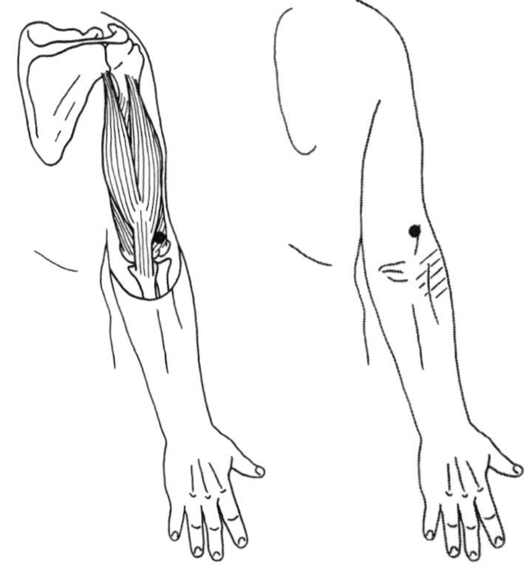

Figure 7.33 Triceps #2 and referred pain pattern in the outer elbow

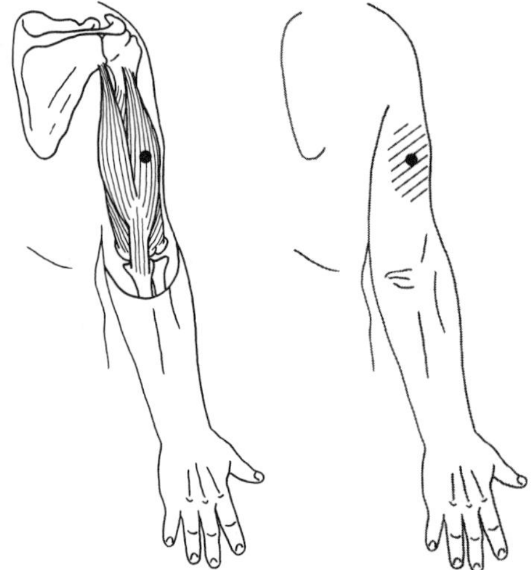

Figure 7.34 Triceps #3 referred pain pattern, an ache in the triceps itself

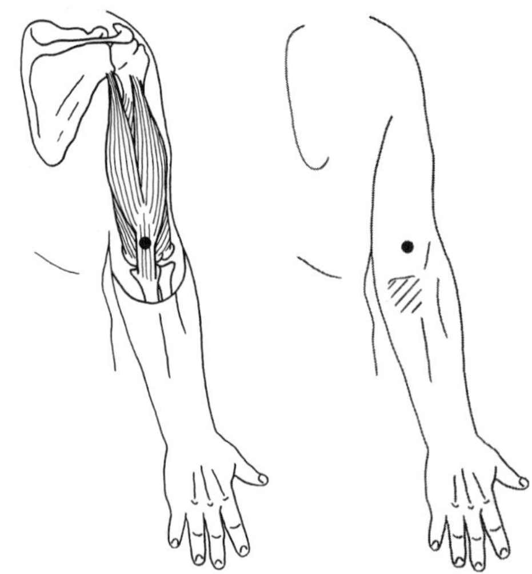

Figure 7.35 Triceps #4 and referred pain pattern in the point of the elbow

Triceps trigger point #2, being very close to the elbow where the muscle is relatively thin, is also easy to miss. It's one of many sources of the pain in the outer elbow known as tennis elbow or lateral epicondylitis (Figure 7.33). Pain may extend some distance down the back of the forearm (Simons, Travell, and Simons 1999, 668-669).

Triceps trigger point #3 causes local pain in the back of the upper arm in the triceps itself (Figure 7.34). It has special importance because it can keep the lateral head tight enough to compress the radial nerve, causing numbness in the back of the forearm and wrist and in the thumb side of the hand. Pain, numbness, or tingling may also occur in the fourth and fifth fingers (Simons, Travell, and Simons 1999, 668-669).

Triceps trigger point #4 makes the *olecranon* (oh-LEH-cruh-non) *process*, or the tip of your elbow, hypersensitive to touch (Figure 7.35). Simply resting the elbow on a tabletop or the arm of a chair can be painful. It can even hurt when the elbow just touches your side (Simons, Travell, and Simons 1999, 668-669).

Triceps trigger point #5 refers pain to the inner elbow and sometimes to the inner forearm (Figure 7.36). It hurts to tap the *medial epicondyle*, the bony knob in the inner elbow. Pain at this site is sometimes called golfer's elbow or medial epicondylitis (Simons, Travell, and Simons 1999, 668-669).

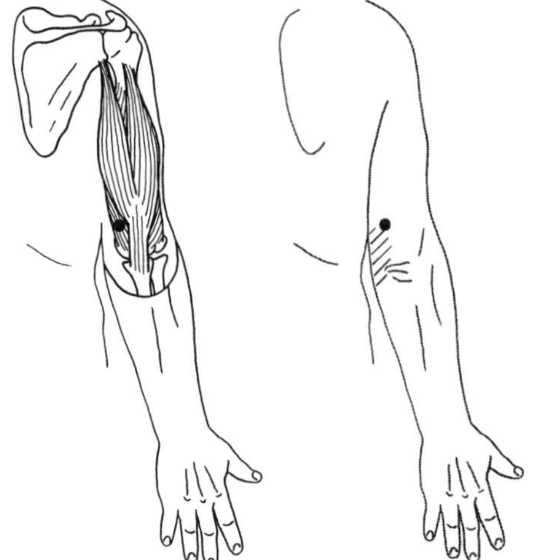

Figure 7.36 Triceps #5 and referred pain pattern in the inner elbow

When active enough, any of these trigger points can cause pain in the fourth and fifth fingers. Any of them can also create an oppressive sense of achiness in the back of the forearm and in the triceps itself. Triceps trigger points can be expected to weaken the elbow and limit it in both bending and straightening (Figure 7.37). Arthritis, tendinitis, epicondylitis, and olecranon bursitis are common explanations for pain referred to the elbow by the triceps when the effects of trigger points haven't been considered (Simons, Travell, and Simons 1999, 674-677).

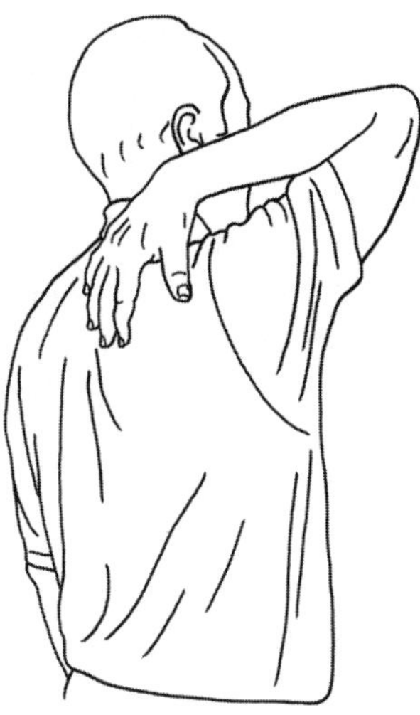

Figure 7.37 Triceps trigger points prevent this

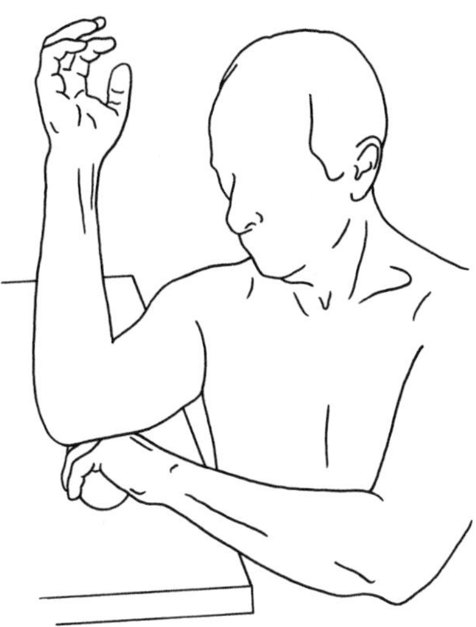

Figure 7.38 Triceps massage with knuckles supported by a ball. (This can also be done against the chest.)

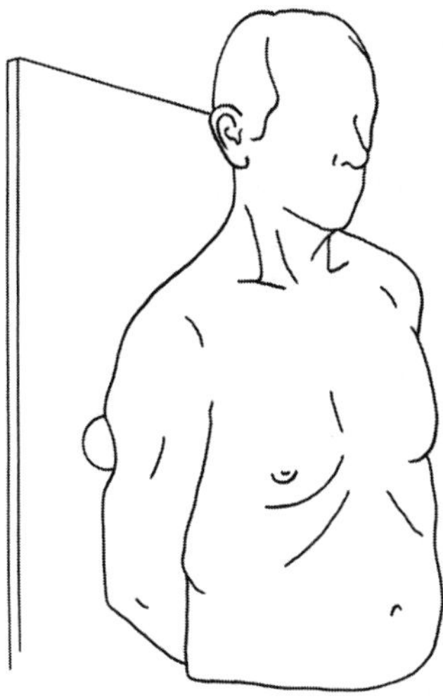

Figure 7.39 Triceps massage with a ball against the wall, with hands together and the elbow bent

Causes

Overexertion in sports or the workplace can create trigger points in the triceps, particularly any strong, repetitive pushing action. Simply holding something down for a long time can make the triceps knot up. Sometimes trigger points in the triceps are satellites of unsuspected trigger points in the latissimus dorsi or the serratus posterior superior (Simons, Travell, and Simons 1999, 677).

Self-Treatment

A convenient and effective way to massage the triceps is with your knuckles, using a tennis ball to give support to your hand (Figure 7.38). This technique works best on a desktop, tabletop, filing cabinet, or even the top of an old-fashioned upright piano. You can also use the ball-and-knuckles trick against your chest or on your knee. You'll have maximum access to all three heads of the triceps and their trigger points using a ball against the wall (Figure 7.39). Clasp your hands behind you and bend your elbow unless stiffness and pain in the shoulder prevents it.

Take special note that the three trigger points in the medial (deep) head are in a line across the back of the arm just above the elbow (Figures 7.33, 7.35, and 7.36). Travell and Simons stress the fact that this deep head is the "workhorse" of the triceps and especially prone to trigger points. Even so, when the triceps is in trouble, you will very likely find that all five trigger points are active.

Partner Treatment

Paired thumbs are an excellent tool for searching out and treating someone else's triceps trigger points (Figure 7.40). It's important to have a very clear mental picture of the structure of the muscle and where each of the three heads lies. The long head is nearest the

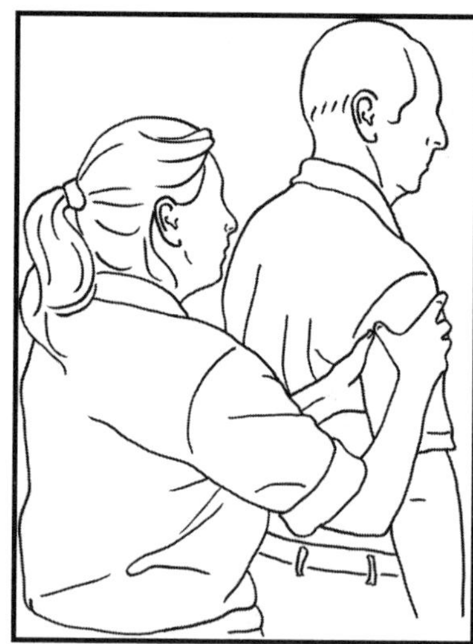

Figure 7.40 Massage of the lateral head of the triceps with paired thumbs, and the long head between the fingers and thumb of the left hand

body. The lateral head is furthest away. The medial head, or deep head, covers the lower third of the back of the upper arm all the way across. You may want to knead the trigger points in the long head by rolling them between your fingers and thumb. The person receiving the treatment can guide you to the exact locations of the tender spots if you can get within an inch or so of them.

Clinical Treatment

Treat the client's triceps with the client facedown. Use paired supported thumbs and stroke away from yourself, using body motion and your weight to do the work (Figure 7.41). For specific treatment of the long head and the medial trigger point in the medial head, use the pincer grip and roll the trigger point between your fingers and thumb (Figure 7.42).

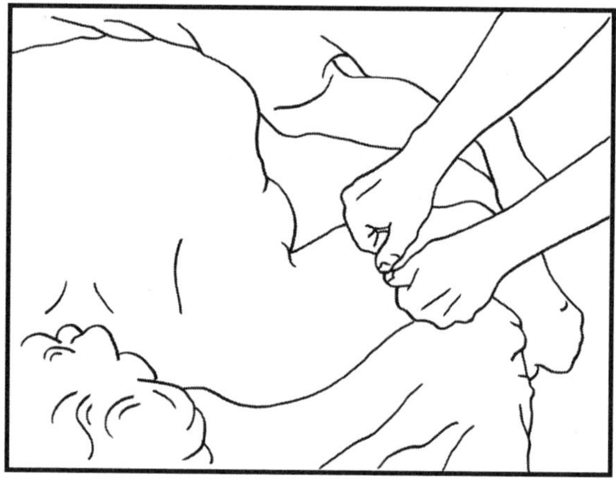

Figure 7.41 Triceps clinical massage with supported thumbs

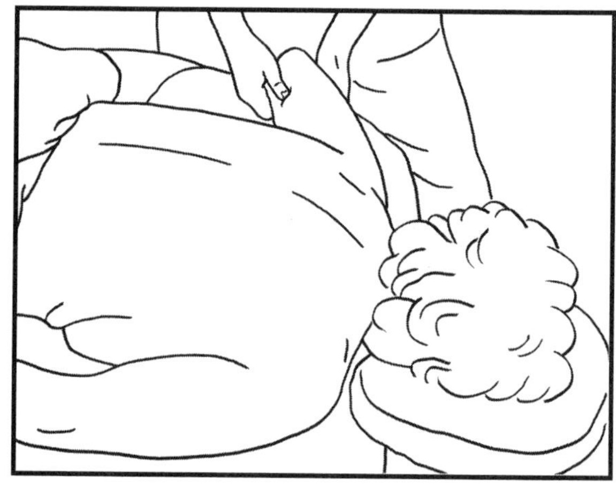

Figure 7.42 Triceps clinical massage, kneading the medial head

Sherry, *age sixty-nine, had recently taken a trip to see her young grandsons. It had entailed carrying her own suitcases and lifting the youngest boy numerous times. By the time she got home, she was suffering numbness in her right thumb and pain in her right biceps and forearm. In addition, things began unexpectedly falling from her hands, and the pain in her shoulder, arm, and hand was keeping her awake at night.*

Trigger points were found in Sherry's rotator cuff muscles, her scalenes, and in all four of her upper arm muscles, including the triceps. All were muscles that had been overtaxed by the unaccustomed heavy lifting that had pulled so strongly on her right arm and shoulder. Three days later she called to report she'd had no pain at all since the massage.

Given Sherry's age and the severity of the muscle strain, it wouldn't have been surprising if her shoulder and arm trouble had eventually progressed to a frozen shoulder. It

was a lesson in how well trigger points respond when given timely and appropriate treatment.

Coracobrachialis

The coracobrachialis lies between the biceps and the triceps on the inner side of the upper arm (Figure 7.43). The muscle is a little larger than your index finger and about twice as long. At its lower end, it attaches about halfway down the upper arm bone. At its upper end, it attaches to the coracoid process, the little piece of the shoulder blade that sticks through to the front of the shoulder. The action of the coracobrachialis pulls the arm tight against the side.

Symptoms

Pain from coracobrachialis trigger points is felt in the anterior deltoid, the triceps, the back of the forearm, and the back of the hand (Figures 7.43 and 7.44). The more active the trigger points are, the more extensive the pain pattern becomes. Under extreme conditions, pain may reach as far as the end of the middle finger. You may not become aware of the involvement of the coracobrachialis in this pattern until more obvious trigger points in the shoulder and upper arm have been deactivated. Trigger points in this muscle can make it difficult to put your arm behind your back or raise it up overhead. A coracobrachialis shortened by trigger points can also squeeze the nerves that supply the arm, causing numbness in the biceps, forearm, hand, and fingers (Simons, Travell, and Simons 1999, 638-644).

Causes

Examples of activities that can strain the coracobrachialis are push-ups, rock climbing, rope climbing, swimming, throwing a ball, and playing golf and tennis. Any job that requires repeatedly pulling something downward can stress the coracobrachialis. The way to continue these activities without pain is to become proficient at self-treatment of the coracobrachialis or any other muscles that are particularly vulnerable. Make it a practice to

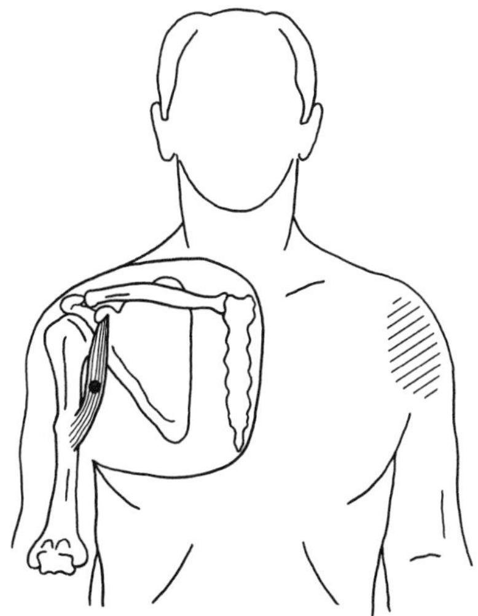

Figure 7.43 Coracobrachialis trigger point and referred pain pattern

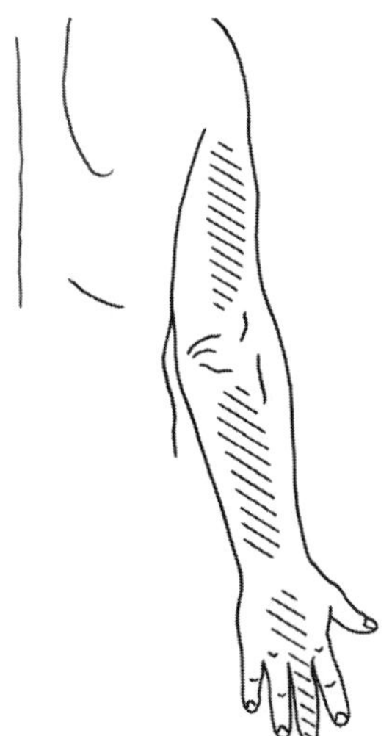

Figure 7.44 Coracobrachialis referred pain pattern

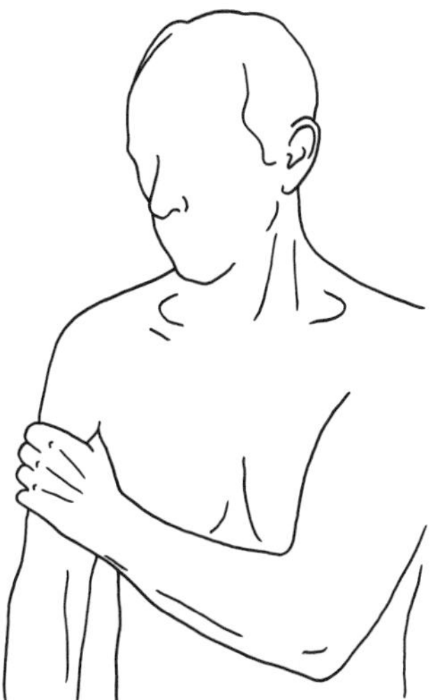

Figure 7.45 Coracobrachialis massage with the thumb

give yourself a little bodywork before and after engaging in anything that puts the muscles under unusual stress. Also be careful about lifting anything heavy with your arms stretched out in front and your palms up.

Self-Treatment

To locate the coracobrachialis, press your thumb against the inner side of the humerus as high up as you can (Figure 7.45). You can feel the muscle contract at this location when you clamp your elbow tight against your side. Massage the trigger points with gentle cross-fiber strokes of the thumb, taking care to stay on the muscle. Major nerves to the arm run alongside the coracobrachialis in this area, so be conservative with your pressure.

Partner Treatment

Use the position shown in Figure 7.46 to treat someone else's coracobrachialis muscles. If you have the person push down on your shoulder repeatedly, you can feel the muscle repeatedly contract, allowing you to zero in on it. The trigger point will be fairly high up on the inner side of the arm. Treat it with several gentle strokes of your fingertips, but even this can be extremely painful if you use too much pressure. This is a muscle that's probably best left to self-treatment, so once you've located the trigger point, you can show your partner how to self-treat it.

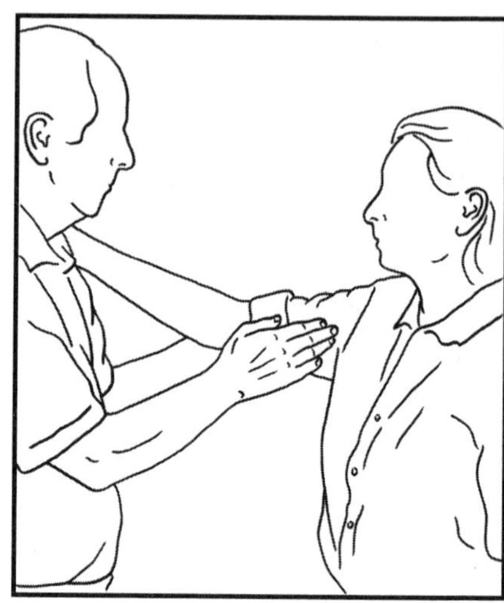

Figure 7.46 Coracobrachialis partner massage with the tips of the fingers

Clinical Treatment

Approach the client's coracobrachialis very cautiously, keeping in mind that much of the neurovascular bundle travels down the inner arm right beside it. This is not a large muscle, so the middle and ring fingers of one hand are quite adequate for the job (Figure 7.47). Feel for the muscle immediately behind the biceps. If you're still unsure of its location, have the client press repeatedly against your other hand in a medial direction (toward the client's own body). Use a few slow strokes to get the healing processes started, then show the client how to self-treat this sensitive area.

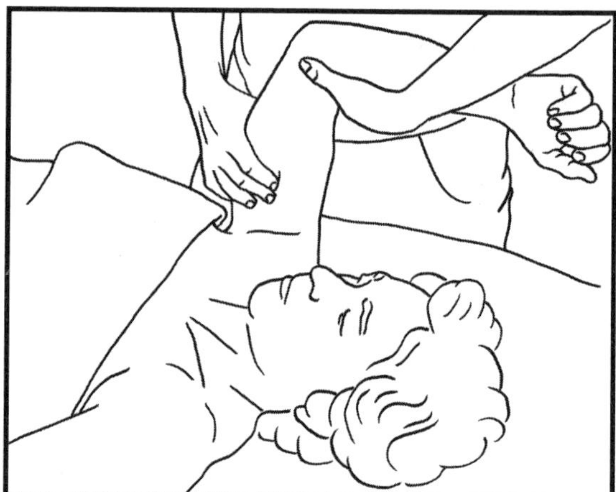

Figure 7.47 Coracobrachialis clinical massage with the index and middle fingers

Chapter 8

Alternative Bodywork Therapies

Stress and Trigger Points

Frozen shoulder tends to occur at times of unusual stress in your life, such as a new responsibility, a family crisis, the loss of a job, or a serious health problem—some threatening change from the ordinary. Even something as common as a fall can leave you in a state of subconscious fear and watchfulness. Anything that increases your emotional stress creates a state of increased physical tension, which is fertile ground for the development of myofascial trigger points. The end result, of course, may not be a frozen shoulder. It can be a spell of low back pain, daily migraine headaches, chronic knee pain, temporomandibular joint trouble, or any other manifestation of myofascial pain syndrome (Simons, Travell, and Simons 1999, 220-221).

You may not be aware of a connection between stress and your shoulder problem, but stress can be a significant part of the situation, and it can definitely interfere with your recovery. This is because stress can make trigger points hard to get rid of. One reason for this is that stress is distracting and very wearing, and that alone can undermine all your best intentions. It's why people go off their diets, and it's why you can go for days without doing your trigger point massage.

Furthermore, stress keeps your muscles tight and in a defensive mode. In this way, stress can be a trigger point perpetuator and is often a primary cause of trigger points in the first place. Stress can also make it hard to get a good night's sleep. If your muscles are exhausted from lack of rest, trigger point massage won't be as effective as it otherwise might be—if you can get yourself to do it at all.

Dealing with the insidious effects of stress should be part of any therapy for a frozen shoulder. Even a minor case of chronic shoulder pain could be a signal that all is not right in your life. Taking action against stress can make all the difference in the treatment of your shoulder trouble, or any other kind of chronic pain.

Obviously, there are dozens of ways of dealing with stress. This chapter is devoted to a number of methods you may not have considered: the alternative bodywork therapies. There are approximately fifty varieties being practiced. As a rule, these aren't systems for self-treatment, as self-applied trigger point massage is. Ordinarily, a practitioner trained in a specific form of bodywork will give you the therapy or guide you through it. Despite the somewhat dubious claims about what the various alternative bodywork therapies actually do, nearly all tend to be soothing to both the body and the emotions. The calming effect of an alternative bodywork therapy may be its major benefit.

None of the alternative therapies can equal trigger point massage in its direct effect on your trigger points. Nonetheless, there may be one or more that may work for you in reducing your tensions and helping to make the treatment of your trigger points more effective. For the most part, alternative therapies have little potential for harm. The biggest problem is that medical insurance generally won't pay for them, even if you would gladly testify in court that they helped you when conventional medicine didn't.

The promotional language for alternative therapies can be very seductive, but you won't be able to judge whether any of them will work for you until you've actually given one a try. In choosing an alternative form of therapy, consider that the method itself may be less important than the personality of the practitioner. It must be someone you intuitively like and trust. This is because most alternative therapies are delivered through physical touch. They have little chance of working for your benefit unless you feel comfortable and safe with the person who is providing the touch. Trust your intuition in this. You'll know in the first session whether the therapy and the therapist are going to be right for you.

The Power of Touch

There is enormous healing power in human touch that science hasn't been able to adequately explain. The merit in the laying on of hands has been spoken of from the very beginning of recorded history. The Greeks, Romans, Egyptians, and other early civilizations all knew its value. The Bible refers to the laying on of hands repeatedly and it's an essential part of faith healing. Most methods of manual therapy can be viewed as systems that formalize human touch and make it socially permissible and safe (nonsexual). The massage and bodywork professions go to great lengths to promote the ethics of safe touch among their practitioners.

Human touch seems to have become a fearful thing in our society today, largely because of the media's preoccupation with sex. "Did someone *touch* you?" is often the first question in an inquiry into suspected abuse, assault, or molestation. The very concept of touch often assumes a connotation of evil. As a consequence, some people rarely if ever feel the touch of another human being, particularly if they live alone, as a great number of people do these days. If you happen to be in that situation, it can seem very abnormal to submit to bodywork of any kind. Men often have more trouble with this than women, but men can gain enormously from hands-on bodywork if they can get past their self-imposed limits.

Placebo Power

Many people enthusiastically attest to the results they've attained with some alternative treatment for their pain. Most alternatives have probably been praised by someone for curing a frozen shoulder. Disbelievers in alternative therapies credit the placebo effect for whatever actual gains that seem to have taken place. But does this necessarily make a placebo a bad thing? On the contrary, belief in a positive outcome is of paramount importance in any kind of therapy. Expectations have great therapeutic value, even when the treatment falls within the bounds of orthodox medical practice. A scientifically valid treatment can be effective on someone who doesn't believe in it, but its effectiveness can be markedly improved when you do believe (Chaitow and DeLany 2000, 93).

Science has become very interested in the placebo effect, not for the sake of excluding it, but for making use of it. Physicians have always relied on the placebo effect. The prescription scratched on an official-looking piece of paper, the framed diplomas on the wall, the white coat and stethoscope—they can all be seen as uses of the placebo effect. The Latinate medical names given to your problem are classic placebos used to impress upon your mind that the doctor has special knowledge. Even the bill you receive contains an element of the placebo. The more you have to pay, the greater confidence you're likely to have that you're getting the best treatment possible.

The amazing thing about placebos is that they appear to help relieve pain in almost everyone on some level. Innumerable studies have shown that sometimes a placebo can entirely stop your pain even in the absence of any other kind of treatment. Sometimes they actually work better than the treatment itself! That's why researchers are so careful to set up double-blind studies, where neither the doctor nor the patient knows what is in the little pill. The number of people who get better with a sugar pill is a demonstration of the power of the placebo.

There is ongoing criticism of bodywork therapies for not having been subjected to double-blind studies. But it's impossible to do an unbiased double-blind study of hands-on treatments because there's no way to keep the experimenter and the subjects in the dark about what's going on. The only reasonable recourse is to honor the placebo effects of touch and consider them a valuable part of the therapy. Fortunately, the placebo effect is becoming an integral component of the new holistic paradigm. New practitioners in all fields are now being taught that the benefits of the placebo effect shouldn't be denigrated. To the contrary, they should be maximized (Jamison 1994, 339-345).

In *The War on Pain*, Scott Fishman, MD, gives evidence that the placebo effect may not be merely a psychological phenomenon. Your thoughts and beliefs have everything to do with the chemistry of the brain, where pain is ultimately registered and evaluated. In reality, thoughts manifest themselves in electrochemical reactions. Dr. Fishman contends that changing your thoughts can make changes in your brain's chemistry. Since the chemistry of the brain intimately affects the chemistry of the rest of the body, it makes perfect sense that your thoughts can have at least an indirect physical effect on your experience of pain. In short, if you believe that a particular treatment is decreasing your pain, it's probably no illusion, and your belief may actually be the critical factor in making it work (Fishman and Berger 2000, 100-121).

The Continuing Role of Self-Treatment

Along with exploring the following alternative therapies, don't give up on self-treatment, even if you seem to be getting nowhere with it. Some people have difficulties with the self-treatment of trigger points, especially those who aren't technically minded. The muscles can be quite mystifying, hidden as they are from view beneath the skin.

It takes a while to weed through the mysteries and develop real skill with self-treatment. Keep coming back to it, doing a little every day if possible. Have the patience to give yourself a chance to learn self-therapy. Self-care is empowering. In time, it can become a valuable life skill that you'll always have—literally at your fingertips. It may take longer to learn than you want, but if you keep trying you will get better at it. Like anything else in life, if you never give up, success is inevitable.

Manual Methods

The wide range of bodywork styles can be overwhelming. To classify the types of bodywork and give some coherence to this confusingly diverse mix, they're divided in this chapter into three categories: purely manual methods, energy therapies, and movement therapies. These therapies can sometimes be useful adjuncts to trigger point therapy, but please observe the cautions below about when specific types of alternative therapy may be contraindicated.

It's very common for therapists to integrate two or more styles of bodywork. Your first choice among manual bodyworkers should be someone who is also highly skilled at trigger point massage. You may be surprised to learn that many chiropractors are taking an interest in trigger point therapy because they've found that it greatly increases the effectiveness of their other methods.

Chiropractic

The word "chiropractic" literally means "done by hand." Its creator, Daniel David Palmer, believed that nerve impingement by subluxations, or small dislocations, in the spinal column caused damage to tissues served by the nerve, resulting in various kinds of disease. His original method was simply a matter of moving individual spinal vertebrae (bone setting) by various ways of twisting and levering the spine. The presumed effect was to improve vertebral alignment, take the pressure off the spinal nerves, and thereby cure a long list of troublesome conditions. Although chiropractic has always been largely concerned with back pain, it has also claimed success with high blood pressure, migraine headaches, gynecological problems, asthma, bed-wetting, earache, dizziness, repetitive strain injury, hyperactivity, indigestion, and infertility.

An Eclectic and Controversial Profession

Over the years, chiropractic has developed great affinity for the holistic, whole body approach. As a consequence, chiropractic these days is rarely pure manipulation of the spine. It often includes a large range of other therapies, such as massage, traction, diathermy, ultrasound, electrostimulation, stretching exercises, acupuncture, acupressure, homeopathy, hydrotherapy, and counseling on nutrition and herbal remedies. So-called Touch for Health, or muscle testing, has become extremely popular in chiropractic.

Some of the manual treatments used in the chiropractic office are very similar to standard physical therapy methods. Chiropractic, however, hasn't earned the acceptance and respectability enjoyed by the physical therapy profession. Because of certain unvalidated practices, chiropractic has been viewed from its beginnings, and even up to the present day, as being poisoned by rampant quackery. One such practice is the ubiquitous use of X-rays, which many people have come to see not only as unnecessary and just another way to pad the bill, but also as a possible danger to their health.

Other questionable practices seem to have arisen in response to justified criticisms. As an example, a heavily promoted, spring-loaded device is now used by many chiropractors to gently thump your vertebrae into place. This method is intended to supercede the traditional way of making a spinal adjustment with the fearful bone-crunching rapid thrust that most identifies chiropractic in the public mind. With this new device, treatment isn't painful and patients aren't required to remove their clothing for adjustments. This makes a visit to the chiropractor fairly uncomplicated and quick. Although the new gadgets are promoted as scientific breakthroughs, there's no evidence that they actually do anything except capitalize on the placebo effect and make chiropractors less liable to lawsuits. Although chiropractic has always been an extremely controversial profession, it seems to have easily as many supporters as it has detractors. Clearly, chiropractic isn't going to go away.

Better Than a Real Doctor?

The reasons that chiropractic continues to survive are worth examination. To begin with, people often go to the chiropractor as a reaction to ineffective and hideously overpriced medical treatment. Some contend that if the medical profession had ever truly lived up to its pretensions, there would never have been a need for chiropractors. Medical doctors insist that chiropractic is not only fraudulent and useless, but that people have been permanently injured and even killed by it. When defenders of chiropractic hear such accusations, they can rightfully point to the fact that many times more people die from prescription drugs and surgical errors each year than have been harmed by chiropractors in the one hundred years they've been around.

The fact is that an enormous number of people feel good about chiropractors and trust them more than they do medical doctors. The chiropractic field may be filled with individuals engaged in fraudulent schemes, but if you believe that your chiropractor has helped you, who's to say you're wrong? If you have pain and whatever happened in the chiropractor's office seems to have made it go away, you're going to be a believer. And why not? Does orthodox medicine, with its sometimes fatal prescription painkillers, ever deliver more?

Chiropractors and Trigger Points

Since some people claim that chiropractic got rid of their shoulder pain, it's something worth looking into. Some of the procedures now used by chiropractors would actually work quite well on the trigger points that cause shoulder problems. Travell and Simons, for example, tentatively endorse therapeutic ultrasound and electrostimulation when applied directly to specific trigger points. These are methods that many chiropractors use. Other methods in the chiropractic bag of tricks, such as acupressure and acupuncture, could also be expected to have a positive effect on a shoulder problem when used primarily for deactivating specific trigger points (Simons, Travell, and Simons 1999, 146-147).

Because they're well trained in anatomy and skilled in hands-on manual treatment, chiropractors have great potential for treating pain with trigger point therapy. The most encouraging development in the field of chiropractic in the last ten years has been its increased employment of trained massage therapists who specialize in treating trigger points. If the trend continues and chiropractors abandon some of their less-effective routines, it could work toward erasing some of the profession's tarnished image. Whichever health care profession makes the best use of trigger point therapy will end up dominating all others in the treatment of pain. Why not chiropractic?

CranioSacral Therapy

CranioSacral Therapy is a system of subtle adjustments applied to the *craniosacral system*, which consists of the cranium, spine, and *sacrum* (the large triangular-shaped bone at the lower end of the spine). The critical premise of the craniosacral system and CranioSacral Therapy is that the cranial bones have the freedom to move and accommodate changes in the volume of the cerebrospinal fluid.

Cerebrospinal fluid is a shock absorber in the craniosacral system and is continuously being renewed. As old fluid is reabsorbed and new fluid flows in, pressure in the system rises and falls at the rate of about 10 cycles per minute. This regular fluctuation produces an extremely slow pulsing called the "cranial rhythm" or "cranial wave." Variations of pressure in the cerebrospinal fluid are believed to have a vital influence on the operation of all the body's other systems, including immune responses and emotions. Manipulation of the bones in the craniosacral system, including the bones of the skull, can change the cranial rhythm and does appear to have curative effects on many conditions (Upledger 1997, 17-19).

The Movement of the Skull Bones

Whether the cranial bones are actually capable of movement has long been the subject of dispute, despite the fact that thousands of therapists have learned to sense rhythmic movements in the cranial bones and modify them when needed. A skilled therapist can feel the sides of the head move in and out almost imperceptibly at the speed of the cranial rhythm. Craniosacral therapists joke among themselves that this is the "skinny-head, fat-head effect." The entire body responds to this rhythm, which can be monitored nearly anywhere on the body but is most easily felt at the level of the shoulders, hips, and feet. Lack of movement at these places indicates constrictions somewhere in the cerebrospinal system, which can cause chronic pain, discoordination, low energy, and emotional and neurological dysfunctions.

Large numbers of osteopathic and chiropractic physicians, physical therapists, and massage therapists endorse the cranial wave theory and practice CranioSacral Therapy. Orthodox medical doctors adamantly deny that the cranial bones are free to move, insisting that the suture joints of the skull fuse and become immobile before adulthood. Interestingly, this medical myth is not a doctrine that is held worldwide. Medical students in Italy, Israel, and other parts of the world are taught that the joints of the cranium permit very slight but detectible movement even into old age. These movements were actually measured electronically in experiments during the 1970s at Michigan State University (Upledger 1997, 142-150). Sadly, orthodox medicine in the United States tends to isolate itself from any evidence that challenges time-honored beliefs. Too often, physicians are handicapped by their education.

Cranial Osteopathy

The cranial wave was first brought to light in the early twentieth century by an osteopath, William Sutherland, who perceived that the skull minutely expanded and contracted at a very slow but measurable speed. He experimented on himself by immobilizing the movement of his own cranial bones and found that it resulted in depression and motor problems. Sutherland also discovered that small movements in the spine and sacrum were synchronous with the cranial rhythm in the skull. He went on to develop a system for manipulating the bones of the skull, spine, and sacrum that seemed to result in improvement in specific conditions and general health. For decades, Sutherland's technique, known as *cranial osteopathy*, was quietly practiced by a limited number of osteopaths and chiropractors until researchers at Michigan State, led by osteopath John Upledger, brought CranioSacral Therapy into full bloom.

Craniosacral Treatment

Training in Craniosacral Therapy involves developing the ability to sense and evaluate the cranial rhythm and constrictions at various locations in the client's body. These constrictions can be released by applying light, sustained pressure to certain places on the head, jaws, neck, spine, and sacrum. Treatment at each place lasts from a few seconds to as long as five minutes, or until a release is felt. The theory is that applying a small force over a long time gets a more effective response from the body than a strong, quick force, as in a traditional osteopathic or chiropractic adjustment. Remarkably, the gentle, motionless touch is so calming that patients frequently go right to sleep.

CranioSacral Therapy encourages the body to make its own adjustments, improving the functioning of the brain and the circulatory, respiratory, neural, hormonal, muscular, and digestive systems. Upledger, the principal developer of the current system, relates very convincing case histories of successful treatment of coma patients, the brain injured, colicky babies, and those with residual back pain after disk surgery. Other examples of problems purportedly treated with success include TMJ dysfunction, headaches, earaches, sinusitis, asthma, facial pain, chronic pain, chronic fatigue, anxiety, nervousness, hyperactivity, attention-deficit disorder, dyslexia, autism, post-traumatic stress disorder, and depression. Several patients tell of good outcomes with shoulder and arm pain (Upledger 1997, 20-36, 45-51).

It's reasonable to speculate that CranioSacral Therapy might serve as a valuable adjunct to trigger point therapy, and vice versa. A few preliminary therapeutic strokes to critical trigger points could make the body give up its craniosacral constrictions much more easily. By the same token, adjustments to the craniosacral system could possibly make trigger points easier to deactivate. In any event, CranioSacral Therapy is fundamentally without risk. As Dr. Upledger says, "the worst thing that can happen is *nothing*."

Medical Massage

If massage were done by a physician or someone supervised by a medical doctor, it could legitimately be called "medical massage." But as practiced today, medical massage is nothing of the sort, and it doesn't carry the endorsement of the medical community. Therapists trained in "medical" massage schools use the same methods taught in conventional massage schools. In both kinds of school, students take medical classes, like physiology and anatomy, which presumably equip them to know when massage is or is not an appropriate treatment.

The same number of hours of instruction and practice are required to become a medical massage practitioner as for becoming a licensed massage therapist: five hundred to a thousand hours depending on the state. That's not very many hours of study compared to the number needed to become a physician, physical therapist, nurse, or even a chiropractor. In truth, the standards of education and proficiency need to be raised in both kinds of massage school. Since the financial motive is predominant for most massage schools, they find it very difficult to flunk anybody out for stupidity or incompetence. It doesn't speak very well for the certification and licensing process, which hinges almost entirely on a student having simply been present for the required hours.

A great many practitioners of medical massage are registered nurses who freely capitalize on their nursing degree to gain status in the field of massage therapy. While it's true that nurses have extensive training in things medical, it doesn't necessarily make their massage more medically effective. The only part of medical massage that could distinguish it from generic Swedish massage is its strong emphasis on joint manipulation and stretching. These are exactly the modes of therapy to be avoided in the early stages of treatment of a frozen shoulder.

The saving grace in the field of medical massage is the growing number of practitioners who incorporate trigger point massage into their routine. Be aware, however, that the medical massage practitioner's overriding concern with enforcing movement in joints could be particularly risky for the vulnerable connective tissue of a shoulder.

Myofascial Release

The object in myofascial release is to stretch the fascia in troubled areas of the body. You'll remember that fascia is the thin, pliable connective tissue that covers muscles and other body elements like a complex, finely woven net. With this bodywork modality, more attention is actually given to the fascia than to the muscles (Chaitow and DeLany 2000, 145-147).

Fascia gives the muscles strength, support, and elasticity. Ultimately, fascia is what gives the body its shape. Interestingly, surgeons thread their sutures through the fascia, not the muscle tissue, when making surgical repairs. The tensile strength is in the fascia, which will hold the sutures, whereas muscle tissue will tear out. Under normal conditions, movement keeps fascia well hydrated and pliable. When movement is limited for whatever reason, fascia tends to lose its water content and become dried out, shrunken, and stiff. Some theories hold that it's the stiffness of the fascia and not stiff muscle that causes stiffness in the joints.

To stretch fascia therapeutically, sustained gentle pressure is applied, usually for several minutes. Multiple releases of the fascia are sought through successive "barriers." Fascia has *viscous flow*, a characteristic that allows it to be slowly deformed into a new shape, which is then retained to a high degree. This is different from elasticity, which lets a material return quickly to its original size and shape.

In myofascial release treatment, gentle forces are applied in various ways, including static compression and skin rolling, in which the skin is pinched and rolled between the fingers and thumb. Muscles are also pushed, pulled, and twisted in directions that will encourage the fascia to soften, lengthen, broaden, and separate. When a barrier is reached and the fascia resists further change, light pressure is maintained for up to five minutes. When the barrier is breeched, the therapist's hands will feel the motion and the softening of the tissue. As with CranioSacral Therapy, results come with gentle pressure applied patiently over time. Just before a release, the therapist will often sense a so-called therapeutic pulse and an increase of heat in the area.

Myofascial release treatments can be carried out with your clothes on. If treatment is done without clothing, no oil is used on the skin so that the hands can have high-friction contact for the sake of the manual stretches. Myofascial release is too nonspecific to be used to directly deactivate trigger points, but the two methods are often combined to amplify the effects of both.

Myotherapy

Manual trigger point therapy was introduced in 1980 by physical therapist Bonnie Prudden with the publication of *Pain Erasure: The Bonnie Prudden Way* (1980). Since then, she and several protégés have taught her method, which she calls *myotherapy*, to practitioners in many fields. Prudden's concept was to make trigger points release by means of ischemic compression (pressing and holding). As a traditional physical therapist, she also placed a strong emphasis on exercise and stretching. Prudden's ideas have had a broad influence in the field of therapeutic massage, and many therapists get very satisfactory results using ischemic compression of trigger points.

The trigger point massage method described in this book improves on Prudden's original method in several respects. With myotherapy, for instance, there's significant risk of applying excessive pressure and causing needless pain in the hope of attaining an immediate result. The distinguishing element in this book's method is to limit treatment of a given trigger point to six to twelve very short strokes, without requiring an immediate release. This approach is much less tiring for the therapist's hands and fingers, with no sacrifice of effectiveness. Trigger points can generally be trusted to release on their own without stretching, as the body heals itself in response to the treatment. Both methods accomplish the same thing in "erasing" your pain, however, if intelligently applied.

Neuromuscular Therapy

Neuromuscular therapy is a form of trigger point therapy that combines Swedish massage, ischemic compression, and myofascial release. This method focuses on softening of both fascia and muscle tissue. Swedish effleurage (gliding strokes) are used to search for trigger points and to generally relax the musculature. Trigger points are treated with the familiar press-and-hold technique. Myofascial release is frequently accomplished while applying pressure to specific trigger points (Chaitow and DeLany 2000, 108-114, 123).

Neuromuscular therapy is taught widely in massage schools and weekend seminars. In practical terms, it's virtually the same as myotherapy. Both approaches could be expected to benefit shoulder problems, provided that the practitioner truly understands how to find and treat trigger points in all twenty-four muscles that may be involved. With both methods, it's important that the therapist be mindful of the risks involved in trying to stretch the rotator cuff muscles before the trigger points have begun to release.

Osteopathy

Osteopathic medicine, or osteopathy, was originally a practice that, like chiropractic, used strictly manipulative techniques for correcting spinal abnormalities thought to cause a wide spectrum of diseases. Over the past century, however, osteopathy has developed into a practice comparable to orthodox allopathic medicine. In addition to traditional manipulation techniques, osteopaths are now permitted to perform surgery and prescribe drugs. Many osteopaths now do very little spinal manipulation.

Osteopaths use a much more diverse set of therapeutic modalities than conventional allopathic physicians, so there may be osteopaths in your community who have begun integrating some form of trigger point therapy into their practice. In addition to treating your shoulder with trigger point massage, an osteopath would be permitted to do trigger point injections. This procedure, which involves injecting procaine (Novocain) directly into trigger points, can deactivate trigger points and bring long-lasting relief. Some insurance plans will pay for a limited number of trigger point injections, since they're considered a legitimate medical treatment for pain. Unfortunately, trigger point massage is rarely covered, even though it's equally effective without being invasive.

Rolfing

Rolfing, a trademarked therapy originated by Ida P. Rolf, is taught only at the Rolf Institute in Boulder, Colorado. Although Ida Rolf called her therapy *structural integration*, it's universally known as *Rolfing* to the public and among certified practitioners. Though practitioners are scarce, Rolfing is well-known because of being unusually deep massage with a reputation for being extremely painful. An initial course of ten treatments is designed to correct long-standing rigidity and tightness in your muscles and the fascia that envelops them.

Ida Rolf believed that the body retains a memory of physical trauma, which is stored in muscles and fascia. In response to trauma, these tissues stiffen, robbing you of your flexibility and range of motion. The muscles then have to work harder to accomplish even ordinary tasks. The resultant stresses quickly exhaust your energies and capacity for self-healing, leaving you vulnerable to chronic pain and many forms of ill health. Emotional traumas supposedly also become entrapped in the inflexible structures. With Rolfing, physical inflexibility and emotional issues are said to resolve at the same time.

Each treatment session is devoted to a particular body area, the first session usually dealing with the neck and upper back. Each area is given a carefully structured treatment. The massage is very penetrating, using the therapist's body weight to apply the pressure, and proceeds with glacial slowness. The extreme slowness of the strokes purportedly minimizes the pain and maximizes the effect. You're directed to make certain movements while the Rolfer works. You're also given movement awareness exercises to do between sessions.

Hellerwork, a therapy derived from Rolfing and very similar to it, gives even more attention to movement education. Neither method is promoted as therapy for specific conditions. Instead, both are presented as "somatic education" for the purpose of improving energy, fitness, self-esteem, self-awareness, posture, and coordination. In the end, however, Rolfing and Hellerwork have the same effects on the muscles as massage and could be considered to be a form of trigger point therapy applied in scattergun fashion. Be aware, however, that the extreme pressure used for Rolfing and Hellerwork could make these therapies risky for shoulder problems unless the therapist is unusually sensitive and responsive to the client.

Sports Massage

Massage designed especially for athletes has been shown to enhance performance and diminish the various kinds of pain associated with sports activity. It's employed before, during, and after participation in sports, with special emphasis placed on injury prevention. Many professional sports teams have professional massage therapists on staff.

In sports, muscles are often chronically overcontracted and overworked, which makes them less efficient, more easily exhausted, and more susceptible to injury. When overused, muscles are deprived of sufficient nourishment and oxygen because of compromised local circulation. Increased circulation is exactly what massage is good for.

Studies show that a 10 to 20 percent increase in muscle strength is possible with regular massage. Other claimed benefits include increased energy, better coordination, and faster healing. Massage augments range of motion, decreases joint stiffness, and reduces recovery time from overtraining. Together, these advantages can extend the careers of professional athletes and benefit amateur athletes as well.

Therapists who specialize in sports massage use an eclectic approach, taking what they need from traditional Swedish massage, neuromuscular therapy, and myofascial release. In general, sports massage is more vigorous and stimulating before a game or workout. This improves efficiency, reaction time, alertness, and endurance and also helps with injury prevention. After a game or workout, efforts are directed toward reducing tension in the muscles and increasing circulation in order to promote tissue repair, elimination of wastes, and quick recovery. It's noteworthy that about 90 percent of the sports massage therapy provided for swimmers is directed to the shoulders.

Personal trainers are taking an interest in self-applied trigger point massage and have begun teaching it to their clients. They've found it to be particularly effective when used right away if pain develops while working out. Because personal trainers take physical conditioning very seriously, their discovery about the value of quick treatment for pain is an important lesson for everyone. Critical shoulder problems, along with similar trouble in other parts of the body, would be very rare if trigger points were treated when they first appear.

Swedish Massage

All forms of therapeutic massage in use today are founded on Swedish massage. In the Western world, Swedish massage in its basic form is the best known and most popular type of bodywork. The fundamental techniques of this modality were established at the beginning of the nineteenth century by a Swede named Per Henrik Ling, thus the name "Swedish" massage. Interestingly, Ling developed the therapy in a search for a cure for his arthritis. Since Ling's problem was fixed by massage, it's likely that his "arthritis" was actually nothing other than myofascial pain.

Oil or massage lotion is almost always used with Swedish massage, and you're expected to remove your clothing to your own level of comfort, although underwear is permitted if necessary. Although Swedish massage is meant to be a full-body treatment, it's sometimes limited to areas above the waist and below the knees for people who are a bit shy. There are five classic strokes that define Swedish massage: *effleurage*, *petrissage*, *deep friction*, *tapotement*, and *vibration*. Each stroke has its own particular effect, but all stimulate circulation.

Effleurage consists of long, smooth strokes along the fibers of whatever muscle is being addressed. Effleurage tends to make you relaxed and sleepy. Many therapists strongly believe that the direction of effleurage strokes should always be toward the heart. The idea is that stroking away from the heart would tend to cause pooling of blood and lymph fluid.

Petrissage encompasses any kind of manipulation that squeezes the muscles between the fingers and thumbs. Basically, "petrissage" means "kneading," but wringing, pressing, rolling, and lifting of the muscle tissue also fall into this category. Petrissage is usually more energizing than effleurage.

Deep friction, or deep tissue massage, is a compressive rubbing that goes deeper into the muscles than either effleurage or petrissage. It also does more to lengthen, spread, and free the fascia. Effleurage and petrissage are done first to prepare the tissue for deep friction.

Tapotement is the rhythmic tapping or striking of the muscles with the fingertips or edges of the hands. Tapotement is intended to loosen and invigorate the muscles. It can feel very good on the legs, arms, and back but not on the neck, chest, or abdomen.

Vibration uses the fingertips or hands in constant contact with the skin, shaking the muscles from side to side. Vibration can be either stimulating or relaxing, depending on speed and duration.

The reason Swedish massage works so well is that it stimulates local circulation and reduces muscle tension. These two effects can improve your sleep, lower your blood pressure, make your joints more flexible, and reduce your level of pain. When Swedish massage helps with pain, it's very likely due to the incidental effect on trigger points. Even therapists who know very little about trigger points know how to work on the knots in your muscles. That's one of the things that makes Swedish massage feel so good. These knots, of course, would almost always be trigger points, and squeezing, kneading, and stroking is exactly what they need. Keep in mind, however, that a full-body, generic Swedish massage wouldn't necessarily meet the very specific needs of a frozen shoulder.

Energy Therapies

According to traditional Chinese medicine, the essential life force called *chi* flows through your body in a system of meridians, pathways, or channels. This notion is central to the rationale of the energy therapies. Theoretically, constrictions in these energy pathways disrupt the flow of chi, causing pain, emotional dysfunction, and disease. The energy therapies allegedly regulate chi and cure your troubles by removing blockages. The flow of chi is readjusted by different means depending on the specific therapy. Yoga and qigong, for example, use breathing. Tai chi uses movement. Do-in uses exercises. Acupressure uses touch, and acupuncture employs needles.

Unfortunately, science hasn't yet found a way to verify the existence of chi or any system of energy meridians. Nonetheless, millions of people believe in chi and have unquestioning faith in the therapies that influence it. The government of mainland China officially endorses chi, along with all the other complex beliefs and practices of traditional Chinese medicine.

Fundamentally, energies therapies are said to restore health and harmony by encouraging your natural healing processes—but the same could be said of the placebo effect. If you believe in the virtues of a placebo, you may find an energy therapy helpful with your shoulder even if science would turn up its nose. The key is in stimulating the body's own healing mechanisms, which is all that any therapy can do—including trigger point massage.

Acupressure and Shiatsu

You can think of "acupressure" as being the Western name for "shiatsu." There may be differences between them in the eyes of practitioners, but they're not essential differences. *Shiatsu*, which means "finger pressure" in Japanese, is one of the oldest forms of natural healing. The Japanese learned finger pressure therapy from the Chinese, and this modality has existed in China for as long as five thousand years.

Finger Pressure Theory

In using acupressure or shiatsu, the therapist applies gentle finger pressure to predetermined, strategic points on the meridians in order to release the flow of chi, the universal energy that courses freely through all healthy living things. Disease, injury, or emotional distress create blockages along the meridians, interfering with the flow of chi. Depending on the meridian they're in, blockages create different symptoms. The list of disorders and symptoms that acupressure or shiatsu claims to cure includes almost anything you can name. Western medicine looks at these therapies as merely esoteric kinds of massage—flaky but essentially harmless unless they keep you from getting "proper" medical treatment.

Finger pressure therapy has evolved into a confusing number of variants in both Japan and China, and all have made their way to the United States, where interest in alternative medicine is so great. The better known forms of Chinese acupressure include tuina, Shen Tao, Jin Shin, Do-in, and qigong. Japanese forms of shiatsu include Zen shiatsu, Namikoshi shiatsu, and tsubo shiatsu. In the United States, the evolution has been carried further, giving birth to macrobiotic shiatsu, barefoot shiatsu, Nippon shiatsu, Ohashiatsu, and—wouldn't you know—New Age Shiatsu, which is a registered trademark.

Treatment

To weed through all this seeming diversity, just remember that all these variations on finger pressure therapy are concerned with the pressing of "points." Some practitioners believe that there must be a giver and a receiver of the therapy. In China, however, self-treatment of points is considered an important part of self-care, at least with the points that can be reached. Each form of acupressure or shiatsu has a different take on the importance of diet, exercise, movement, and thought. Additionally, some use the application of heat or cold or immersion in water as a complement to finger pressure.

It might appear that finger pressure therapy is the same thing as the ischemic compression, or press-and-hold technique, used in older forms of trigger point therapy. However, considerably less pressure is used with acupressure and shiatsu, and it's not necessarily directed at trigger points. The pressure used in shiatsu and acupressure is always comfortable, never painful. No oil is used and you remain clothed. No massage tools are used, and there are no long, gliding strokes, although the therapist may sometimes rub points in tiny circles. The massage table is positioned low to the floor, or you may be on a mat on the floor itself.

Regarding any benefits for your shoulder, acupressure and shiatsu do provide the calming reassurance of structured human touch, which in itself may stimulate the healing process. If the therapist also has a sophisticated knowledge of trigger points and referred pain, you may find acupressure or shiatsu helpful.

Acupuncture

Acupuncture developed from acupressure and has exactly the same uses. In both kinds of therapy, treatment is directed at carefully selected points for the purpose of allowing free flow of the elemental life force, promoting general good health, and treating specific conditions. Acupuncture has gained widespread acceptance in both the East and the West. The World Health Organization identifies about one hundred ailments that can be treated with acupuncture.

These days, more than a few medical doctors, physical therapists, osteopaths, and chiropractors in the United States and Europe practice acupuncture. The field is very unevenly regulated, however, and some states don't require a degree or training of any kind. Western doctors usually use acupuncture for pain relief and to combat addictions. In China, it's actually used for surgical anesthesia. Although it's been tried for that purpose in the United States, the results have been very inconsistent.

Before beginning treatment, the acupuncturist will want to assess your specific problems and the general condition of your health. Along with asking an extensive list of questions, the practitioner will examine your tongue and evaluate as many as twelve pulses in your wrist. With traditional Chinese acupuncture, treatment entails inserting very fine needles, which are left in for twenty minutes to an hour. The needles may be wiggled, twiddled, pumped, or flicked to increase the stimulation of the points. Western practitioners leave the needles in for only a few seconds. Although there are over five hundred recognized acupuncture points, only about one hundred are commonly used.

Acupuncture clearly doesn't work on everyone. It may be that a positive response requires a psychological affinity for the treatment's esoteric aspects. You need a good rule of thumb for judging whether an alternative therapy like acupuncture is going to work for you. If you don't see clear improvement in five treatments or less, you'd be wise to move on and try something else.

Many acupuncturists are finding that their therapy provides more relief from pain if they integrate treatment of trigger points with techniques that address chi and the meridians. Others who aren't so wedded to Eastern philosophy believe that any positive effects from acupuncture are explained by its effects on trigger points. One team of researchers found a 71 percent correspondence between trigger points and the acupuncture points used for the relief of pain. The acupuncturist's search for blockages often takes the form of manually feeling for tender spots, which is exactly the same criterion for finding trigger points (Simons, Travell, and Simons 1999, 41-42; Melzack, Fox, and Stillwell 1977, 3-23).

Travell and Simons view acupuncture as comparable to the dry needling of trigger points that they found effective. An advantage that dry needling has over procaine injections is that it has no deadening effect. With the muscle tissue retaining its sensitivity, other trigger points can be located in the area. On the other hand, trigger point injections have the advantage of leaving less residual soreness (Chaitow and DeLany 2000, 155; Lewit 1979, 83-90).

Acupuncture may help you with a frozen shoulder or simple shoulder pain, provided that it's directed at the specific trigger points causing your shoulder pain. Keep in mind that residual soreness after an acupuncture session may prevent self-applied trigger point massage for several days.

Applied Kinesiology

Kinesiology is the scientific study of the muscles and body movement from the standpoint of normal function, injuries, dysfunction, rehabilitation, and the enhancement of athletic performance. Physicians who specialize in sports medicine have a vital interest in kinesiology.

In the middle of the twentieth century, kinesiology became a subject of interest for a number of chiropractors who invented a new treatment, *applied kinesiology*, which in the ensuing years has become a very popular cure-all. The convoluted theory behind applied kinesiology is that imbalances in muscle strength might be an indicator of the state of a person's health. An elaborate system of muscle testing was concocted, along with a routine for strengthening weakened muscles with one form of rubbing or another. The restored balance in muscle strength would presumably rejuvenate the function of glands and internal organs, which would in turn dispel a wide range of diseases and dysfunctions.

Kinesiology Gone Wild

Applied kinesiology has expanded into an astonishing variety of new systems, all based on essentially the same principles but with alluring new names, including Touch for Health, wellness kinesiology, biokinesiology, foundation kinesiology, advanced kinesiology, educational kinesiology, professional kinesiology, health kinesiology, Christian kinesiology, and hypertonic muscle release. These various forms of applied kinesiology are practiced by osteopaths, chiropractors, massage therapists, physical therapists, and dentists. A person with no formal training whatever can call themselves kinesiologists as long as they don't infringe on a trademarked name. In most places, no licensing is needed. Practitioners of applied kinesiology claim it will improve your general health, reveal nutritional deficiencies, maximize mental and physical performance, cure addictions, banish allergies, reduce anxiety, put an end to eating disorders, tranquilize hyperactivity, heal repetitive strain injuries, alleviate stress, and get rid of back pain.

Those Old Meridians Again

The most common mode of treatment in applied kinesiology is to briskly rub certain sore places on the back and chest, which have been given the impressive name *neurolymphatic reflex points*. Many therapists are inclined to believe that these points lie on the meridians, but others simply search around for tender spots to rub. The theory is that rubbing stimulates the reflex points and opens the "energy circuit" to the gland or internal organ that caused the problem. The muscle is tested before and after rubbing to see if it has strengthened.

Muscle testing can be an impressive show. The apparent increase in strength from stimulation of the neurolymphatic reflex points can seem very real and be quite convincing. The problem is that the before-and-after muscle testing involves the person trying to move an arm or leg in a particular direction while the therapist pushes back. This is where the placebo effect comes into play. There's too much potential for conscious or unconscious cheating when both parties have a strong desire to see something happen. Whether changes in muscle strength actually occur is very much open to question. Even if they do occur, it may not have anything to do with the application of kinesiology.

Those Old Trigger Points Again

The reality about neurolymphatic reflex points is that they're in the same areas where you would expect to find very common trigger points. Considering that neurolymphatic reflex points might actually be myofascial trigger points and nothing more, it's only logical to speculate that any true change in muscle strength could have something to do with the nature of trigger points.

Keep in mind that one of the characteristic effects of a trigger point is that it causes referred weakness in other muscles. When you treat the trigger point, the referred weakness goes away. This is a more cogent rationale for the effects of muscle testing than anything having to do with these otherwise undetectable and inexplicable neurolymphatic reflex points.

You may encounter people who enthusiastically assure you that applied kinesiology cured their frozen shoulder. It's really not in your best interest to disbelieve them. They'll vigorously defend their beliefs anyway, and they might actually be right. They're only reporting a personal experience, a case history, that they believe to be authentic. Anecdotal case histories are where science begins after all. If they can tell you exactly what was done to treat their problem, it would be worth trying it for yourself to see what happens. The applied kinesiology therapies do no harm, and you may get an unexpected cure.

Reiki

Reiki, the best known of the energy modalities, is based on 2,500-year-old Tibetan writings about the Buddhist ability to heal the body, mind, and spirit by redirecting universal life energy, which (as rumor has it) permeates all living things. Reiki practitioners aim to channel this energy through themselves and into you for the purpose of breaking open energy blockages and encouraging self-healing. In the Reiki philosophy, stifled or misdirected energy is what causes pain and disease.

The channeling of energy is achieved by the practitioner holding their hands in a series of twelve different positions for several minutes near major organs and glands. There are four positions each for the head, back, and abdomen. The placement of the hands is very gentle, and depending on the practitioner's style, the hands may not even touch you at all. You remained fully clothed, no oil is used, and perfect silence is maintained.

Reiki is more a philosophy for living than a therapy, and it holds high standards for its practitioners. They're expected to cultivate a mind-set that will encourage them to take responsibility for their own health, be kind to everyone, assume a positive attitude about all things, and use their powers for helping others. Practitioners of Reiki don't claim to cure specific diseases, and you shouldn't have too much hope that Reiki will directly affect your shoulder problems. Even so, Reiki's calm, peaceful approach is usually quite effective in reducing tension and anxiety, which can improve the effectiveness of any trigger point treatments. Furthermore, if universal life energy is a reality, all the advertised benefits of Reiki may land in your lap. On the other hand, if universal life energy is only a figment of the imagination, maybe the placebo effect will help, provided you can suspend your disbelief for a few sessions.

Movement Therapies

The classic advice given to people with shoulder trouble is to keep the shoulder moving at all costs, and when it comes to conventional therapy for a frozen shoulder, treatment consists largely of forcing you to move your arm. The implied promise is that movement will help you retain your range of motion and keep your shoulder from freezing up. You may have discovered by now that it doesn't really work like that. Sadly, the promulgators of the movement ethic understand very little about what's really going on with your shoulder.

In reality, myofascial trigger points in your shoulder and upper back are probably the reason for your trouble with movement. Until you begin to get your trigger points under control, movement isn't going to be helpful. In fact, movement is guaranteed to be downright unpleasant. However, once you begin to make progress with the pain caused by trigger points, you should indeed begin a program of cautious, nonforced movement. Conventional physical therapy would then be appropriate, and certainly less painful. At that point, you might also like to try one of the following alternative therapies. To lower your risk of a setback, plan to do a bit of self-applied trigger point massage before and after any movement session.

Eastern Systems

Most of the systems of stylized movement now used for toning the body and maintaining health were developed centuries ago in China as martial arts. The better known forms, such as Shaolin, qigong, and tai chi, are practiced daily by millions of Chinese. Along with a number of derivatives, these three most popular systems are also practiced throughout the Western world, although with decidedly less dedication and devotion than in China.

The Eastern systems use very slow, controlled, unforced movement to strengthen and stretch muscles in all parts of the body. Yoga, a similar system of therapeutic movement originating in India, requires that you move into certain postures and positions and hold them for a length of time. In contrast, the Chinese modalities generally encourage graceful, continuous, fluid movement.

Eastern systems of therapeutic movement have potential for helping rehabilitate a frozen shoulder, provided that you first let your trigger point therapy begin to do its work. With a shoulder problem, be aware that any of the movement therapies can give you more pain and possibly a serious relapse if you go at them too early or too ambitiously.

Alexander Technique

The Alexander Technique is not actually a therapy, in that it doesn't treat specific conditions. Instead, it involves mind-body reeducation for improved alignment of the head, neck, and spine, which results in more efficient breathing, reduced muscle strain, and improved general health.

The basis for the Alexander Technique is the belief that chronic physical problems, muscle pain, and breathing difficulties are the result of misuse of the body, manifested in bad posture and inefficient movement. During Alexander lessons, you're taught to become more aware of habitual patterns of strain. You then learn and practice new and better ways to move. Although individual lessons are the customary format, group classes are offered, too.

The Alexander Technique was introduced in the early 1900s by Frederick Matthias Alexander, an Australian actor, who developed the method to correct vocal problems he was having in his own stage performances. As a consequence, the Alexander Technique is very popular among artists performing in music, theater, and dance. In the last forty years, the method has become popular throughout the world and has benefited people in all walks of life. The medical community generally endorses the Alexander Technique because it seems to foster better health with virtually no risks.

In a course of Alexander lessons, you learn to realign your head, neck, and spine for ease, balance, and release of tension. Head, neck, and spine position are considered to be the primary control because they govern the way the rest of the body functions. Patterns of misuse of your body in the form of tension and bad posture come to feel normal as the years go by, primarily because proprioception (sensory self-awareness) diminishes, perhaps as part of the aging process.

Your reeducation involves two steps. First, you increase your visual and sensory awareness of bad patterns of posture and movement. Then you replace the old patterns with new ones. The Alexander teacher observes you, guides your attention to inefficient postures and movements, and gently helps you correct them. Part of the process is consciously practicing simple, everyday actions. You're encouraged to think through the new movement in advance, picturing your body relaxing, lengthening, and moving freely.

It's probable that body misalignments and habitual muscle tension have contributed to your shoulder difficulty. It may be that after you've begun to make progress with your trigger points, Alexander lessons could be a valuable part of your rehabilitation. The Alexander Technique's freer and more natural posture and movement style might also help prevent another serious shoulder problem from arising.

Feldenkrais Method

The Feldenkrais system of controlled exercises doesn't aim to treat particular conditions. It's best seen as a rehabilitation modality that, in conjunction with physical therapy, is helpful in overcoming injuries and joint disorders. The object is to change poor posture and habitual, overcompensating movement patterns that place unnecessary strain on the body.

Physicist and judo expert Moshe Feldenkrais was born in Russia but lived most of his adult life in Israel. He developed his methods in the process of rehabilitating himself after a serious soccer injury to his knee that left him with recurrent crippling pain. Inspired by Alexander's ideas, Feldenkrais believed that you must raise your awareness of unconscious habits before change can begin. That awareness would include sharpened perception of movement, feeling, sensations, and thoughts. Changing any one of these would institute change in the others. Changes in movement would be the most direct because movement is observable and more open to conscious control.

The Feldenkrais Method is very much like a Western style of tai chi, except that much of the work is done while lying on the floor, whereas you do tai chi while on your feet. Like tai chi, Feldenkrais aims at building natural, graceful movement that is free-flowing and effortless. This is done by repeatedly performing small, fluid movements to reprogram your nervous system, making you better coordinated and more flexible and balanced. There are psychological and emotional benefits as well, which bring increased energy and improved self-esteem.

There are two ways to work with the Feldenkrais Method. The first, Functional Integration, is done with a private teacher in one-on-one lessons. The second, Awareness Through Movement, is conducted through group study. Nothing is forced in Feldenkrais, and there's very little pain because you work within your own limits, extending them only as your body adjusts to the new patterns. Self-help programs in the Feldenkrais Method are available online and in a number of books. It's recommended, however, that you begin this study with a teacher, who will analyze your difficulties and guide you through the fine points of the new movements. As with all movement therapies, this is a program to take up only after your pain has become significantly reduced and you've begun to get some of your shoulder movement back.

Chapter 9

Physical Therapy for the Shoulder

A big change is underway in the field of physical therapy. Within the next few years, this third-largest of the health care professions (after doctors and nurses) intends to have professional autonomy. This means that physical therapists aim to be licensed to diagnose medical conditions that are within their scope of practice and to screen for disease that needs to be referred to a physician. Most importantly, they want everyone to have direct access to physical therapy and to be covered by insurance without needing a referral from a physician (Gray 2004, 359).

In Australia, a physical therapist can be your primary care provider. Educational programs are being adapted to make this happen in the United States and other countries as well. A primary objective is to make a doctorate in physical therapy the entry-level requirement for licensing by the year 2020. These are worthy aspirations that demonstrate an interest in upgrading the physical therapy profession. There's also much talk of the need for better research and the improvement of treatment modalities, although like most movements toward change there's a good bit more talk than action. And there's always the inevitable resistance of those who prefer the comfort of traditional practices and the status quo.

Trigger Points—Knocking at the Back Door

Comfortably established members of the physical therapy profession would prefer that everyone adhere to the official *Guide to Physical Therapist Practice* (American Physical Therapy Association 2003, 15-18), which describes "preferred therapist practice patterns" and seeks to promote the standardization and use of traditional, supposedly proven methods. In actual practice, however, physical therapy is very diverse and each practitioner tends to develop a favorite mix of techniques, proven or *unproven*. A number of the less conformist practitioners include unsanctioned alternatives, like CranioSacral Therapy, acupressure, acupuncture, Reiki, myofascial release—and now, at long last, trigger point therapy.

Many physical therapists are taking continuing education classes to learn trigger point therapy and making it an integral part of their treatments. They're doing this, not because it has been officially approved, but because therapists have found in practice that it works very well. Some physical therapy schools are even beginning to teach trigger point therapy in a tentative way as a part of general classes in manual therapies. This interest in trigger points has been a long time coming, considering that the benefits of trigger point therapy have been known since the early 1940s, when Janet Travell first began writing about it.

Hopefully, the physical therapy profession as a whole will eventually come to recognize and employ trigger point therapy as a primary treatment for pain as more and more individual practitioners experience its simplicity, directness, and effectiveness. At the present time, however, trigger point therapy has not attained the official recognition and acceptance by the leadership of the physical therapy profession that it deserves. Incredibly, nowhere in the 744 pages of the *Guide to Physical Therapist Practice* (American Physical Therapy Association 2003) does it even mention myofascial pain, trigger points, or any form of trigger point therapy.

Academic physical therapists are still dragging their feet regarding trigger points and myofascial pain. The professorial mind-set is to wait for studies of this "unproven" method of therapy to come out, even though trigger point therapy has actually been subjected to more scientific scrutiny than some of the methods traditionally used by physical therapists (Simons, Travell, and Simons 1999, 11-235; Chaitow and DeLany 2000, 65-84; Irwin 2004, 3-10).

The Emperor Has No Clothes

The physical therapy profession is sorely in need of an honest new look at its treatment methods. Traditional physical therapy methods too often fail in the treatment of pain, primarily because they're founded so exclusively on the stretching and strengthening of muscles. These failures are rarely acknowledged, discussed, or subjected to scientific study. A frozen shoulder is a good example of where conventional physical therapy can go terribly wrong, not only failing to help, but even making the problem worse. It's a mistake to assume that because a frozen shoulder seems stiff and weak it needs stretching and strengthening.

The reality is that stiff and weak shoulder muscles are generally a result of myofascial trigger points, which can become very resistant to release when the muscles are bullied with stretching exercises that have the explicit intention of forcing your arm and shoulder to move. Physical therapy, especially aggressive physical therapy, frequently intensifies a shoulder problem, as many patients would attest.

Unfortunately, many therapists trained in the old methods will always believe that stretching and strengthening is the correct thing to do for a frozen shoulder, because that's what they were taught in school. If there's a flaw in the plan to make all physical therapists into "doctors," it's the risk that this will encourage an even stronger and more defiant assertion of long-held but indefensible academic adherence to traditional methods.

Those physical therapists who are learning about trigger points are finding out that conventional stretching exercises can be precisely the *wrong* thing for a frozen shoulder. It's not that stretching per se is bad. The error has been using stretching too soon and too insistently and not facing up to its dangers and negative effects. Stretching and strengthening can have an effective and appropriate place in rehabilitation of a frozen shoulder, but not if you neglect the trigger points.

The solution, of course, is to meld the two concepts, bringing trigger point therapy into the everyday practice of physical therapy. In the right balance, this could be a powerful combination. The fundamental idea is that trigger point therapy should come first if you hope to make stretching and strengthening work safely.

The Role of the Public

Too many physicians and physical therapists still consider trigger point therapy an alternative treatment with unproven results. Nothing could be further from the truth. Of all the many kinds of physical therapy for pain, trigger point therapy has the strongest basis in science, thanks to the large number of studies by Janet Travell, David Simons, and many others. Trigger point therapy is unique among the many kinds of treatment for pain because it delineates the precise physical cause of pain, the myofascial trigger point, and goes right to it. Trigger point therapy gets rid of your pain by addressing its *cause*. Not even pharmaceutical drugs treat the cause of your pain. They only affect the *sensation* of pain (Simons, Travell, and Simons 1999, 11-93; Chaitow and DeLany 2000, 65-84).

Public demand will make all the difference in bringing trigger point therapy into the realm of physical therapy. When patients begin asking for trigger point therapy in sufficient numbers, they will get it. Physical therapists should be expected to be masters of trigger point therapy, and any practitioner (physicians included) who claims to treat a frozen shoulder should be able to find and effectively treat the trigger points in all twenty-four muscles that may be involved. The specific mode of treatment—trigger point massage, spray and stretch, trigger point injections, dry needling, and so on—matters less than simply being able to treat these specific trigger points in a confident and reliable way. Trigger point therapy, particularly in the form of trigger point massage, is just not that hard.

Thousands of ordinary citizens have mastered self-applied trigger point massage and have successfully treated their own pain. Among health practitioners, the community of massage therapists was the first to widely recognize the value of trigger point massage, and many of them have developed a high degree of skill with it and have practiced it for twenty years or more. Physical therapists and medical doctors should be expected to acquire at least equal facility, if not greater. Unfortunately, only public expectation that they do so will make it happen. Inertia and allegiance to the status quo within the physical therapy and medical professions will otherwise prevent this from happening for decades to come.

Physical Therapy Research

Physical therapists who use trigger point therapy in their practice are having to bring it in through the back door, without evaluation and approval by leaders in their field. There appears to be little interest in investigating trigger point therapy. Surprisingly, there aren't even many high-quality randomized trials of well-established, traditional manual therapies for pain, like stretching and exercise (Freiwald et al. 1998a, 267-272). This suggests that researchers believe that the established methods are good enough. There is no basis for this belief except that the methods are in fact established and familiar to all. The fact that they often don't work and can even aggravate someone's pain seems to be of little concern.

The elephant in the room that nobody ever talks about is the almost total lack of studies specific to stretching, the preeminent physical therapy method for pain. The effectiveness of stretching as it relates to the lengthening of healthy athletic muscles has been studied extensively, but only recently has a frank examination of the therapeutic use of stretching begun. One study by a group of Dutch researchers found that patients actually recovered sooner *without* stretching (Diercks and Stevens 2004, 499-502). A group of Taiwanese doctors found that acupressure worked better in reducing pain than physical therapy did (Hsieh et al.

2004, 168-176). The unavoidable inference in both studies was that stretching in many cases could actually be an impediment to recovery instead of an aid.

One reason for the reluctance to do an unbiased examination of stretching as therapy for pain is that it's firmly entrenched in academic programs, where old ideas tend to be passed from generation to generation virtually unquestioned and unchanged. Once an idea gets into a textbook, scientific interest seems to die.

As a treatment modality for pain, stretching has long enjoyed widespread acceptance, not just in physical therapy but in all fields of health care (Freiwald et al. 1998b, 54-59; Spring, Schneider, and Tritschler 1997, 981-986). Intuitively, stretching seems like the right thing to do, the natural thing, and it often is when you're in good physical condition and aren't suffering from myofascial trigger points. But few people ever challenge the glib assertions of stretching's effectiveness for pain, even though it requires turning a deaf ear to the complaints of patients. The many studies that attempt to evaluate conventional physical therapy methods are seriously flawed and of doubtful value because they include multiple treatment modalities in their experiment designs and never study specific treatments, such as stretching, in isolation (Sullivan, Kues, and Mayhew 1996, 359-364; Beyers and Bonutti 2004, 321-323).

The Lack of Scientific Validation

The most basic rule of research is that you must do everything you can to limit the number of variables. You have no hope of knowing what really works if you don't study one thing at a time. But that's not how physical therapy research is done. The integrated approach is used, where the risk of failure is diluted by distributing it over several diverse kinds of treatment. Each researcher has his or her own recipe of special ingredients to try out, but single therapies are hardly ever tested in isolation, where there might be a chance for drawing valid conclusions. Combinations of therapies may be advantageous for treatment—something might work if you're lucky. But testing combinations of treatments isn't good science if you really want to find out whether a specific kind of treatment really works.

The lack of scientific validation of traditional physical therapy methods is bothersome. A search of PubMed and the archives of the journal *Physical Therapy* for the last ten years revealed that the primary focus in scientific studies on this topic is "easy science." Physical therapy research consists overwhelmingly of overly meticulous measurement (clinical evaluation) of physical problems, assessment of the prevalence of pain in various demographic groups, and the development of means for prevention of physical problems. While these are undoubtedly useful studies, the long-established forms of physical therapy—exercising, stretching, joint and soft tissue mobilization, hydrotherapy, cryotherapy, and electrotherapy—have gone largely unexamined, even though they clearly fail to solve pain problems for many people. Too often a study is clearly being done by researchers who have a financially motivated interest in promoting particular method or an expensive, new therapeutic gadget.

You may be surprised to know that trigger points and myofascial pain are seldom mentioned in physical therapy's professional journals, indicating that there's very little interest in researching or understanding trigger points in the academic world of physical therapy. This is unacceptable in light of the research that does exist. The work of Travell and Simons strongly suggests that trigger point therapy holds great potential for making physical therapy truly effective for the entire range of myofascial pain problems, and yet academic physical therapists continue to ignore it. This is a tragedy not only for physical therapy patients who continue to suffer needlessly, but also for physical therapists, who suffer from the same kinds of myofascial pain as their patients (Simons 2005).

Physical Therapists Have Pain Too

A poignant aspect to the existing physical therapy research is that certain studies indicate as many as two-thirds of practicing physical therapists suffer pain related to their work at some time in any given year (Bork et al. 1996, 827-835; Holder et al. 1999, 642-652). In addition, as many as 17 percent of physical therapists ultimately leave the profession because of chronic pain and other work-related disabilities (Cromie, Robertson, and Best 2000, 336-351). This could be some of the best evidence that traditional physical therapy methods are seriously defective, as physical therapists seem to have as much difficulty making their methods work on themselves as on their patients.

Physical therapists who experience chronic pain have a golden opportunity to do meaningful, informal experiments with trigger point therapy. By developing skill at self-applied trigger point massage, they could not only intimately explore a method that might benefit their patients, they might also extend their professional lives. Self-treatment could be used as a preliminary study of the broader concepts in trigger point science. Personal experience in self-treatment could generate tentative measurable observations that could then be subjected to verification in controlled studies in physical therapy clinics. Perhaps some of the therapists who are bringing trigger point therapy into their practice through the back door will see the importance of doing this research and take the initiative in getting it done, ideally in an academic setting.

Physical Therapy Methods

Despite the fact that current physical therapy methods fail for some people, they do succeed for others. None of the above discussion is meant to keep you away from physical therapy or put you in a quandary about it. You may be considering physical therapy for your shoulder problem, perhaps based on a doctor's recommendation. If you choose to try it, be sure to ask whether the physical therapist makes use of trigger point therapy. It will make all the difference. It would also be good to understand in advance something about the different physical therapy methods commonly used for the treatment of shoulder problems, along with the pros and cons of each. Some of these methods may be helpful, especially if employed at the proper time in the healing process—after your trigger points have been attended to.

There are a number of physical therapy methods for frozen shoulder that are generally administered by the therapist without the patient's active participation. These include such things as stretching maneuvers, joint mobilization, soft tissue mobilization, and electrotherapy. In addition to such office procedures, patients are almost always given self-treatment programs to be done at home. These programs usually consist of simple stretches and exercises, presumably fitted to the particular needs and abilities of the patient. The patient is expected to take considerable responsibility for their outcome by stretching and exercising in a dutiful manner. Self-treatment is empowering when it works. However, many people suffering from a frozen shoulder find these physical therapy home programs quite impossible because of the added pain they cause. Stretching, of course, is the heart of the problem.

Stretching

There's no question that stretching succeeds with many patients. Otherwise, it would have been discontinued long ago. Unfortunately, when therapists look only at the successful outcomes of stretching, they fall into the trap of believing that stretching should be good for everyone. They have trouble accepting that many people in pain simply can't tolerate stretching. When patients protest that stretching hurts too much, the zealous practitioner insists that *more* stretching be applied, reiterating the old saw about no pain, no gain. At this point, patients who can't tolerate stretching stop doing their homework or just drop out of physical therapy altogether. This of course makes it easy for the therapist to blame the treatment failure on patient noncompliance.

Despite these criticisms, and even if you have had trouble in the past with stretches and exercises, you may find that you can manage some of the physical therapy routines after trigger point therapy has begun to cut your pain and allow your muscles to lengthen. Nonetheless, keep in mind that as a treatment for myofascial pain, trigger point therapy is a stand-alone modality. Stretching and exercising aren't a requirement for full recovery. They might speed the return of your range of motion if you use them as a follow-up to trigger point therapy, but strength and range of motion usually return naturally with normal activity after your trigger points have been deactivated and your pain is gone.

The bottom line is that if stretching or exercise hurts, don't do it. The intelligent strategy is to first minimize your pain with trigger point massage. Then, if you choose to do stretches and exercises, do them in moderation and be ready to cut back if they seem to revive the problem. In examining the various methods of physical therapy described below, you'll see that nearly all employ stretching to some extent.

Spray and Stretch

The reason physical therapy so often fails to solve shoulder problems is the hyperirritability of myofascial trigger points. In *Myofascial Pain and Dysfunction: The Trigger Point Manual*, Travell and Simons offer a solution for this problem with their method of *spray and stretch*. The governing principle of this technique is that a brief application of extreme cold to the skin overlying a trigger point distracts the central nervous system enough to allow a moderate stretch of the muscle without it reacting defensively. Equally important is the application of moist hot packs immediately afterward to prevent cooling of the muscle. In the *Trigger Point Manual*, the spray and stretch treatment for each muscle is well illustrated and thoroughly explained (Simons, Travell, and Simons 1999, 126-138).

Although spray and stretch has been shown to be a decided improvement over conventional stretching exercises, the method has not been widely accepted and applied in the field of physical therapy. Conventional stretching exercises persist, perhaps only because they are simple procedures that everyone can grasp, and because they're so deeply embedded in the culture of physical therapy (Simons 2001).

Travell and Simons call spray and stretch their "workhorse method," but the method entails several stringent requirements to prevent making the problem worse. First, therapists must be certain they're stretching the muscle containing the trigger point that's referring the

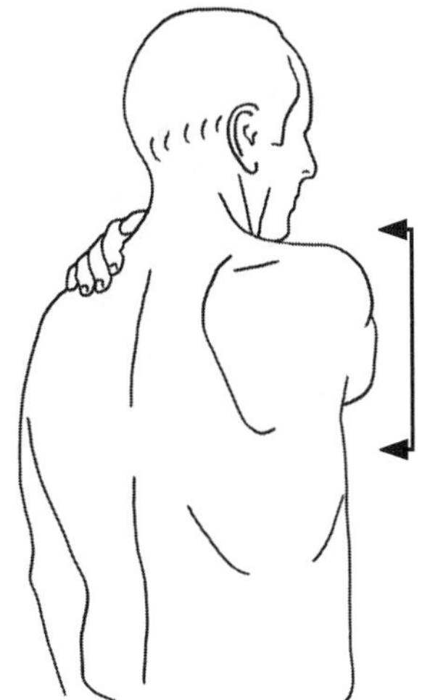

Figure 9.1 The area to be iced or sprayed includes all of the shoulder blade.

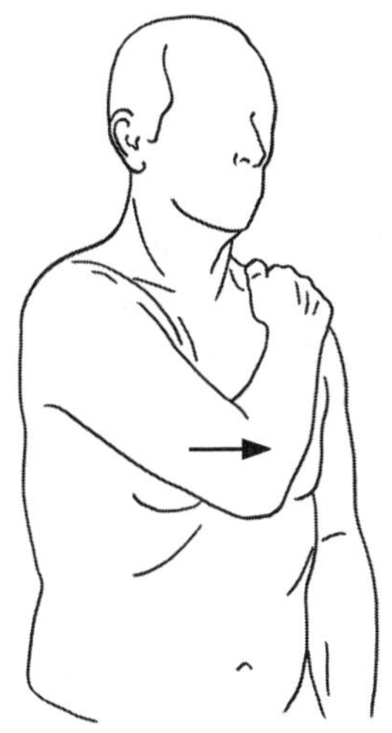

Figure 9.2 The position used to stretch the muscles behind the shoulder

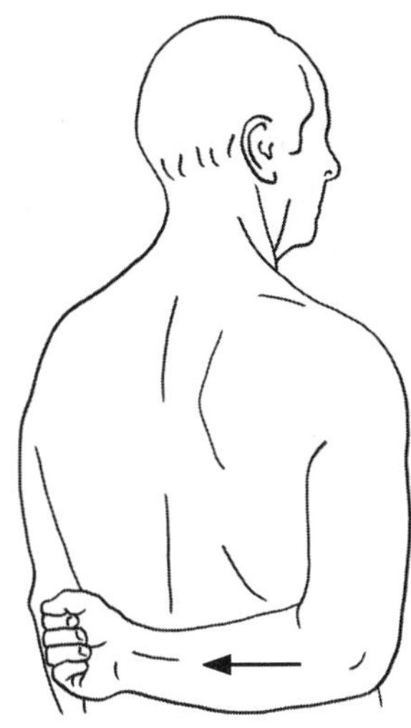

Figure 9.3 The position used for stretching muscles in the top and front of the shoulder

pain. If they focus on the place that hurts, they may apply the method to the wrong muscles. The spray and stretch method requires the therapist to be well educated about trigger points and their referral patterns.

Second, before stretching the shoulder muscles, it's essential to chill the skin that overlies their trigger points and all the areas of referred pain (Figure 9.1) with ice or a refrigerant spray. In chilling the skin, it's vital for the therapist to work quickly. If the cooling agent is applied for too long, the underlying muscles will get cold, which will inhibit the stretch rather than facilitating it, and the result will be more pain.

The Travell and Simons system for stretching individual shoulder muscles is very detailed, but it can be boiled down to just three movements of the arm, which are done with the therapist's assistance. Note that some of the muscles are stretched by more than one kind of movement. Moving your arm across the front of your body (Figure 9.2) stretches the supraspinatus, infraspinatus, teres minor, middle trapezius, posterior deltoid, and rhomboid muscles. Putting your arm behind your back (Figure 9.3) lengthens the supraspinatus, infraspinatus, teres minor, pectoralis major, coracobrachialis, and anterior deltoid muscles. Outward rotation with your arm out to the side (Figure 9.4) stretches the subscapularis, pectoralis major, pectoralis minor, and serratus anterior.

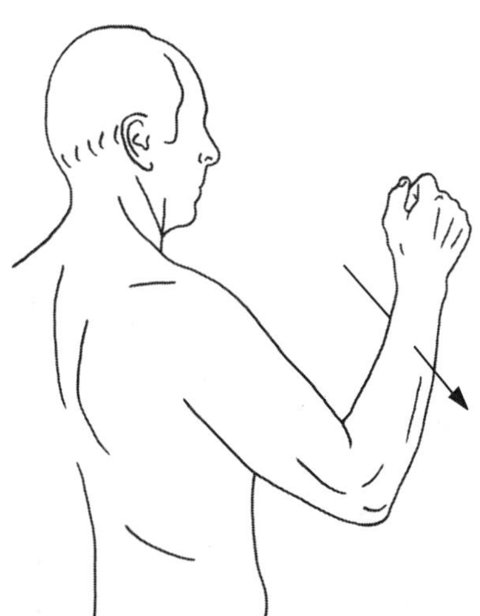

Figure 9.4 Outward rotation of the arm stretches the pectoralis major, pectoralis minor, subscapularis, and serratus anterior.

After stretching, a third requirement is that the therapist must immediately rewarm the cooled skin with moist hot packs to keep it from drawing heat out of the muscles. If movement was limited by the trigger point before treatment, a fourth step calls for gentle movement through the attainable range of motion several times to let the body know that it's now possible to move more freely.

Even with these elaborate safeguards, stretching remains hazardous for many people, and Travell and Simons specifically warn that the stretch must not be forced. They advise merely taking up the slack and stopping short of the pain threshold. Attempting to stretch a muscle whose trigger points resist release may strain the muscle's attachments and cause the muscle or its connective tissue to tear. This is because the taut bands of muscle fiber on either side of the trigger point are already stretched to their limit. Because of the restrictions they put on stretching, these taut bands in muscles may be a critical factor in ligament and tendon injuries (Simons, Travell, and Simons 1999, 127-135).

Another reason some physical therapists are reluctant to use spray and stretch is ecological concern about the vapocoolant spray Fluori-Methane. It contains two chlorofluorocarbons, a type of chemical believed to be a major contributor to the degradation of the atmosphere's ozone layer. A temporary medical exemption has been given to the Gebauer Company to continue producing the product for medical uses, but the exemption could unexpectedly expire at any time. This would put therapists in a bad spot if they were depending on Fluori-Methane in their daily practice.

Ice and Stretch

In response to concerns about the use of Fluori-Methane, Travell and Simons came up with *ice and stretch*. This alternative to spray and stretch works nearly as well and eliminates both the cost of the Fluori-Methane and its potential damage to the ozone layer.

Ice is used to shock and distract the nervous system in the same manner as the vapocoolant spray, needing only a few strokes to quickly chill the skin over the trigger point and its referral area. Then you gently stretch the muscle as you would in spray and stretch, stopping short of the point where it gets painful. Ice and stretch is actually suitable for self-treatment of any muscle you can reach with a bag of frozen peas, and a friend or relative could help you with places you can't reach.

In place of frozen peas, you can use one of the commercially available ice bags intended for the self-treatment of inflammation. Some people prefer to freeze water in a polystyrene cup or a soft drink can. This is fine, but these items should be put in a plastic bag to help keep condensation off the skin. Wet skin promotes cooling of the muscle, which you must avoid at all cost. It helps to keep blotting the skin with a paper towel.

Just as with the spray and stretch method, you must warm the skin again immediately after the gentle stretch. A heating pad over a damp cloth or a hot shower will do it. Then move your arm carefully in all directions to get back the sense that you can dare to move it. It's not wise to attempt ice and stretch, however, without first getting your pain under control. Trigger point massage should be continued as the primary form of therapy. Ice and stretch is not a substitute.

Proprioceptive Neuromuscular Facilitation

The contrived and somewhat pretentious term *proprioceptive neuromuscular facilitation* (PNF) encompasses various methods designed to make stretching work better. Some forms of PNF use active movement against resistance by the practitioner. In other forms, stretching is combined with voluntary contraction and release in the target muscles. Various tactics are used along with stretching to help force a result. These include post-isometric relaxation, contract-relax, reciprocal inhibition, muscle energy technique, strain-counterstrain, myofascial release, controlled breathing, and eye movement. These gambits all add to PNF's complexity but not necessarily to its success (Simons, Travell, and Simons 1999, 153-154; Chaitow and DeLany 2000, 368-371).

In *Facilitated Stretching*, a small book that attempts to simplify PNF, author Robert E. McAtee recognizes the risks in stretching. He repeatedly cautions that "stretching should be pain-free . . . if pain persists, don't use PNF until you know the cause of the pain" (McAtee 1993, 15). This is good advice and an unusual degree of candor coming from someone who could only be called a very enthusiastic stretcher.

McAtee points out that isometric contractions can make muscles resistant to stretching and that cramps may also occur. Preliminary contractions are meant to make stretching work by causing the muscles to reflexively relax after the contraction, but there's some doubt whether this actually happens. Electromyographic measurements indicate that the muscles are actually more active after contracting than before. In other words, the preliminary contraction leaves the muscles tighter than they otherwise would be, an effect opposite the one intended (Moore and Hutton 1980, 322-329; Condon and Hutton 1987, 24-30).

McAtee believes that PNF is needlessly complex and that it works no better than plain stretching. He adds that you should expect any kind of stretching to cause delayed-onset soreness the next day and advises minimizing this effect by being satisfied with small gains (McAtee 1993, 10-15). Unfortunately, being satisfied with small gains is almost diametrically opposed to human nature.

Active Isolated Stretching

Active isolated stretching is an even more aggressive form of stretching. The patient makes full-range, fluid movements that go briefly (about two seconds) past the limits of the restriction. The movements may or may not be assisted by the therapist. An overly ambitious therapist can easily overdo this technique, taking you dangerously close to *ballistic stretching*, in which you repeatedly bounce against the stretching barrier. This is stretching at its most extreme and most hazardous.

There are significant risks to active isolated stretching if you're not careful. You can experience microtrauma in muscles and tendons, extreme soreness, and reflexive spasming (Chaitow and DeLany 2000, 154). This method should be reserved for athletes and others who are in good physical condition and free of myofascial pain. The reaction of your trigger points to active isolated stretching can throw you into a severe pain crisis that can last for days or weeks, even when followed with competent trigger point therapy.

Muscle Energy Techniques

In using *muscle energy techniques* to cope with a shoulder problem, the patient makes small, active arm movements with mild effort against resistance provided by the therapist. The movement begins at or near the place where movement is stopped by restriction. The object is to move the arm to a new barrier with a minimum of forced stretching. The patient continues pressing against the counterforce for up to twenty seconds. Patients are directed to use no more than 20 percent of their strength, a very small amount of force. But even with this small force, muscle energy techniques can cause increased pain. Sometimes it can be made less hazardous by doing trigger point massage before and after the treatment, but only if you and the therapist stretch very conservatively.

Joint Mobilization

In *joint mobilization*, the therapist slowly and carefully moves the patient's arm through its full range of motion. Sometimes called *gliding mobilization*, this procedure is intended to increase freedom of movement in soft tissue and joints. A technique is also employed for separating the bony surfaces of the joint *(distraction)* and moving one surface in circles relative to the other (*oscillation*) to stretch the connective tissue. The patient remains passive, providing neither assistance nor resistance, although in a variation of this technique the patient does participate actively in the movement.

Joint mobilization won't release your trigger points or cause the spontaneous breaking of adhesions. It is, however, an effective means for gradually regaining your range of motion after trigger point massage has begun to succeed. An extreme form of joint mobilization is *manipulation under anesthesia*, in which the arm is forcibly moved through what would be its normal range of motion with the intention of breaking adhesions in the joint. Manipulation under anesthesia is rarely needed when nonforced joint mobilization is used along with soft-tissue mobilization and trigger point massage.

Integrated Neuromuscular Inhibition

A complex technique, *integrated neuromuscular inhibition* involves the therapist moving your arm to stretch specific shoulder muscles while pressing and holding their trigger points. It begins with you holding your arm near its movement barrier in a position of ease for thirty seconds and then contracting the target muscle for ten seconds. The therapist then initiates a gentle stretch as you relax. This is called a *passive* stretch because you don't participate in making the movement. The problem with this method lies in its dependence on the questionable "contract-relax" effect, and in the ever-present ambition to attain a measurable result. Nevertheless, because of the attention paid to trigger points, this technique may produce small improvements in range of motion if used by the therapist with particular sensitivity. Any increase in pain is a signal to desist.

Positional Release

Positional release is similar to the osteopathic method of *strain-counterstrain*. In treating your shoulder, the therapist places your arm in its most pain-free position, then holds this position of comfort for ninety seconds. Pressure is often held on the trigger point that's been causing the pain and restriction. Finally, the arm is moved in a slow, painless return to the strained position in which pain was felt. This method aims to accomplish a spontaneous release of restricted tissue and a reduction in pain without stretching. This can be an effective form of trigger point therapy, but be aware that therapists who believe strongly in stretching will be tempted to unnecessarily corrupt the positional release method with their favorite weapon.

Soft-Tissue Mobilization

When the physical therapist kneads, spreads, and stretches the muscles and connective tissue of the shoulder by hand, the insurance company will be billed for *soft-tissue mobilization*. This manual technique employs elements of myofascial release, but the actual process is very much like the petrissage (kneading) technique of Swedish massage. The objective of soft-tissue mobilization is to reverse the changes in connective tissue caused by immobilization so that the arm and shoulder will move more freely. Soft-tissue mobilization is also used for making scar tissue more pliable.

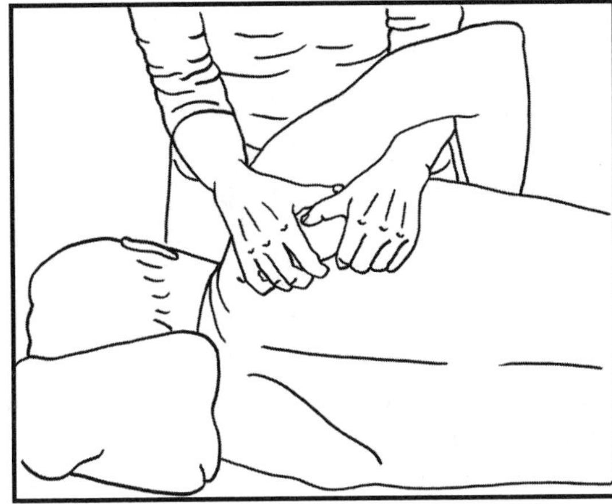

Figure 9.5 Scapular mobilization for stretching the muscles that attach to the shoulder blade

This method also includes *scapular mobilization*, in which the therapist moves the shoulder blade through its normal movement patterns while kneading the muscles that attach to it (Figure 9.5). Other terminology for this process is *interscapular muscle release* and *scapulothoracic release* (Simons, Travell, and Simons 1999, 489-490; McMahon and Donatelli 2004, 424-431). When you have a frozen shoulder, scapular mobilization can easily be overdone. Call a halt if the therapist seems to be jerking and tugging on your shoulder blade with too much vigor.

Electrotherapy

Electrotherapy is known by a wide variety of names, including high-voltage galvanic stimulation, electrogalvanic stimulation, electrostimulation, microcurrent stimulation, microampere stimulation, electro muscle stimulation, electro-acupuncture, and interferential current therapy. In everyday speech, all versions of electrotherapy are simply called "e-stim."

Theoretically, e-stim works by fatiguing the muscle tissue with small, rapid spasmodic contractions, presumably causing the muscle to reflexively relax after the stimulation ends. This again relies on the debatable contract-relax effect. In some cases, the actual effect may be to irritate critical trigger points, particularly if too much e-stim is used. On the other hand, the passive muscle exercise provided by e-stim does increase general circulation in muscle tissue. The rapid contractions may also cause the release of painkilling endorphins. E-stim uses at least 150 volts, which makes it somewhat uncomfortable, and it can take up to fifteen minutes per muscle. This is roughly sixty times as long as it would take to treat the same muscle with trigger point massage.

The high-tech aura of this treatment may contribute to the placebo effect in decreasing pain, but e-stim is too nonspecific to reliably hit the targeted trigger point. Even so, electrotherapy is used in some form by virtually all physical therapists as a part of the mixed-modality or comprehensive pain management approach. The scattergun approach to therapy isn't based on strict science, but now and again something works.

Transcutaneous electrical nerve stimulation (TENS) is a highly successful form of electrotherapy that works by directly interfering with pain signals in the central nervous system. TENS is very effective in relieving pain while the unit is active, but it has no effect on the cause of the pain and has no place in the treatment of trigger points and chronic myofascial pain.

Vibration

Ultrasound, which is vibration above the range of human hearing, is used for deep heating of muscles before stretching. It's used extensively in physical therapy, but it doesn't override the ability of trigger points to keep a muscle tight. A good trigger point massage therapist would have no need of ultrasound.

Infrasonic vibration, which is below the range of human hearing, is applied to your muscles by means of various handheld electrical vibrators that operate at between 8 and 14 hertz. You can pay a lot of money for a chair that accomplishes nothing more. This well-known and popular method for the treatment of sore muscles produces a sense of relaxation but has a negligible effect on myofascial trigger points. As a consequence, you should expect any reduction of your shoulder pain to be only temporary.

Hydrotherapy and Cryotherapy

Most physical therapists use *hydrotherapy* in the form of moist heat at some point in their treatments for pain. Warm water produces muscle relaxation and increased circulation to the area and presumably aids in getting muscle fibers and connective tissue to lengthen. Heat has no specific effect in causing trigger points to release, but it can irritate them if too much heat is used or if it's kept in place too long.

Cryotherapy, or the chilling of muscle tissue with ice, has its uses in physical therapy for the reduction of inflammation and swelling. It's most effective right after an injury, and it can have a temporary deadening effect on pain. Cold, however, is a classic cause and perpetuator of trigger points, so whenever ice or another chilling substance is used in the treatment of myofascial pain, it should always be followed immediately with moist heat.

Physical Therapy as Self-Treatment

For shoulder pain and stiffness, physical therapists and doctors often prescribe stretching and strengthening exercises to be done at home. Your homework is considered to be a large factor in how soon you regain flexibility, strength, motor control, and endurance in your shoulder. A responsible practitioner will warn you to procede with caution and take care not to overdo your self-therapy. There are others, however, who still mistakenly urge you toward doing your therapy aggressively.

Remember that trigger points shorten and weaken the muscles that operate the shoulder. This makes trigger points the initial cause of much shoulder pain, instability, and impairment, as well as many injuries to the shoulder's ligaments, tendons, and other connective tissue. When a muscle is resistant to stretching, you can strain or even tear muscle attachments if you persist in stretching, and the rotator cuff is particularly at risk.

This important rule always applies: If a stretch or an exercise hurts, *don't do it.* Wait until the pain is gone. And don't be misled by promises of relief to be gained by medication. You should never do stretches or exercises under the illusory influence of a painkiller. Your pain is still there, trying to warn you to be careful, but its voice is being silenced by the drug. It's amazing how easy it is to overdo stretching and strengthening exercises, even when your natural warning system is unimpaired by painkillers. Sadly, it's not unusual for well-intentioned therapy for a frozen shoulder to send someone to the emergency room in such intense pain that they readily agree to surgery they may not really need.

Active Stretching

There are two kinds of stretching. *Passive stretching* is when a therapist moves your arm and shoulder. *Active stretching* is when you make the movements yourself. If you choose to do stretching as therapy for your shoulder, it's best to keep it under your own control. Remember that stretching is not a necessity. If trigger point massage succeeds in getting rid of your pain, your strength, flexibility, and range of motion will return naturally over time with normal activity. The only advantage of stretching is that it might speed things along—provided that it doesn't set you back by being done carelessly or overzealously.

The stretching techniques described here are all well-known, and you've probably seen them illustrated in many other places. It's worth looking at them again, however, with a view to understanding what they actually do. With any of the stretches, take your time and do only a little bit at first. Then wait for a few hours or until the next day to see how your shoulder reacts before doing more.

Codman Exercises

These most familiar shoulder exercises were introduced over seventy years ago in a textbook on the shoulder by Ernest Codman, a Boston doctor who had made the shoulder his life's work. Dr. Codman called his therapy "stooping" exercises because the patient leans over to do them. He recommended swinging the arm in circles and making "pendulum-like movements," believing that the weight of the arm helps stretch the contracted tissue of the joint and prevent adhesions (Codman 1934, 202-203).

Unfortunately, Dr. Codman apparently gave little thought to the muscles, and of course he lived too early to have any conception of myofascial trigger points. In actual use, the Codman exercises' pendulum movements (swinging the arm in straight lines) tend to inflict sudden jerks on the muscles at the ends of the swings, causing muscle stretching to occur abruptly. This can have the effect of making the muscles tighten defensively instead of lengthening. Moving the arm in circles, however, causes a smoother and gentler lengthening of the muscles and allows you to concentrate on relaxing them (Figure 9.6).

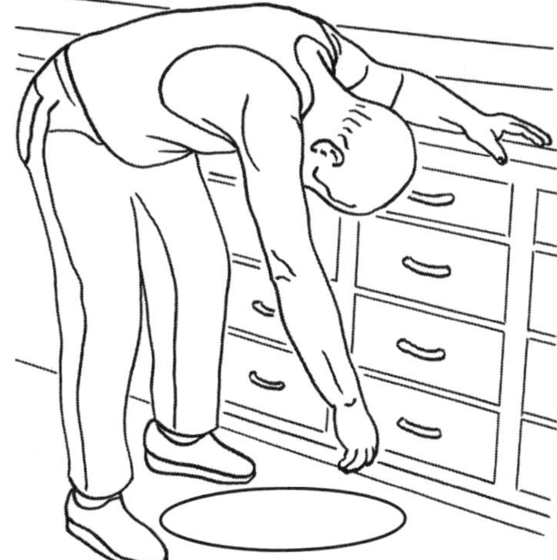

Figure 9.6 Codman circles for gently stretching the shoulder muscles and connective tissue

It's worth remembering that with the weight of the arm pulling it downward, the muscles of the shoulder must still maintain some degree of tension to keep the joint from pulling apart. You shouldn't hold a weight in your hand while doing Codman circles because it causes the muscles to tighten even more, rather than loosen.

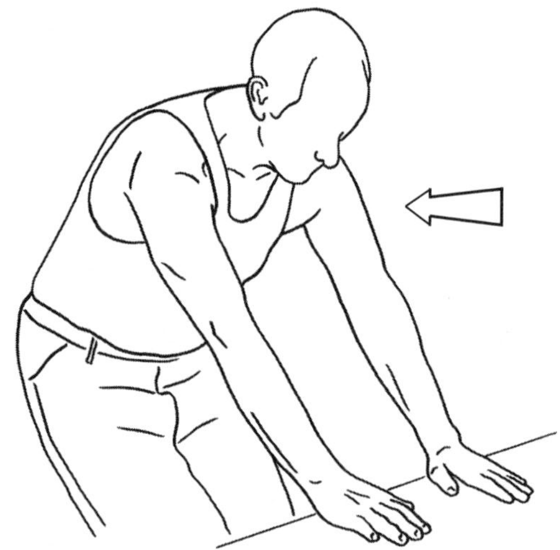

Figure 9.7 Raising the arm using a kitchen counter, desk, top of a filing cabinet, tabletop, or bookcase

Raising the Arm

The power for normal movement to raise the arm comes from the trapezius, deltoids, supraspinatus, serratus anterior, and biceps. Trigger points in these muscles cause pain and weakness that can make it hard for them to contract. Raising the arm also necessitates lengthening many of the muscles that operate the shoulder: the subscapularis, infraspinatus, teres minor, teres major, latissimus dorsi, pectoralis major, pectoralis minor, triceps, and coracobrachialis. Trigger points in these muscles, of course, tend to prevent lengthening by giving you pain.

You can remove much of the stress and strain from all these muscles by using something other than these muscles to raise your arm. A kitchen countertop or desktop is a handy means of doing this (Figure 9.7). With your hands in place, just slowly back away from the counter. Don't support any of your weight on your hands, as this will contract the muscles you want to stretch.

The common walking cane, usually about three feet long, is the classic implement for lifting your arm to stretch a stiff shoulder. You could also use a piece of plastic PVC pipe or a curtain rod of that length. You might think of just getting a three-foot dowel rod from the hardware store, but don't do that. Dowels are unsanded and unfinished, so they'll give you splinters. A cut-off broomstick or mop handle, however, does have a finish on it, making a very handy, cheap, and versatile tool for shoulder therapy. Pulley systems are available for raising your arm, but they don't do the job any better than a simple three-foot piece of broomstick. To stretch different groups of muscles, raise your arm in three distinctly different directions (Figures 9.8, 9.9, and 9.10). People who can tolerate stretching have cured their own frozen shoulder using broomstick therapy and nothing else. The trick is to go at a snail's pace and be very, very patient.

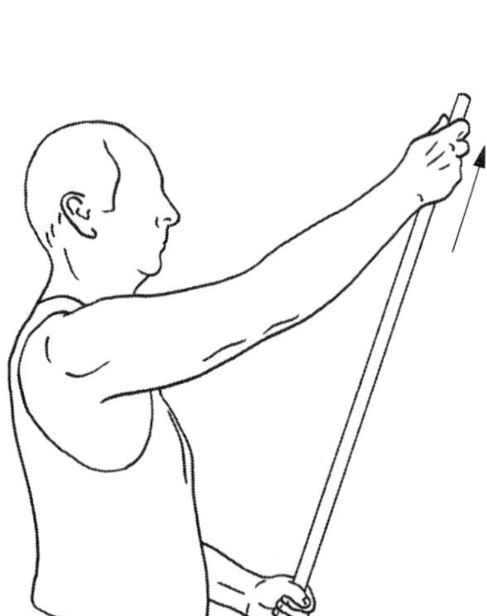

Figure 9.8 Raising the arm forward with a broomstick

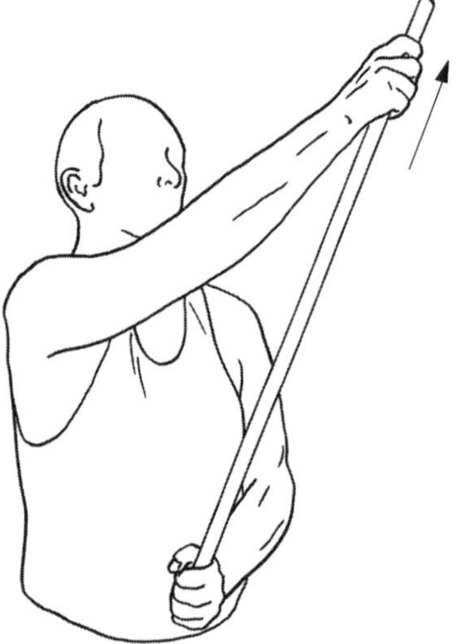

Figure 9.9 Raising the arm across the body with a broomstick

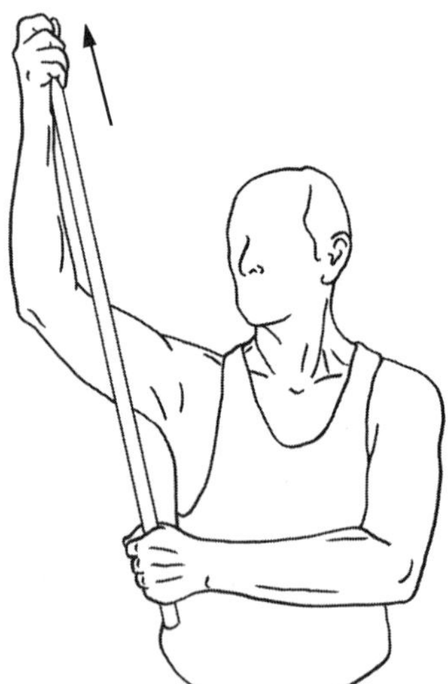

Figure 9.10 Raising the arm to the side with a broomstick

Rotator Muscle Stretches

The four muscles that rotate your arm need special attention since they're almost always at the heart of the problem with a stiff or frozen shoulder. As shown in Figures 9.2, 9.3, and 9.4, three basic positions are used when the therapist does the stretching for you, but you can also do these stretches unassisted. The safest and gentlest stretch for the supraspinatus, infraspinatus, and teres minor is done by reaching across and placing your hand on your opposite shoulder, using a little help from the opposite hand (Figure 9.11). The middle trapezius, posterior deltoid, and rhomboid muscles are also stretched with this maneuver.

A more demanding stretch of the supraspinatus, infraspinatus, and teres minor muscles is accomplished by using a broomstick to pull the arm into internal rotation, adduction, and extension behind your back (Figure 9.12). This also stretches the pectoralis major, anterior deltoid, and coracobrachialis muscles. More demanding yet is to pull your arm up behind your back with a broomstick or towel (Figures 9.13 and 9.14). In addition to the muscles already named, this will stretch the triceps. Figure 9.15 shows a nearly normal range of motion for this stretch.

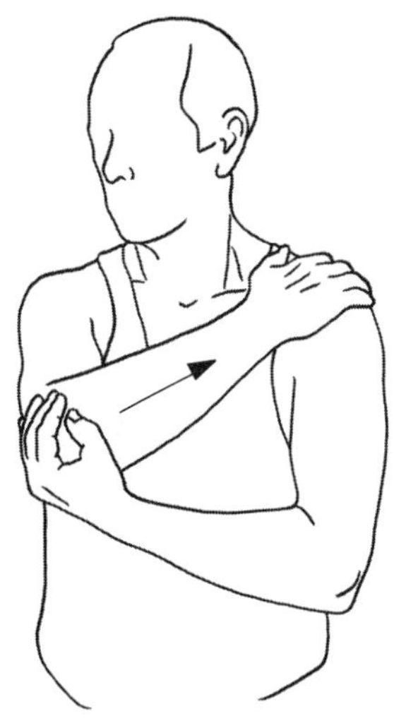

Figure 9.11 Stretching the supraspinatus, infraspinatus, and teres minor muscles

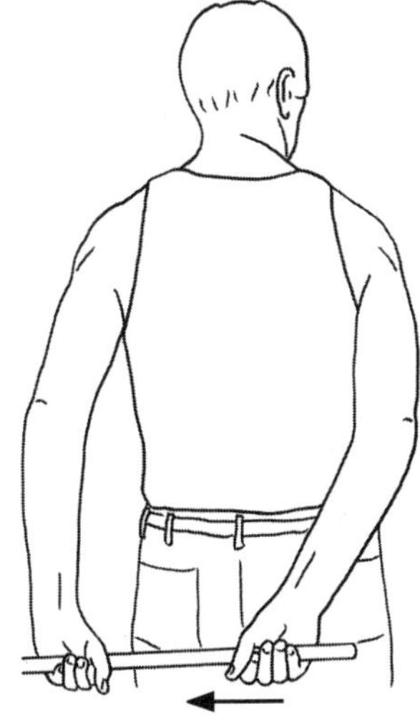

Figure 9.12 Stretching the supraspinatus, infraspinatus, and teres minor muscles

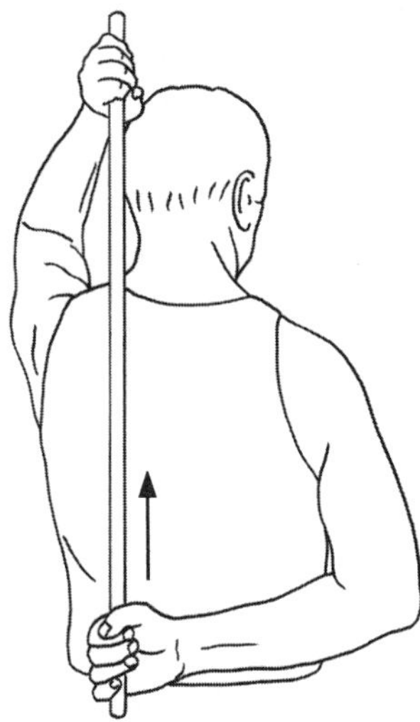

Figure 9.13 Lifting the arm behind the back with a broomstick

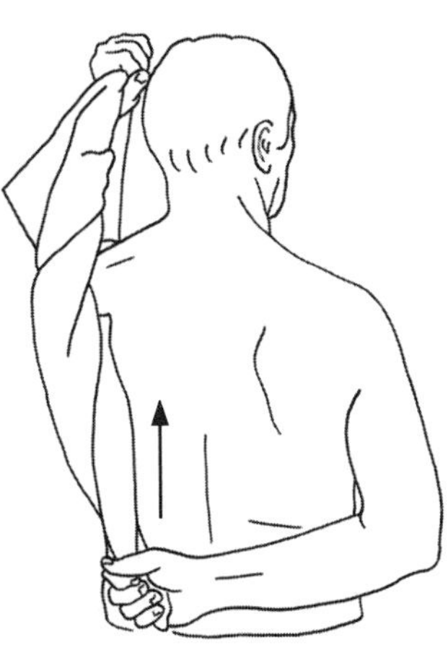

Figure 9.14 Lifting the arm behind the back with a towel

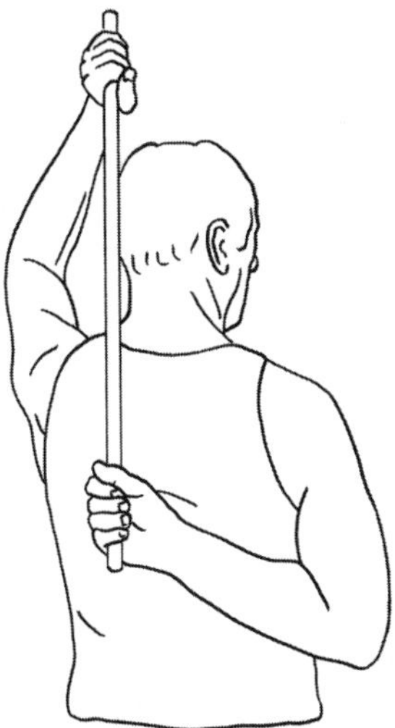

Figure 9.15 Approaching the normal range of motion

The Doorway Stretch

The best stretch for the infamous subscapularis muscle is simply to lean into a doorway with your hands on the doorjambs. You can do the same thing in a corner, but a doorway gives you a better grip. In preparation for the doorway stretch, it's a good idea to use a broomstick to push your arm into outward rotation for several sessions (Figure 9.16). This lets the subscapularis get used to the idea. Both of these stretches lengthen the pectoralis major, pectoralis minor, serratus anterior, and coracobrachialis, along with the subscapularis.

With the doorway stretch, the position of your hands on the doorjambs has an effect on how much each muscle is being stretched (Figure 9.17). Begin in the lowest position, with your hands level with your shoulders. It may take days or even weeks before you can get to the highest position, but if you're patient with yourself, you will ultimately be able to lean into the doorway with your hands all the way up. For safety, keep one foot under you in the doorway.

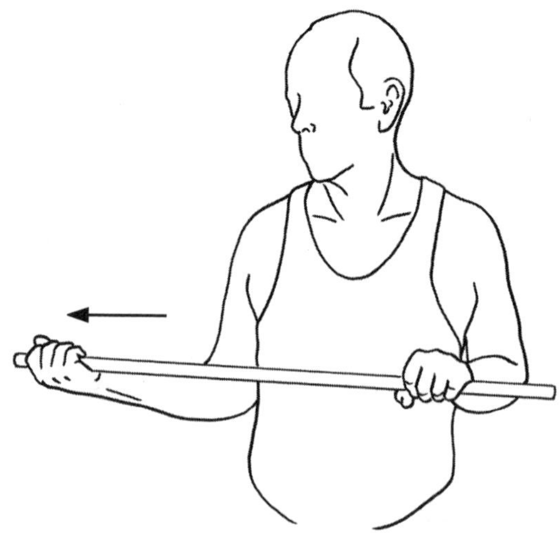

Figure 9.16 Pushing the right arm into external rotation with a broomstick while keeping the right elbow tight against the side

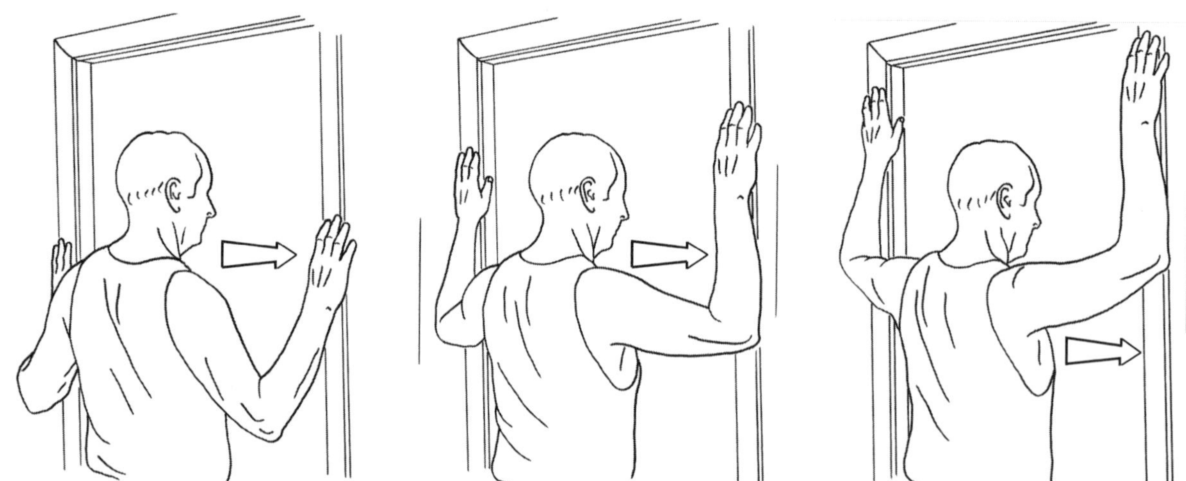

Figure 9.17 Stretching the subscapularis, pectoral, and serratus anterior muscles by leaning into a doorway with the hands in successively higher positions

Strengthening Exercises

There's no question that the inactivity imposed by shoulder pain causes some degree of deconditioning and weakening of the muscles. A large portion of this weakness is only temporary, however, when trigger points are the cause. Most of your strength returns just as soon as the trigger points have been deactivated unless you've been kept from using your arm for an extended length of time.

Unfortunately, many physical therapists think more like physical trainers than therapists and view any sign of muscle weakness as something that needs to be immediately corrected. Just as with stretching, some patients respond very well to strengthening exercises and get considerable pain relief and improved flexibility. But these lucky people set an impossible standard for the many others whose muscles respond negatively to strengthening exercises.

At the same time, it would be an error to avoid all exercise of your arm and shoulder out of fear that it might cause pain. A good rule with exercise is to stay within your comfort zone. You can work right up to the edge of pain, but be ready to back off at the first twinge. Also, wait until trigger point massage has mostly taken the pain away and you've begun to feel comfortable with careful stretching of the muscles. Be especially conservative the first few days of exercise. Make a conscious commitment to do less than you think you can. With exercise, nothing will get you into trouble faster than trying to do too much too soon.

Strengthening the Rotator Muscles

If you go to a physical therapist for help with your shoulder, standard procedure is to give you a length of rubber tubing and a program of exercises to do with it. You might get a nice little brochure illustrating the exercises. You're more likely to get a photocopied sheet with a selection of exercises cut and pasted from one book or another. The cut-and-paste version can look pretty cheap, but it does have the advantage of being "just for you," so hopefully it won't include exercises you shouldn't be doing. It would be nice to believe the therapist has crafted this set of exercises for your specific situation, but you should use your own discretion. Trust your intuition and your own sense of what's right for you and what you can handle.

The rubber tubing also comes as flat latex strips, and both types are usually color coded to indicate their strength. To provide something to pull against, you tie a large knot in the end and trap that end between a closed door and the door frame. Or you can tie the end to a doorknob. You maintain a firm grip on the other end by wrapping the tubing or strip around your hand. Inexpensive elastic "sports cords" (available online or in large sporting goods stores) come with handles and door anchors already attached.

Rubber tubing or elastic bands, which allow you to exercise against resistance, are used for internal rotation and external rotation exercises. Rotating your arm inward requires contraction of your subscapularis, pectoralis major, anterior deltoid, coracobrachialis, and biceps muscles (Figure 9.18). Rotating outward requires contraction of your infraspinatus, teres minor, posterior deltoid, rhomboids, and middle trapezius (Figure 9.19).

An ever-present hazard with rubber material is that it degrades with time, making it subject to breaking at just the wrong moment. The tubing can snap and hit you, ordinarily not a terrible danger unless it hits you in the eye. Perhaps worse, an unexpected break can cause you to make an abrupt uncontrolled movement that could be extremely painful or even damaging to your shoulder.

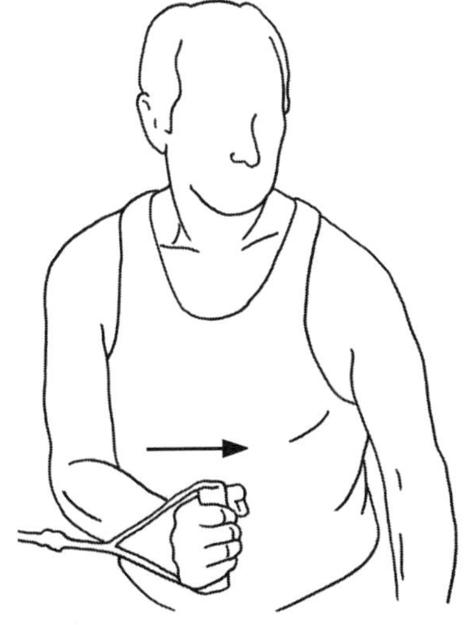

Figure 9.18 Inward rotation against rubber tubing resistance

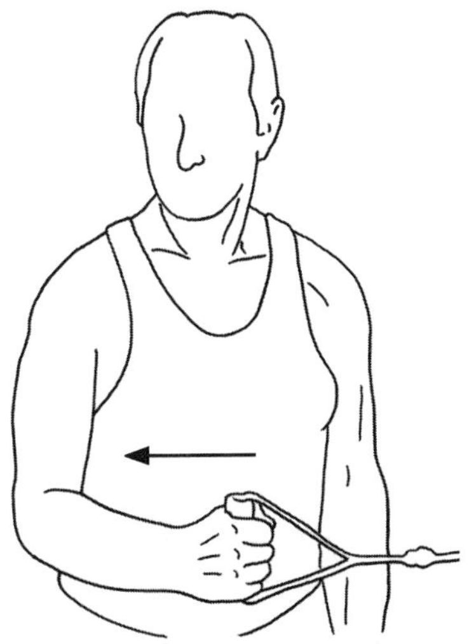

Figure 9.19 Outward rotation against rubber tubing resistance

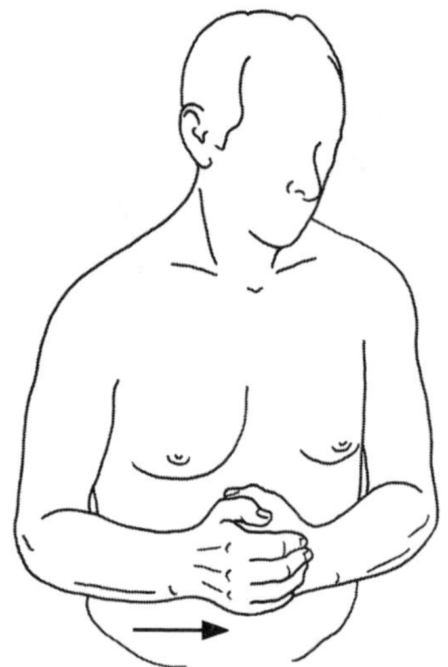

Figure 9.20 Inward rotation of the right arm against resistance, keeping the elbow tucked in

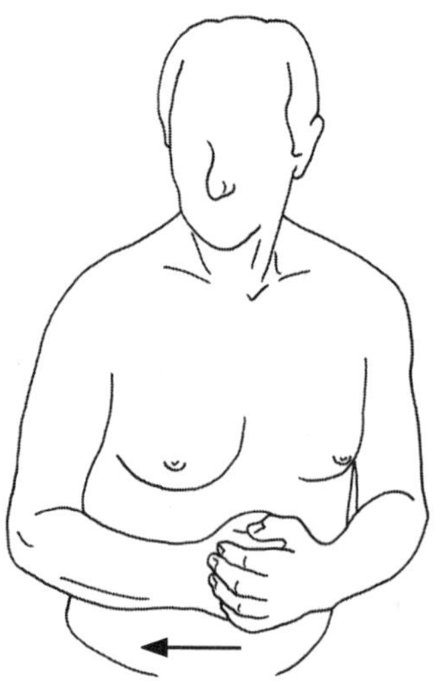

Figure 9.21 Outward rotation of the right arm against resistance, keeping the elbow tucked in

If you don't want to wear goggles and be constantly on guard when you exercise, you can dispense with the rubber tubing and provide your own resistance to both inward and outward rotation. This *isotonic* method of exercise has the advantage of giving both arms a workout at the same time. While you're contracting the inward rotation muscles of your bad arm, the outward rotators of your good arm provide the resistance, which puts everything entirely under your own control (Figure 9.20). You can use as much or as little force as you like. As always, begin gently and experimentally and see how your shoulder reacts.

The same principles are in effect when you work your outward rotators (Figure 9.21). These two exercises are not only the safest way to strengthen the rotator cuff muscles, they're also extremely effective, even for the athletically inclined. The principle of isotonic contraction is exactly what gave old-time bodybuilder Charles Atlas his strength and wonderfully sculpted physique.

If you'd prefer to use a measurable force in exercising your rotators, you can lie down and use a small weight (Figure 9.22). The illustration shows a three-pound dumbbell, which is certainly too heavy to begin with. A one-pound weight would be better at first. A can of soup, at three-quarters of a pound, is better yet. Note that the upper arm is positioned at roughly a right angle to the body. This exercise alternately contracts the inward and outward rotator muscles. The motion resembles how you would beat your chest with one fist, if you were that kind of person.

You can strengthen the subscapularis pretty much in isolation by moving the weight in another direction (Figure 9.23). Begin with your forearm vertical, with the weight in its

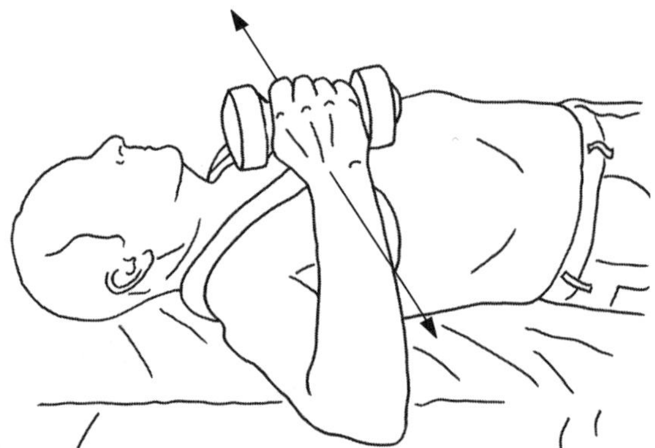

Figure 9.22 Strengthening with internal and external rotation of the arm, bringing the dumbbell all the way across your chest

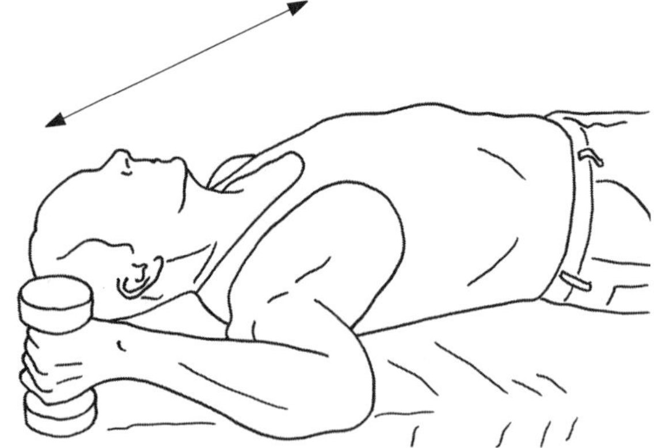

Figure 9.23 Subscapularis strengthening with a dumbbell

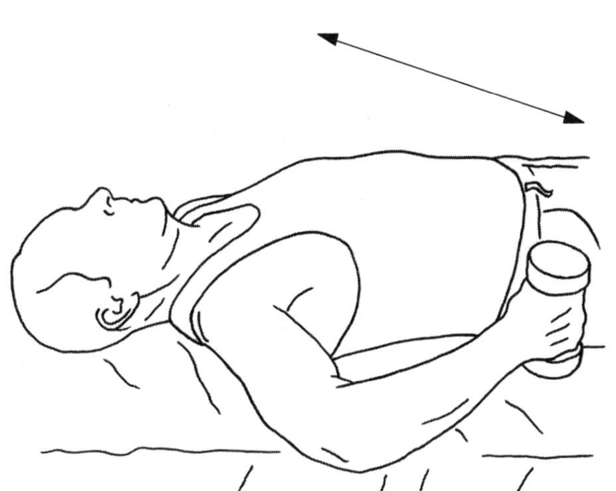

Figure 9.24 Infraspinatus and teres minor strengthening with a dumbbell

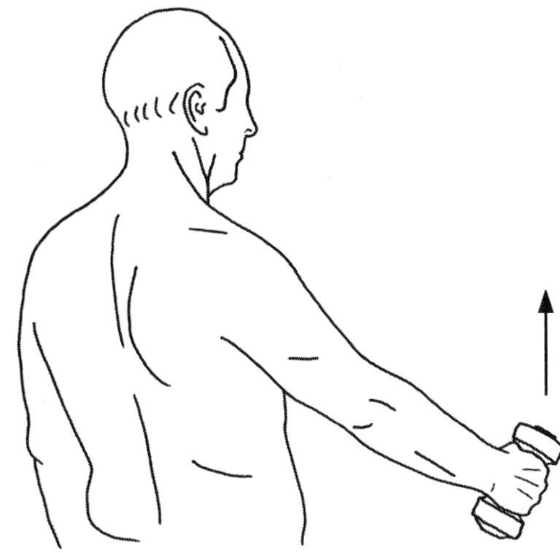

Figure 9.25 Supraspinatus strengthening with a dumbbell, moving the arm up and down halfway between the front and the side

highest position. Then slowly lower the weight down beside your head. To complete the movement, bring the forearm back up to vertical. To begin more conservatively, do this exercise without a weight, employing only the weight of your arm.

To strengthen the infraspinatus and teres minor, lower your arm in the other direction to end up with the weight beside your hip bone (Figure 9.24). Obviously, you can alternate these two exercises, letting the weight down in one direction and then the other.

To give special attention to the supraspinatus, you can exercise it by simply raising your arm while standing up (Figure 9.25). The arm is raised neither to the front nor to the side, but halfway in between. Begin without a weight and move your arm only a foot or so. This is the range in which the supraspinatus is most active, since it's the muscle that initiates the upward movement of the arm. The deltoids and trapezius join in as you bring your arm higher.

This upward movement of the arm is what causes the so-called impingement syndrome, experienced as a sharp pain in the top of the shoulder joint. This happens when the three rotator muscles other than the supraspinatus have been weakened by trigger points and aren't keeping the ball in the socket. Any action of the supraspinatus then jams the head of the humerus up against the acromion and the intervening bursa. If attempting this maneuver is painful, don't do this exercise until the subscapularis, infraspinatus, and teres minor are healthy enough to keep the joint properly articulated. Impingement syndrome doesn't originate as a problem in the joint. It begins as a problem with the muscles.

Strengthening the Other Shoulder Muscles

If you do an extensive amount of work to strengthen your rotator muscles, it's a good idea to work on the other muscles that operate the shoulder and arm as well, just for the sake of keeping things in balance. Raising a weight to the rear will contract the triceps, posterior deltoid, latissimus dorsi, and teres major (Figure 9.26). You can make it a conservative effort or a vigorous workout, depending on the weight you use and the distance you try to move your arm. Be smart and begin without the weight, and don't try to reach for the moon.

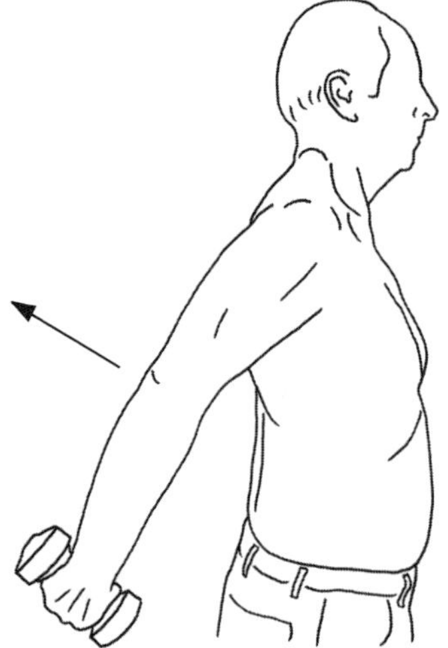

Figure 9.26 Strengthening the triceps, posterior deltoid, latissimus dorsi, and teres major with a dumbbell

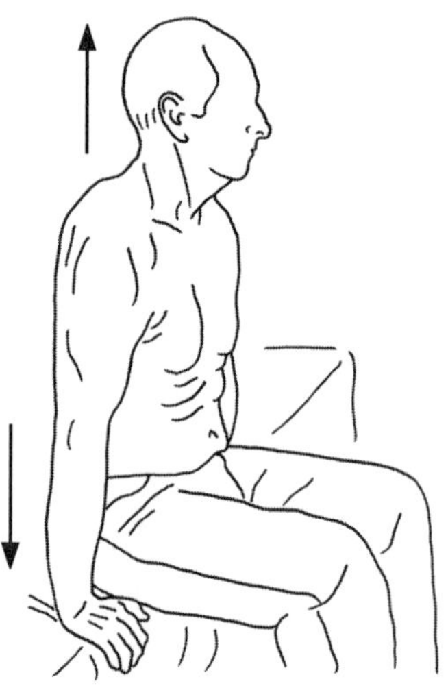

Figure 9.27 Latissimus dorsi strengthening with body lift

Simply pushing down and lifting yourself off the edge of your bed a few times can give a number of muscles a surprisingly strenuous workout (Figure 9.27). Even if you don't succeed in getting clear of the bed, the effort will contract the latissimus dorsi, teres major, subscapularis, pectoralis major, pectoralis minor, lower trapezius, serratus anterior, and rectus abdominis muscles.

One last gambit that can do a lot of good for almost every muscle involved with the shoulder is the familiar shoulder roll. You can do this in one fluid, continuous movement, which is a good safe exercise, especially if you do it slowly. Alternatively, you can break it down into three components and savor what happens when you move your shoulders in distinctly different directions. Begin by protracting both shoulders forward to contract the pectoralis major, pectoralis minor, and serratus anterior (Figure 9.28). This lengthens all the muscles behind the shoulder at the same time.

Next, raise your shoulders up toward your ears (Figure 9.29). This contracts the upper trapezius and levator scapulae muscles while lengthening the lower trapezius, latissimus dorsi, and teres major. Finally, pull both shoulders back to contract the middle trapezius and rhomboids (Figure 9.30). As you do this, you'll have a pleasurable sense of stretching in the pectoralis major muscles. The pulling on your ribs under your arms is due to the stretching of the serratus anterior, in case you wondered.

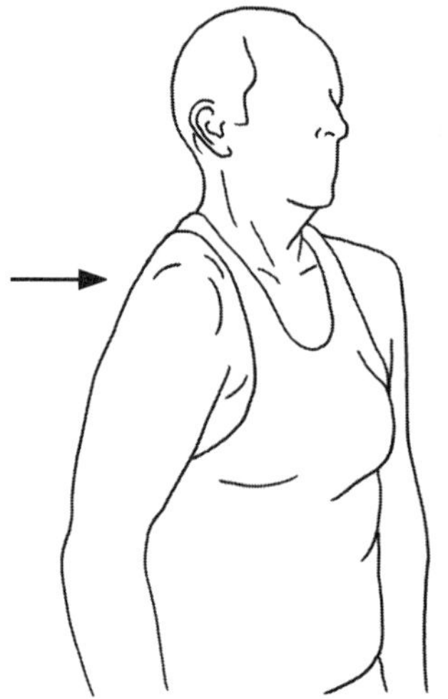

Figure 9.28 Pectoralis major and pectoralis minor strengthening with shoulder protraction

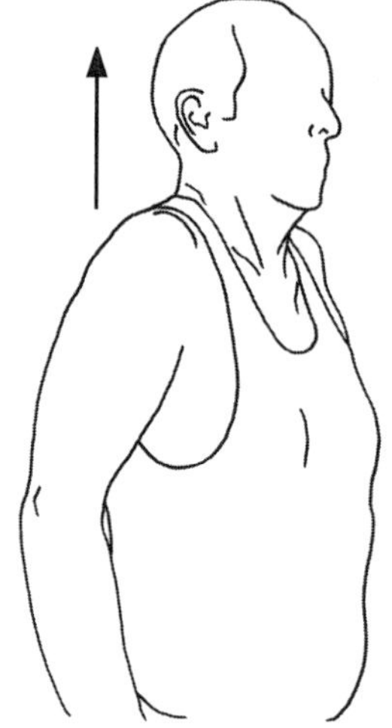

Figure 9.29 Upper trapezius and levator scapulae strengthening with shoulder elevation

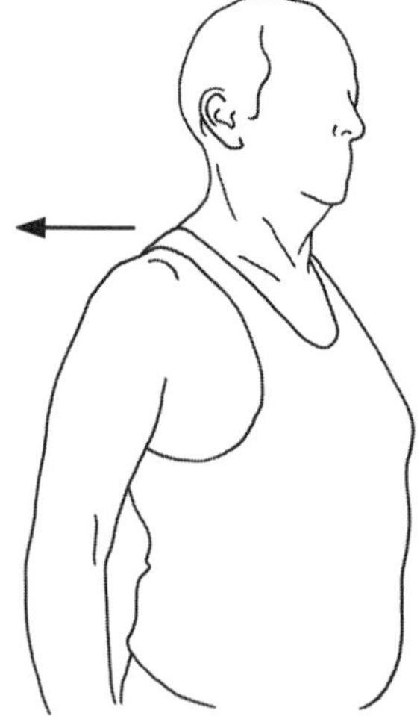

Figure 9.30 Middle trapezius and rhomboid strengthening with shoulder retraction

Summing Up Physical Therapy

If trigger point massage stops your pain and allows movement, it's very unlikely that you need physical therapy, any kind of extensive testing, or expensive medical treatment. The bottom line is that, after the pain is gone, most people will regain full range of motion naturally within a few weeks with normal activity. Most of the time, trigger point massage will stop the pain.

Rehabilitation of your shoulder after surgery or a serious accident involving broken bones or torn tissue may be a different matter. In such a case, a physical therapist or occupational therapist with extensive experience helping the disabled could be an indispensable ally. Even so, the most gifted and knowledgeable therapist or physician still functions under a handicap if they lack a working knowledge of myofascial trigger points and the effects they can have on your muscles. It wouldn't be a bad idea to give them a peek at this book.

Chapter 10

Medical Management of the Shoulder

From the standpoint of conventional medicine, the treatment of a frozen shoulder takes three possible pathways: painkillers, physical therapy, or surgery. The medical approach often uses all three as standard procedure. This routine is so well established that it's rarely questioned, although many people who have undergone medical management of a shoulder problem would contend that there needs to be a better way.

Painkilling drugs can be quite appropriate when they make life tolerable while the body heals from trauma or disease, but their adverse side effects have become a matter of increasing concern. Too often, they're viewed by both physician and patient as a cure for the problem, when in reality they provide only temporary relief and a false sense of security that can keep you from actively pursuing a genuine cure.

Physical therapy, though helpful for some people, is clearly unsuccessful for many others and sometimes detrimental. Aggressive physical therapy is a common prescription for the treatment of a frozen shoulder and sounds like strong medicine. In practice, "aggressive physical therapy" is code for aggressive stretching, a desperate measure ordered when conservative treatment has failed. As discussed in the previous chapter, stretching for shoulder problems should be used with great care because of its potential for damaging the vulnerable muscles and tendons of the rotator cuff.

Surgery is perhaps the state of the art of modern medicine, and along with skillful diagnosis, it's what many doctors do best. Indeed, when your shoulder has suffered genuine physical injury, such as a broken bone or a complete tear in a muscle, tendon, or ligament, surgery may be your only choice. When surgery turns out well, it can be a wonderful thing. But you should be aware that a surprising number of doctors admit that surgeries commonly done for frozen shoulder and for other shoulder injuries may not really be necessary in many cases (Arroyo and Flatow 1999, 36-37).

There's no denying that modern medicine at its best is full of wonders and to a large extent deserves the faith of the public and the high status it has attained. Surgery for the shoulder in particular is very highly developed, and new physicians are better trained than ever before. The procedures are sound in principle and usually successful in the hands of a highly skilled physician. However, distressing failures of shoulder surgery are a real risk when surgeons have attained only mediocre technical abilities or are downright incompetent. Surgery is so heavily promoted and has become so popular that many people undoubtedly agree to it when it may not be necessary.

Many doctors believe that even a torn rotator cuff, an inflamed bursa, or a shoulder joint filled with adhesions can very often heal itself with conservative treatment. An ethical physician usually wants patients to try conservative treatment for three to six months before considering surgery or costly tests like CAT scans and MRIs. It's too bad that so few physicians realize that conservative treatment for an afflicted shoulder could be significantly improved if trigger point therapy were simply added to standard physical therapy.

If the doctor fails to take trigger points and myofascial pain into account when considering all the possible causes of shoulder pain and disability, medical treatment can be unnecessarily risky, prolonged, expensive, and ineffective. The nearly invariable medical assumption is that the cause of shoulder pain and stiffness is in the complex tissues of the shoulder joint, so the joint becomes the exclusive object of attention. Rarely does it occur to the doctor that myofascial trigger points affecting operation of the shoulder joint could be the origin of many of the problems that show up there. As a consequence, most physicians still refer to shoulder afflictions such as frozen shoulder as "enigmatic," even though this is no longer true because of the light Janet Travell and David Simons have shed on this issue (Simons, Travell, and Simons 1999, 544-546, 604-606).

Medical Diagnosis of the Shoulder

Many of the mysteries and enigmas regarding the origins of shoulder problems are explained by the trigger point phenomenon. But even the latest medical textbooks on the shoulder rarely even mention myofascial pain and trigger points. When given any consideration at all, it's usually just two or three paragraphs that at best reveal a superficial understanding, and sometimes the information is downright erroneous. Given this situation, today's physicians graduate from medical school largely ignorant of one of the most important causes of pain and disability. Unless physicians have made an independent study of myofascial pain, this gap in their knowledge can undermine their ability to accurately diagnose a painful shoulder.

That said, medical diagnosis can be very proficient when it comes to checking for serious disease in internal organs, such as the heart, gallbladder, or lungs, which are known to refer pain to the shoulder. In fact, a primary reason for seeing a doctor is to rule these things out or to catch them before they've caused too much harm. If your trigger points are hard to get rid of or seem to come back right away without your having done anything to aggravate them, it's worth making sure you don't have an internal problem.

Visceral Disease Affecting the Shoulder

Some of the organs that can cause pain in the shoulder area are the lungs, heart, liver, pancreas, gallbladder, kidney, stomach, colon, and large intestine. Structures such as the diaphragm, esophagus, and aorta can also refer pain to the shoulder (Gray 2004, 365-376). Other potential causes of shoulder pain include such systemic diseases as gout, syphilis, gonorrhea, sickle-cell anemia, hemophilia, rheumatic disease, and metastatic cancer. Specific diseases that may give you shoulder pain are angina, pericarditis, aortic aneurysm, breast cancer, tumors of the spine, hiatal hernia, ruptured spleen, peptic ulcer, upper urinary tract infection, lung cancer, pulmonary tuberculosis, pneumothorax, tuberculosis, and Pancoast's tumor when it affects the brachial nerve plexus that serves the shoulder and arm (Cappel et al. 2001, 78-79).

You shouldn't let these lists of nightmares keep you awake at night, because none of them are nearly as common a cause of shoulder pain as myofascial trigger points. But you need to be aware of these possible other causes. It wouldn't be good to be preoccupied with trigger points for an extended period of time and allow something serious to go untreated.

Nerve Injuries Affecting the Shoulder

Pain in the shoulder can be caused by nerves in the neck and shoulder area that have been injured by accidental overstretching, compression, or blunt force trauma. Inadvertent damage to nerves during surgery is another cause. Unfortunately, it's not uncommon (Jensen and Rockwood 1997, 116-121). Electrophysiologic examination is needed to determine whether nerve injuries are causing the problem. However, even when nerves have been damaged, they usually don't require treatment because nerve tissue in muscle is very good at regenerating and healing itself over time. When symptoms from a nerve injury persist beyond six months and continue to diminish a person's quality of life, surgery is often attempted. But the success of these surgeries is extremely variable, and they sometimes result in serious complications and even death (Kozin 1999, 847-880).

Trigger points in certain shoulder muscles can cause compression of nerves that pass through or near them. When nerve injury or entrapment causes shoulder pain but isn't competently diagnosed, the symptoms may be misinterpreted and mistakenly treated as disorders of the glenohumeral joint, including impingement syndrome and rotator cuff tear. The skilled diagnosis and treatment of the trigger points involved could shorten recovery time for most shoulder symptoms from nerve compression and prevent unnecessary suffering and adverse outcomes from medical treatment (Simons, Travell, and Simons 1999, 558).

Medical Examination of the Shoulder

Physicians use four methods to gather information about the condition of your shoulder: visual assessment, palpation (touch), movement testing, and imaging studies such as X-rays, ultrasound, computerized axial tomography (CAT scans), and magnetic resonance imaging (MRI). Finding out the location and intensity of your pain is very important, but it can only be determined based on your verbal reports and body language. One of the fundamental problems in medicine is that pain can't be directly perceived or measured by an outside observer.

Doctors who diagnose and treat myofascial pain get a little closer to understanding your pain by expanding the palpation aspect of the examination to include a hands-on search for trigger points. It's extremely helpful to be able to put your finger right on the spot that produces the pain. Incorrect conclusions can be drawn about a painful spot, however, if the doctor is unaware of trigger points or has decided not to believe in them. If an opinionated but uninformed professor in medical school maligns the whole idea of trigger points, it can poison a young doctor's thinking for a lifetime. This blocks out an entire branch of medicine that could contain the solution to a number of the mysteries regarding the shoulder.

Visual Assessment and Palpation

A considerable amount of valuable information can be collected with a methodical inspection of your shoulder's appearance. The examiner first assesses your general posture, with special attention to the symmetry of your shoulders. The bad shoulder is compared with the good one from both front and back, looking for differences in height, contour, and positioning.

Fullness or enlargement of the front or back of the shoulder can indicate a dislocation of the glenohumeral (ball-and-socket) joint, which may be accompanied by an injury to the rotator cuff or glenoid labrum (Wirth, Orfaly, and Rockwood 2001, 109, 147-149). It's important to know that a shoulder dislocation can be caused and maintained by trigger points if they disturb the balance of strength in the rotator cuff muscles. Conversely, the strain imposed by a dislocation can promote the development of trigger points. In regard to an unstable shoulder joint, the condition of the shoulder muscles is of paramount importance and the possibility of trigger points should always be considered (Simons, Travell, and Simons 1999, 545-546).

The physician also looks for enlargement of the acromioclavicular joint, on top of the shoulder (Figure 10.1, letter A). Pain when this area is pressed may be a sign of a sprain, separation, dislocation, or arthritic growth (Wirth, Orfaly, and Rockwood 2001, 109). A tender, bony bump can be good evidence of a genuine joint problem, but pain by itself could be from a trapezius trigger point that lies right behind the joint. Trauma or disease of the acromioclavicular joint shouldn't be the only things that come to mind (Simons, Travell, and Simons 1999, 278-281).

The examiner also feels for tenderness in the subacromial bursa, under the outer edge of the acromion (Figure 10.1, letter B). If it hurts to press there, the doctor may too hastily conclude that you have bursitis or a rotator cuff tear (Wirth, Orfaly, and Rockwood 2001, 110). These conditions are indeed a possibility, but doctors should be aware that an extremely tender attachment trigger point in the supraspinatus muscle is often found at the same spot (Simons, Travell, and Simons 1999, 538).

In the medical view, tenderness in the biceps tendon in the groove in the front of the head of the humerus (Figure 10.1, letter C) is due to bicipital tendinitis (Wirth, Orfaly, and Rockwood 2001, 110). To be sure, in extreme situations the biceps tendon can become inflamed and swollen, but tenderness in the front of the shoulder is most often nothing more serious than a trigger point in the anterior deltoid, which covers the biceps tendon. It can also be referred tenderness from biceps or infraspinatus trigger points (Simons, Travell, and Simons 1999, 552-553, 623, 649).

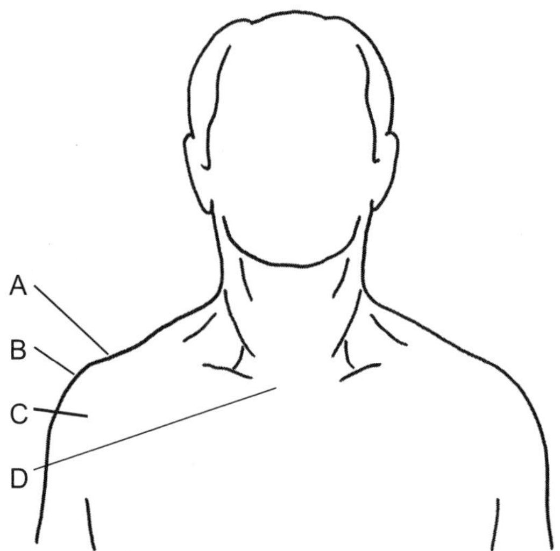

Figure 10.1 Anterior view for examination of the shoulder showing places of possible trouble; see the text for details.

Tenderness and a bony prominence just beside the top of the breastbone can be a dislocated sternoclavicular joint (Figure 10.1, letter D). This is an unlikely place for a trigger point or referred myofascial pain, but a sternoclavicular dislocation could cause trigger points to develop in the sternocleidomastoid, subclavius, and pectoralis major muscles. This would be a factor to consider if instability of the joint became an issue after the dislocation was reduced. A collarbone fracture could affect these same muscles (Chaitow and DeLany 2000, 298).

A sunken look in the trapezius, deltoid, supraspinatus, or infraspinatus is worthy of concern (Figure 10.2, letters E and F) because it may be a sign of atrophy due to disuse after a nerve injury or rotator cuff tear (Wirth, Orfaly, and Rockwood 2001, 109-110; Cappel et al. 2001, 81-82). Trigger points aren't usually the cause of muscle atrophy except in rare cases when they're responsible for long-term inactivity because of chronic pain (Mense and Simons 2001, 214).

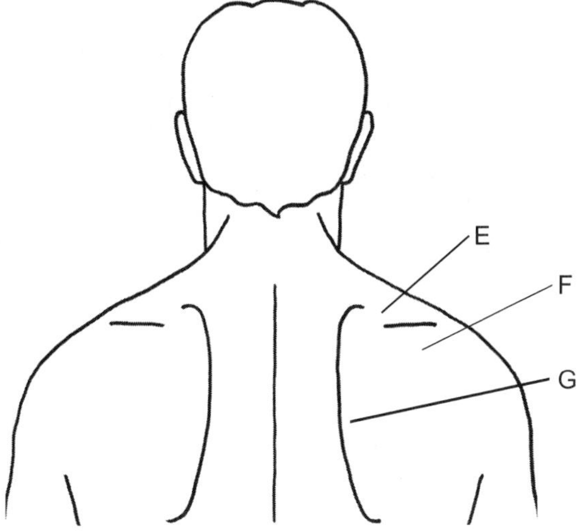

Figure 10.2 Posterior view for examination of the shoulder showing places of possible trouble; see the text for details.

Prominence, or "winging," of the inner border of the shoulder blade (Figure 10.2, letter G) can be evidence of weakness in the serratus anterior muscle, which occasionally may be due to paralysis from a nerve injury (Wirth, Orfaly, and Rockwood 2001, 112). Short of that extreme situation, doctors often speculate that such weakness is from strain or age-related inactivity and prescribe physical therapy for strengthening. However, trigger points that weaken the serratus anterior and shorten the pectoralis minor are the usual cause of shoulder blade winging, in which case exercise is inappropriate and conventional physical therapy could make these trigger points worse (Simons, Travell, and Simons 1999, 847, 890).

Strength and Movement Tests

There are more than sixty kinds of strength and movement tests that can be used in the systematic assessment and evaluation of the shoulder (Cappel et al. 2001, 76). Unfortunately, the accuracy of these tests is diminished when arm movement and muscle contraction are inhibited by myofascial pain (Wirth, Orfaly, and Rockwood 2001, 107).

Many practitioners acknowledge that strength and movement tests lack reliability and validity but still contend that they're the best noninvasive kinds of testing available. The use of these tests continues, as do the inferences drawn from them (Cappel et al. 2001, 92-93). Regrettably, there is little awareness among practitioners that trigger points can be the primary cause of muscle weakness and restricted range of motion. Trigger points can also be the unsuspected source of false positives in common tests for the six most common shoulder diagnoses: arthritis, tendinitis, bursitis, adhesive capsulitis, impingement syndrome, and rotator cuff injury (Simons, Travell, and Simons 1999, 544-546). A look at how trigger points might affect specific tests could help clarify this issue and possibly make diagnosis more accurate.

Range of Motion Tests

When the examiner tests your range of motion by asking you to reach up as high as you can and you have to raise your shoulder in order to lift your arm, you will show the *shrug sign* (Figure 10.3). You do this by contracting the trapezius muscle on top of the shoulder and leaning to the opposite side. Physicians are likely to attribute the shrug sign to a

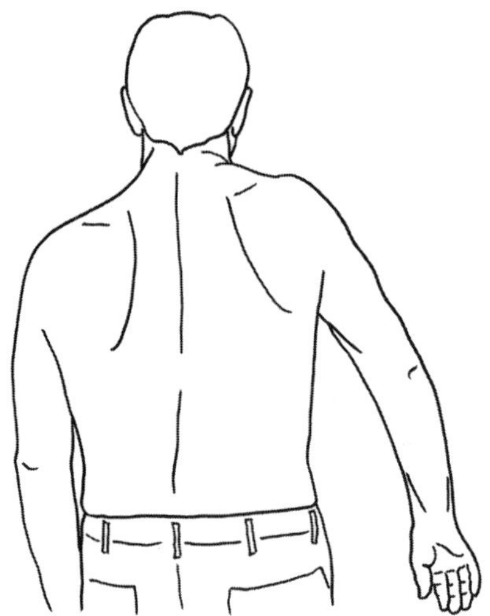

Figure 10.3 The shrug sign: lifting the shoulder in an effort to lift the arm

rotator cuff tear or adhesive capsulitis and prescribe treatment based on that assessment (Wirth, Orfaly, and Rockwood 2001, 142). Rotator cuff tears are always a possibility, but pain from trigger points in the supraspinatus, lower trapezius, and deltoid muscles can make you dislike lifting your arm and make you cheat by raising your shoulder (Simons, Travell, and Simons 1999, 542, 599).

Apley's scratch tests, originated by A. Graham Apley, a British orthopedic physician, are a quick way to determine the limits of three basic arm movements that require maximum inward and outward rotation and adduction of the arm (Figures 10.4, 10.5, and 10.6). These tests are almost laughable because trigger points in rotator cuff muscles can make it quite impossible to scratch your back in any of the three ways. Nonetheless, the inability to scratch your back is likely to bring a quick diagnosis of adhesive capsulitis, arthritis, tendinitis, bursitis, impingement syndrome, inflammation, or rotator cuff injury, along with a routine prescription for an anti-inflammatory drug and physical therapy (Wirth, Orfaly, and Rockwood 2001, 111-113).

Any of these medical diagnoses of the shoulder are possible, but it may be that none of them are correct. Apley's scratch tests aren't very helpful in making a specific diagnosis unless you take into account what role trigger points are playing in limiting these movements. Other tests for range of motion have the same flaw.

Trigger points in any of the four rotator cuff muscles can make it difficult to inwardly rotate your arm to reach up behind your back (Figure 10.4). Outward rotation for reaching your back from above is impeded by subscapularis and pectoralis major trigger points (Figure 10.5). You won't be able to reach across to scratch your back from the opposite side if you have trigger points in your infraspinatus, teres minor, teres major, triceps, or latissimus dorsi muscles (Figure 10.6). In any of these situations, trigger points in other muscles in the shoulder complex are probably also involved. With these kinds of restricted range of motion, trigger point massage is likely to be much more appropriate therapy than painkillers, anti-inflammatories, surgery, or programs of stretching.

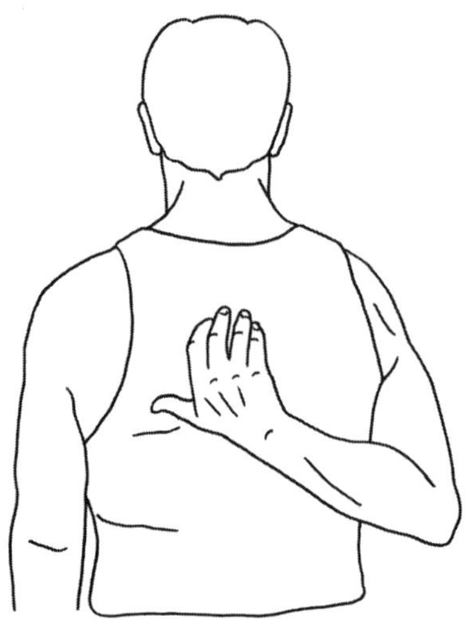

Figure 10.4 Apley's scratch test for inward rotation

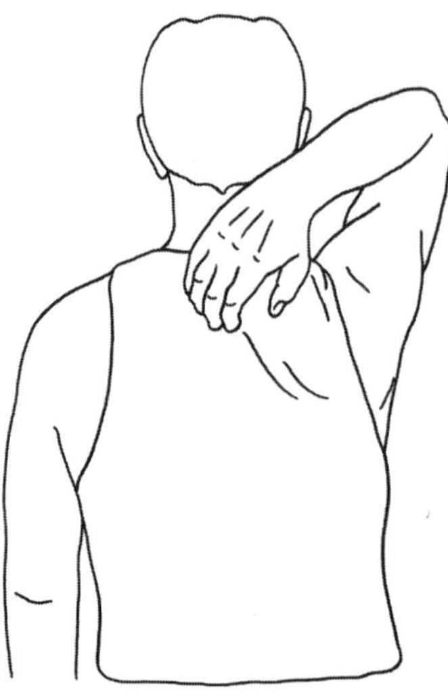

Figure 10.5 Apley's scratch test for outward rotation

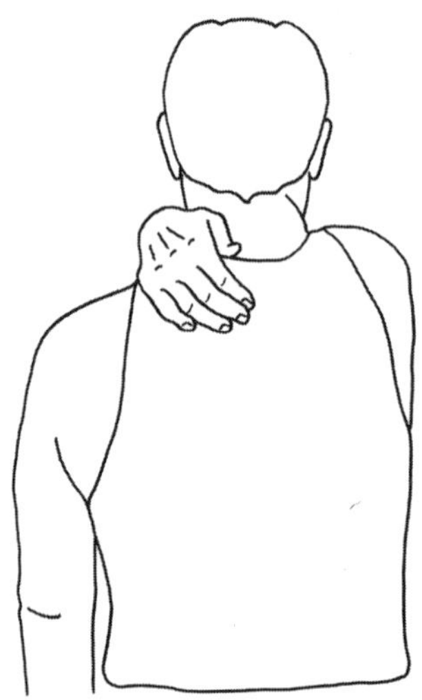

Figure 10.6 Apley's scratch test for cross-body adduction

Impingement Tests

In the *Neer impingement test,* the examiner raises your arm to see if you experience pain in your shoulder joint from compressive forces between the head of the humerus and the underside of the acromion (Figure 10.7). Since you don't make the movement yourself, the shoulder muscles don't contract. *Yocum's impingement test* and the *Hawkins impingement test* accomplish the same thing with different positions of the forearm (Figures 10.8 and 10.9). Any pain caused by these tests is said to indicate a rotator cuff tear or excessive compression of the subacromial bursa and other tissues (Wirth, Orfaly, and Rockwood 2001, 113; Donatelli et al. 2004, 115-116). A high degree of reliability and validity is claimed for these tests, but they all put the arm into near maximum inward rotation, which puts a maximum stretch on the infraspinatus. Trigger points in this muscle will respond by sending a sharp stab of pain to the front of the shoulder. This factor can cause the physician to mistakenly conclude that there's serious trouble in the joint when it's actually nothing worse than referred myofascial pain.

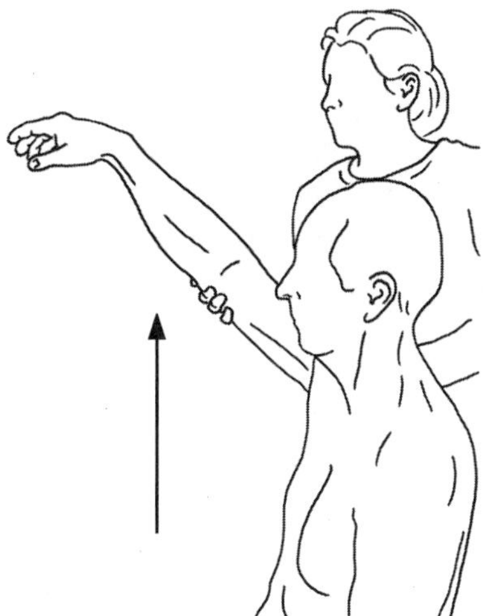

Figure 10.7 Neer impingement test. The examiner's left hand is holding the shoulder down.

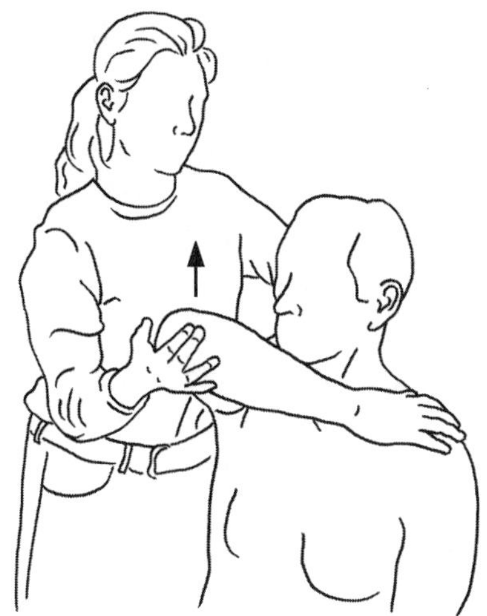

Figure 10.8 Yocum's impingement test. For maximum inward rotation, press upward on the elbow while pressing down on the shoulder.

The *cross-body adduction test,* also called the *crossover impingement test,* puts stress on the acromioclavicular joint (Figure 10.10). Sharp pain in the joint, which is in the top of the shoulder, could be a sign of a sprained or torn ligament or arthritis (Wirth, Orfaly, and Rockwood 2001, 113; Cappel et al. 2001, 98). But this position stretches the infraspinatus and shortens the pectoralis major, both of which could send pain to the shoulder, giving a false positive for the test unless you and the examiner are very exacting about the precise location of the pain (Simons, Travell, and Simons 1999, 556).

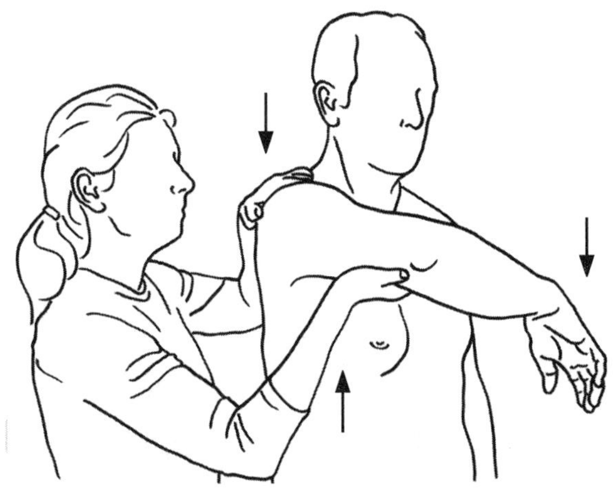

Figure 10.9 Hawkins impingement test. The examiner raises the elbow, then the patient inwardly rotates the arm.

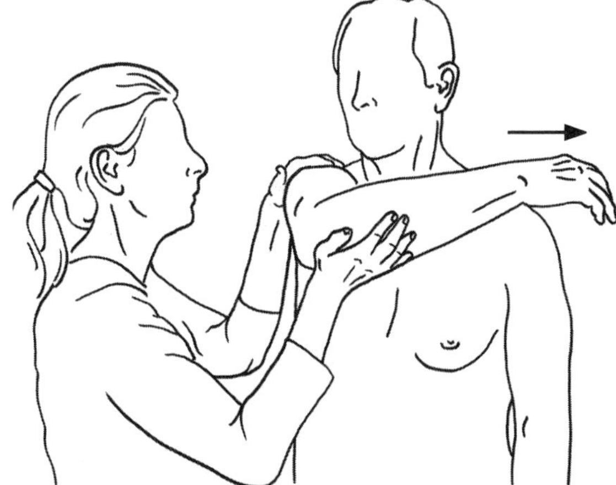

Figure 10.10 Cross-body adduction test for acromioclavicular joint impingement

Rotator Cuff Injury Tests

The *drop arm test* is for determining whether there may be a full-thickness rotator cuff tear (Figure 10.11). The examiner raises your arm somewhat above a 90 degree angle from your body and then lets go. You then begin to lower your arm slowly. The leverage of the deltoid is poor at this angle, so it can't hold the arm up by itself and needs the help of the supraspinatus. If your arm approaches 90 degrees and suddenly drops uncontrollably, there may be a tear in the supraspinatus tendon that prevents the muscle from holding the weight of the arm (Donatelli et al. 2004, 115-116). This test would seem to produce evidence of a serious problem, except that trigger points can cause the same effect.

The *supraspinatus isolation test*, often called the "empty can" test because of the position of the hand, is very much like the drop arm test, except that the examiner presses down on your arm as you try to keep it up (Figure 10.12). This is assumed to be a measure of the strength of the supraspinatus as it may relate to a partial tear in its tendon (Donatelli et al. 2004, 117; Cappel et al. 2001, 99). But active trigger points in the supraspinatus and deltoid can be expected to weaken both muscles considerably, and they'll also produce intolerable pain when challenged by this test (Simons, Travell, and Simons 1999, 114).

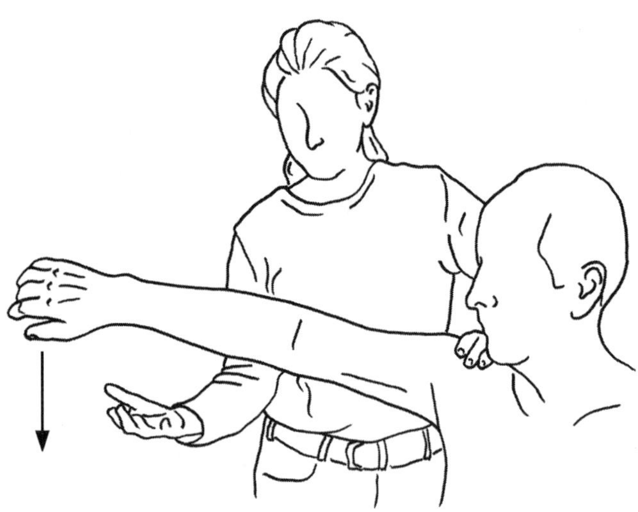

Figure 10.11 Drop arm test. The patient slowly lowers the arm to see if the arm will drop because of a rotator cuff tear.

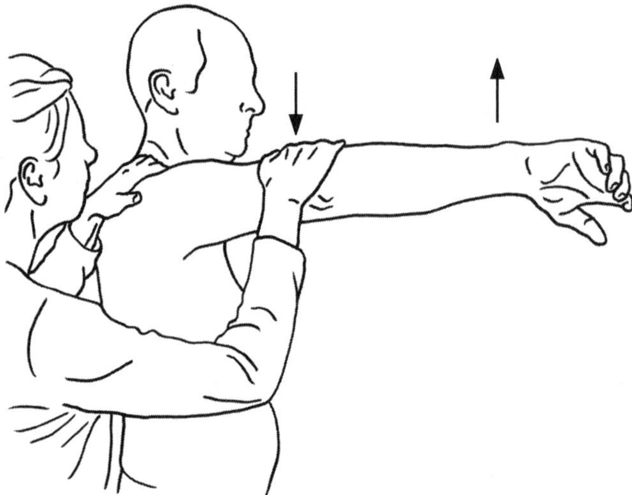

Figure 10.12 Supraspinatus isolation test for muscle strength. The examiner pulls down while the patient resists.

The *external rotation test* compares the outward rotation of your bad shoulder with the good one (Figure 10.13). The inability of your arm to rotate all the way out to the side is taken as an indication of weakness in the infraspinatus and teres minor muscles and possibly a massive rotator cuff tear, specifically a tear in the infraspinatus tendon (Gerber 1999, 82-83; Wirth, Orfaly, and Rockwood 2001, 111). The *external rotation lag sign* is also a test of infraspinatus strength and tendon continuity, but more clearly demonstrated (Figure 10.14). The examiner pulls your arm into near maximum outward rotation. You're asked to keep your arm in outward rotation as the examiner lets go of your wrist while still holding your arm at the elbow. The test is presumably positive for infraspinatus tendon trouble if your arm springs away from the examiner back toward center (Donatelli et al. 2004, 120-121). These tests could indeed detect muscle weakness and rotator cuff tears, but

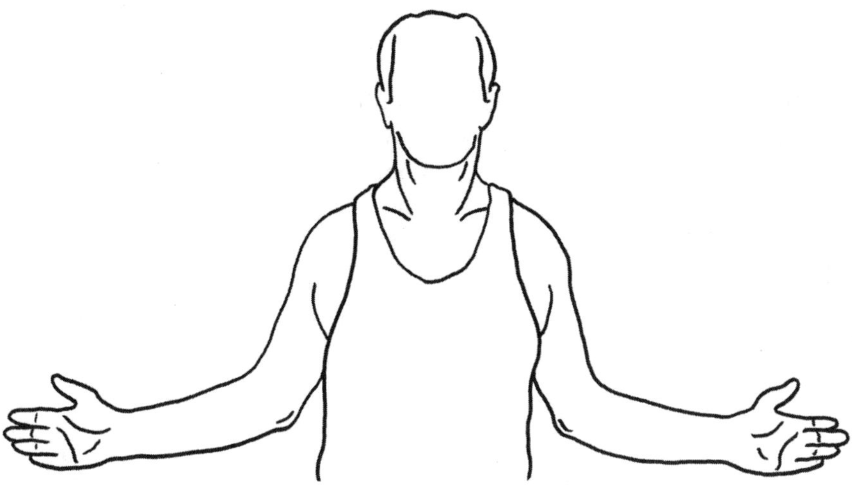

Figure 10.13 External rotation test (outward rotation), comparing the range of motion in the bad shoulder to the good one

the combined effects of infraspinatus and subscapularis trigger points would also make it difficult to move your arm into outward rotation and keep it there (Simons, Travell, and Simons 1999, 596-599).

Gerber's lift-off test is supposed to detect subscapularis weakness or a tear specifically in the subscapularis tendon (Figure 10.15). The examiner places your hand in the small of your back and then pulls it away and asks you to hold it there. The test is positive for a tear if your hand immediately returns to the small of your back. If you're able to hold your hand away from your back, the examiner pushes your hand as you try to resist. A normal subscapularis will hold your hand in place. If it gives way, it demonstrates subscapularis weakness (Wirth, Orfaly, and Rockwood 2001, 112; Donatelli et al. 2004, 119). Again, trigger points in the supraspinatus, infraspinatus, and subscapularis muscles could cause these same effects, rendering the test unreliable for detecting a rotator cuff tear (Simons, Travell, and Simons 1999, 542, 556, 596).

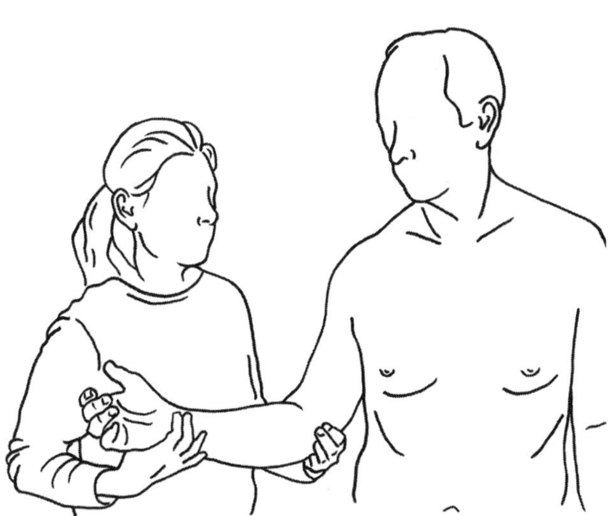

Figure 10.14 External rotation lag sign test for infraspinatus strength and tendon tear. The examiner pulls the arm into outward rotation, then the patient tries to hold it there.

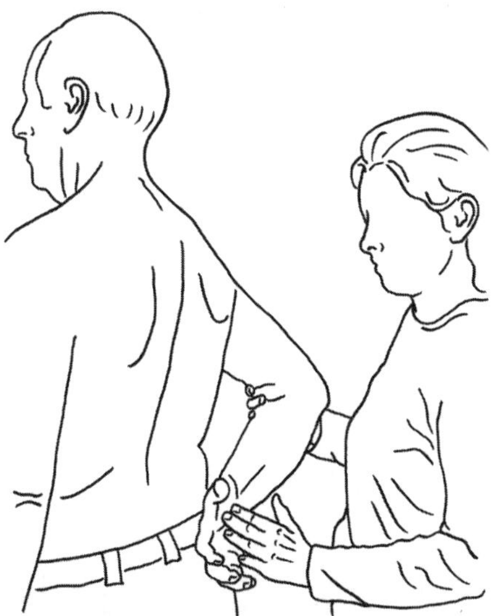

Figure 10.15 Gerber's lift-off test for subscapularis strength and tears

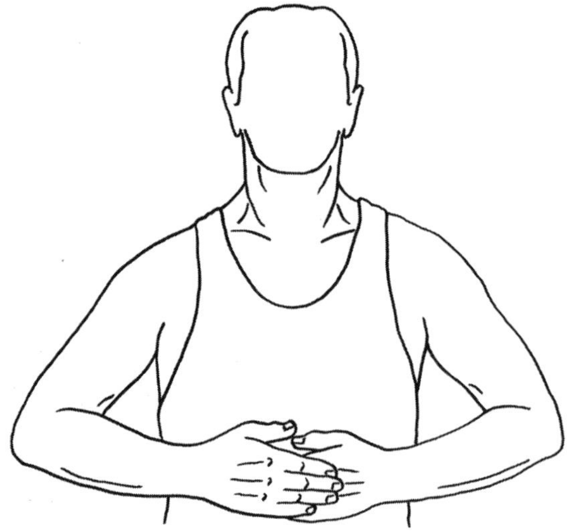

Figure 10.16 Abdominal compression test for comparing inward rotation in both arms

The *abdominal compression test* is used for evaluating the subscapularis when it's too painful to place your hand behind you (Figure 10.16). You press on your abdomen with both hands while you bring both elbows forward into the same plane. This puts your arms into near maximum inward rotation. If one elbow won't come forward, it demonstrates weakness in the subscapularis muscle on that side (Williams 1999, 112). But the restricted movement can be a sign of trigger points in the infraspinatus that prevent full inward rotation, and subscapularis trigger points can be the cause of weakness in the muscle.

Joint Instability Tests

Your glenohumeral joint (the shoulder's ball-and-socket joint) can be dislocated by sports injuries, auto accidents, and falls. Dislocations can lead to frozen shoulder, especially in older people. A shoulder *subluxation*, or partial dislocation, can exist for a long time unrecognized. Instability tests are important because shoulder dislocation causes injury to connective tissue in the front and back of the joint (Cappel et al. 2001, 102-103).

Dislocations and subluxations can strain or tear the rotator cuff and damage the glenoid fossa (the socket) by stretching the surrounding capsule and tearing the glenoid labrum, the rim of the socket (Figure 10.17). *Anterior dislocation* (in a forward direction) can cause a *Bankart lesion*, in which the anterior glenoid labrum has torn loose. Recurrent anterior dislocations in an unstable shoulder occur when the arm is lifted and outwardly rotated. *Posterior dislocations* (in a backward direction) make it impossible to outwardly rotate the arm. Once the capsule is damaged or torn, the humeral head has difficulty staying in the glenoid fossa; that is, the ball easily pops out of the socket. Physicians use the *sulcus test* to see if there's too much laxity in the joint. In the test, the examiner pulls down on the arm while feeling the *sulcus*, or gap, under the acromion for excessive downward movement of the head of the

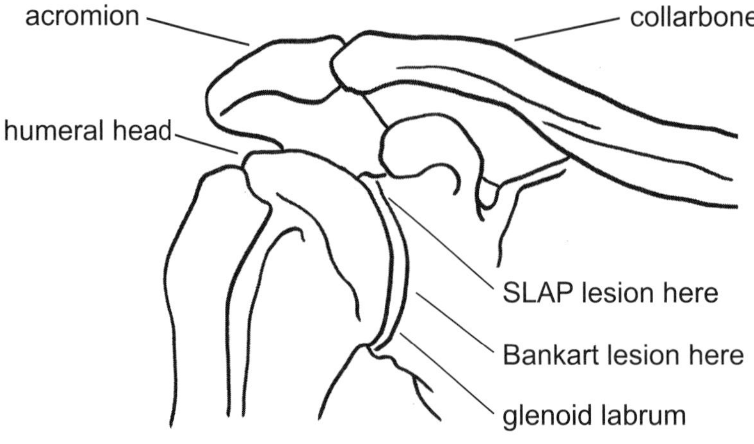

Figure 10.17 Glenoid labrum injuries

humerus (Figure 10.18). Physical therapy is usually recommended for strengthening the rotator muscles, especially the subscapularis. Dislocations that constantly recur may require surgical repair of the labrum and joint capsule (Wirth, Orfaly, and Rockwood 2001, 147-150).

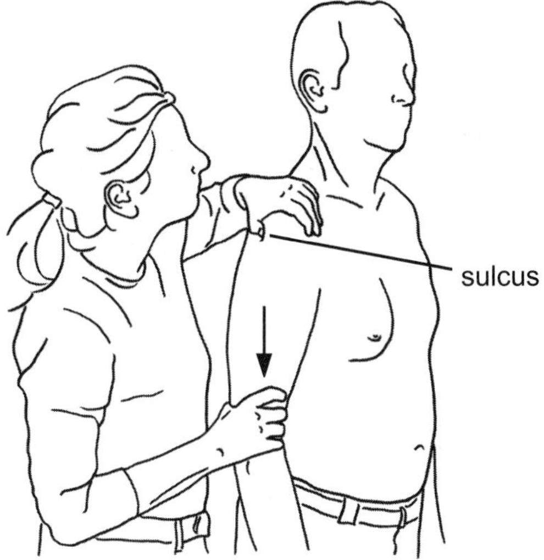

Figure 10.18 The sulcus test checks for laxity between the acromion and the head of the humerus.

Shortening of the subscapularis and imbalance of muscle strength caused by trigger points contribute to subluxation of the humeral head. This means that trigger points can keep the ball-and-socket joint partially dislocated. Chronic subluxation in an upward and forward direction could be the primary cause of impingement syndrome, which in turn may be the ultimate reason for most rotator cuff tears, especially in the supraspinatus tendon, the one most often damaged (Simons, Travell, and Simons 1999, 545-546, 599).

The *apprehension test* detects shoulder instability in the forward direction (Figure 10.19). The examiner puts your arm into outward rotation with your upper arm at 90 degrees and the elbow bent. This is the movement that tends to dislocate an unstable shoulder. Your guarding against further movement and expression of fear is called the *apprehension sign* (Wirth, Orfaly, and Rockwood 2001, 114). The reliability of this test is undermined by the extreme pain you may feel with your arm in this position when you have a frozen shoulder and extremely active subscapularis trigger points.

The *glenohumeral load and shift test* actively moves the humeral head forward, back, and downward in the socket to see if there's excessive movement (Figure 10.20). The forward or back movement can actually dislocate the shoulder when the joint is sufficiently lax. Unless the looseness of the joint is extremely obvious, the test is quite subjective and relies very much on the experience and skill of the examiner. Interestingly, some investigators find little

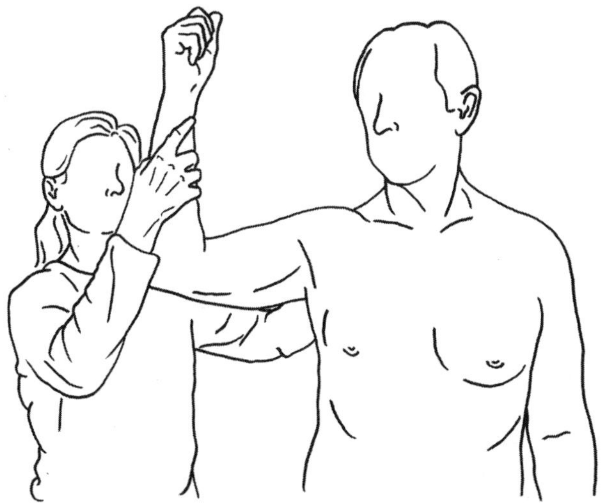

Figure 10.19 Apprehension test. The examiner pulls arm into maximum outward rotation checking for anterior shoulder instability.

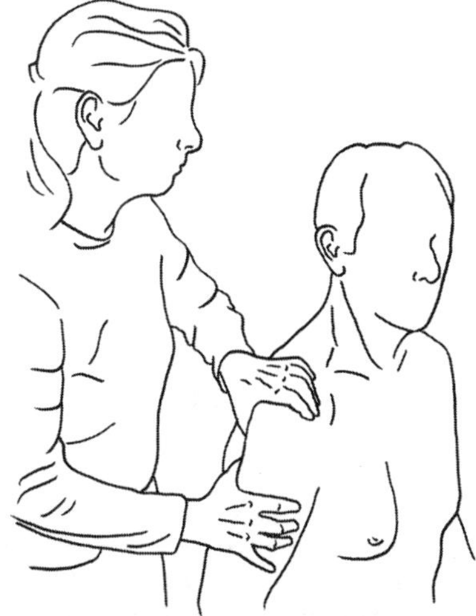

Figure 10.20 Glenohumeral load and shift test. The examiner's left hand holds the shoulder still while the right moves the humerus forward and back.

difference in laxity between a normal shoulder and a chronically unstable shoulder that required surgery (Donatelli et al. 2004, 109; Cappel et al. 2001, 91, 103-105).

Glenoid Labrum Injury Tests

The *crank test*, also called the *compression-rotation test*, is used to detect an anterior glenoid labrum tear, or Bankart lesion (Figures 10.17 and 10.21). The examiner applies force on your elbow toward the glenohumeral joint and then moves your arm in a circle as though cranking it. A painful locking sensation indicates a disruption in the labral rim of the socket. This injury is the most common reason for recurrent shoulder dislocation.

A similar maneuver, the *clunk test*, can also help determine whether the labrum has become detached from the glenoid fossa. The examiner presses the humeral head into glenoid cavity while moving the arm in a circle (Figure 10.22). A positive sign is pain and a catch (Donatelli et al. 2004, 111; Cappel et al. 2001, 100-101). Neither the crank nor the clunk test may be possible with a frozen shoulder because of the required position of the arm.

The *biceps load test* is for identifying a SLAP lesion (superior labrum anterior-to-posterior tear), which is a detachment of both the glenoid labrum and biceps tendon along the top of the glenoid rim. The examiner holds your wrist and elbow while you contract your biceps against resistance (Figure 10.23). The test is positive if you feel pain deep in the joint. A SLAP lesion can be the cause of a painful catching or popping in the joint (Donatelli et al. 2004, 112-114). Because of the position of your arm, subscapularis trigger points would undoubtedly cause some percentage of false positives.

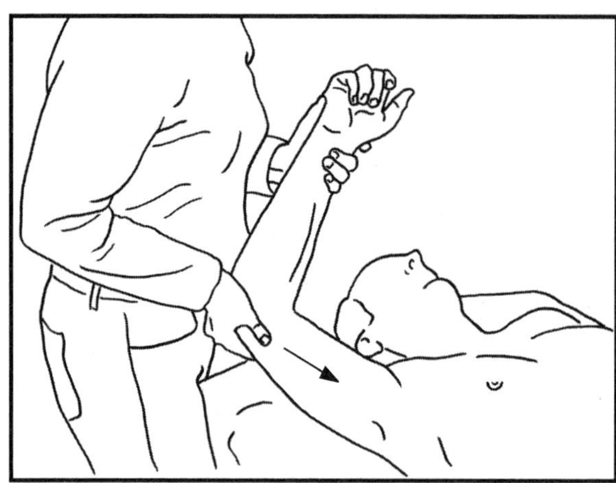

Figure 10.21 Crank test for an anterior labrum tear. Pressure is applied at the elbow while rotating (cranking) the arm.

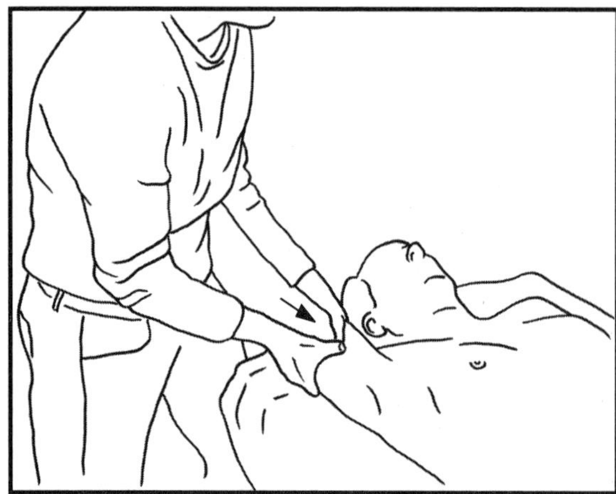

Figure 10.22 Clunk test for a Bankart lesion. The ball is pressed into the socket while the arm is moved in a circle.

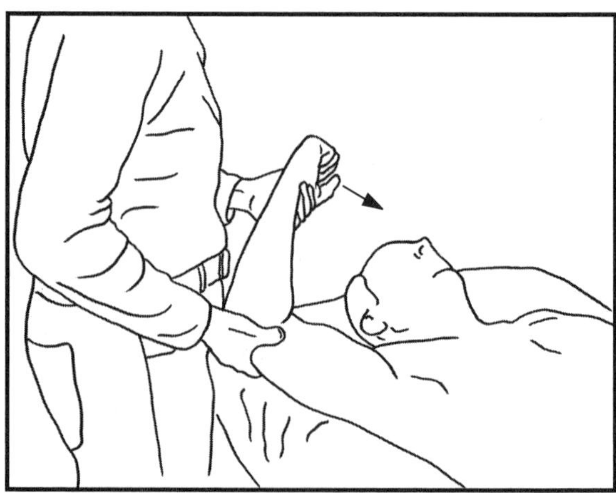

Figure 10.23 The biceps load test (for a SLAP lesion) causes pain when the biceps contracts against resistance.

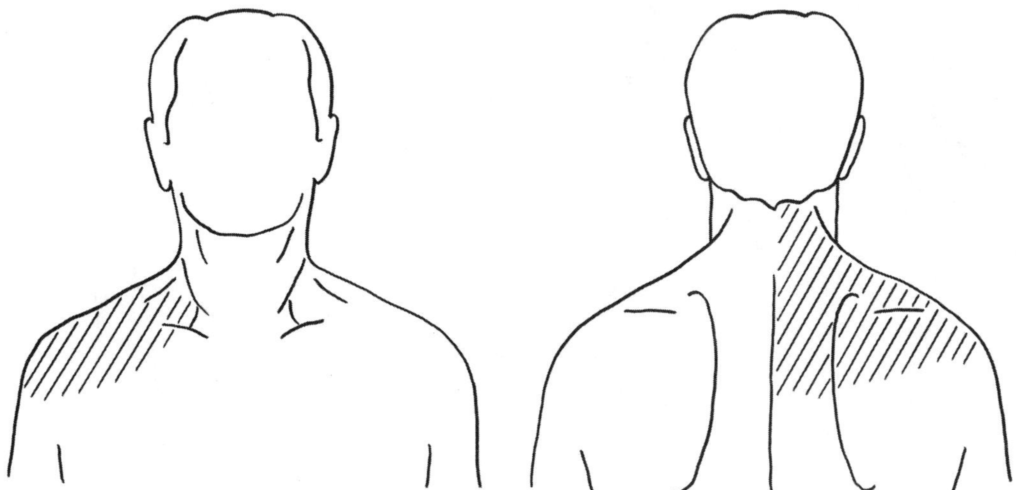

Figure 10.24 Composite referred pain pattern from cervical nerve roots C5, C6, C7, and C8 when compressed by a herniated cervical disk on the right side

Nerve Impingement Tests

When cervical nerve roots are compressed by arthritic spurs or herniated disks in your neck, they can refer pain to your neck, upper back, upper chest, and shoulders (Figure 10.24). This is commonly spoken of as having a "pinched nerve" in the neck. The pain, which can be a constant dull ache, a sense of burning, or a sharp and electrical kind of pain, is similar to referred myofascial pain from scalene trigger points. A pinched cervical nerve root can also cause numbness, tingling, and weakness in the arms and hands, also just like the scalene trigger points. Because symptoms caused by the scalenes and cervical nerve impingement cover many of the same areas, this calls for exacting tests to differentiate the two. One difference is that scalene trigger points often make the hands swell, whereas a disk problem doesn't. Constant pain from either source tends to create satellite trigger points in shoulder muscles and can ultimately lead to a frozen shoulder.

Spurling's cervical compression test can often determine whether your shoulder pain is from cervical nerve impingement. In the test, you lean your head back, then rotate and tilt it toward the painful shoulder while the examiner presses down on the top of your head (Figure 10.25). This places added pressure on the disk that can reproduce or accentuate the pain and neurological symptoms if the disk is to blame. A skilled physician can conduct this test with your head in various positions to selectively provoke a reaction at different spots in your neck (Snider et al. 2001, 533-542). Spurling's test is a very good one, but it isn't foolproof. Certain positions of the head can cause pain from scalene trigger points, leading a doctor unfamiliar with the possible myofascial sources of the symptoms to a mistaken conclusion (Simons, Travell, and Simons 1999, 504-515).

The *cervical decompression test* is a way to confirm the results of Spurling's test. The examiner pulls up on your head to relieve pressure on the cervical disks (Figure 10.26). If this relieves your shoulder pain, it presumably further implicates a compressed disk as the cause of the problem (Chaitow and DeLany 2000, 173). If cervical decompression fails to relieve your pain or makes it worse, it may be because lifting the head stretches the scalenes, which can incite their trigger points to deliver a shot of pain to your shoulder, upper back, or chest. An alert physician will be aware of this possibility and may want to do tests for thoracic outlet syndrome.

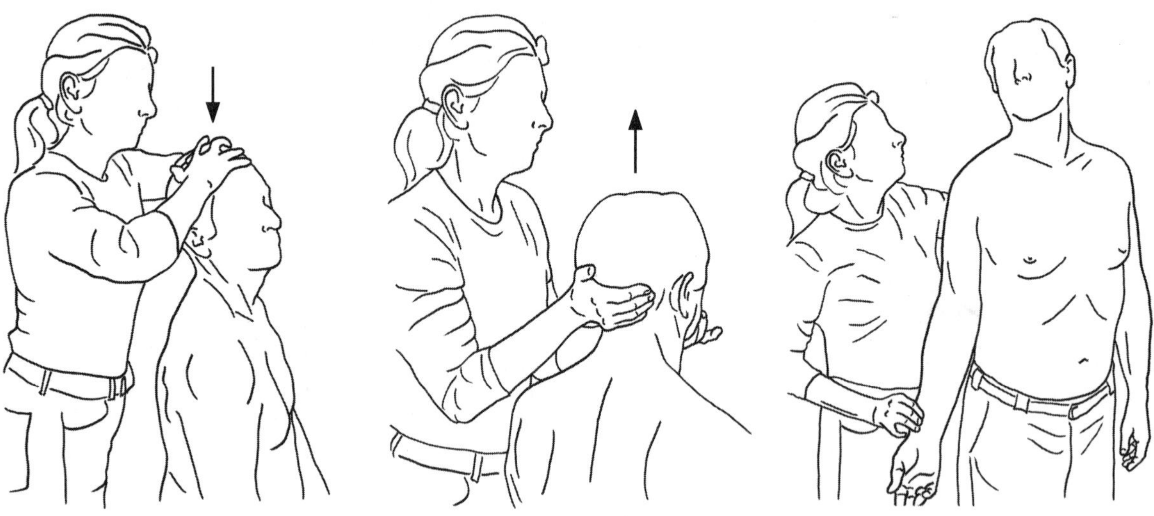

Figure 10.25 Spurling's cervical compression test

Figure 10.26 Cervical decompression test; pulling the head upward

Figure 10.27 Adson's test for pulse obliteration from a scalene strain

Thoracic Outlet Syndrome Tests

Thoracic outlet syndrome is also called *scalenus anticus syndrome* when involvement of the scalenes is recognized. As discussed in chapter 5, shoulder, arm, and hand symptoms can be caused by compression of the arm's neurovascular bundle between the first rib and the collarbone. Scalenes shortened by trigger points cause this by pulling up on the first rib. When physicians don't accept the importance of myofascial trigger points, they tend to get caught up in looking for a cervical rib (an extra top rib) or some other bone or ligament abnormality in the front of the neck. A number of clinical tests are used for diagnosing structural causes of thoracic outlet syndrome, despite having up to a 50 percent incidence of false positives (Cappel et al. 2001, 93-94).

Adson's test is the most common test for thoracic outlet syndrome (Figure 10.27). The examiner monitors your pulse at the wrist to see if it disappears when the scalenes are stressed by various positions of the head and arm. In the version illustrated here, the position of the arm and head would tend to compress the subclavian artery that serves the arm. In the traditional medical view, this would suggest some kind of bony obstruction, which is sometimes the case (Apley and Solomon 1997, 48). Even so, scalene trigger points are by far the most common cause for this pulse obliteration. Scalene shortening can be verified by the two following tests.

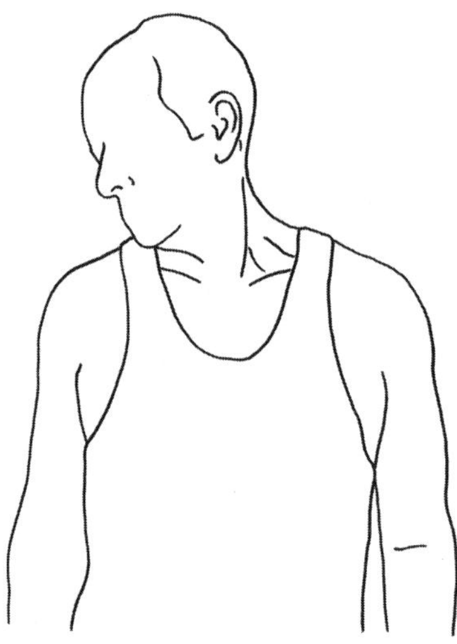

Figure 10.28 Scalene cramp test to accentuate symptoms

The *scalene cramp test* can reproduce or accentuate symptoms from scalene trigger points. This is done by turning your head as far as you can toward the symptomatic side and trying to touch your shoulder with your chin (Figure 10.28). This movement maximally shortens the scalenes, making the trigger points increase their pain referral. This test may not make a clear difference if you're already in severe pain (Simons, Travell, and Simons 1999, 511).

The *scalene relief test* is a way to confirm the cramp test. Putting your arm above your head indirectly raises the collarbone away from the first rib, taking the pressure off the brachial nerves and stopping the pain (Figure 10.29). The test is positive for thoracic outlet syndrome and scalene involvement if your symptoms decrease or disappear (Simons, Travell, and Simons 1999, 512). This test can't be done, of course, when you have a frozen shoulder and can't raise your arm. A much more direct and reliable test would be to simply search the scalene muscles for trigger points, something that can be done very quickly with finger pressure without moving either your head or your arm. This can render all other thoracic outlet tests unnecessary.

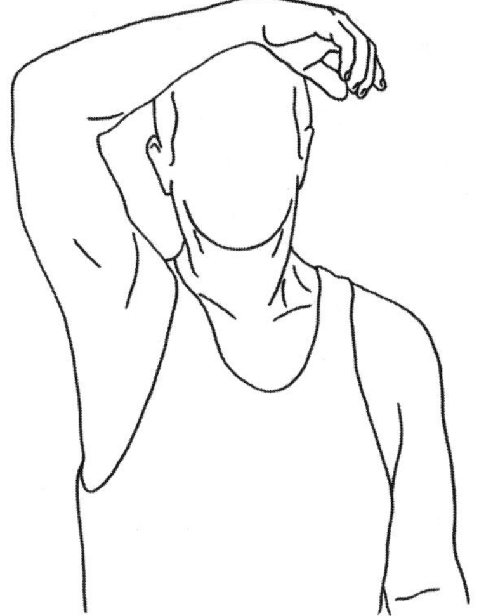

Figure 10.29 Scalene relief test to alleviate symptoms

Imaging Studies

Many people feel annoyed and disappointed when their doctor orders expensive technological tests and prescribes equally expensive treatment without even doing a hands-on examination. Doctors sometimes appear uncomfortable with the physical examination of patients, or in too much of a hurry to bother. Some physicians admit that hands-on diagnosis is a dying art, primarily because technology has taken over and medical schools no longer allow enough time for medical students to develop palpation skills (Apley and Solomon 1997, vii).

It's true that imaging studies like X-rays, MRI, ultrasound, and CAT scans are able to detect physical and structural abnormalities that can remain hidden to visual inspection and the doctor's touch. But these technological tools aren't perfect in their ability to see physical or structural trouble, and they certainly can't tell the doctor why an abnormality is there or what caused it. Very often, lab tests come back negative and MRIs and CAT scans don't show anything at all, despite serious symptoms. The doctor is then left guessing and, grasping at straws, may try a change of medication or prescribe another round of physical therapy. Even worse, when the machines don't come up with the answer, the doctor and your insurance company may begin to see you as a psychological case or a malingerer. Some physicians have fallen into the habit of ascribing all mysterious symptoms to fibromyalgia and labeling patients as essentially incurable.

Arthroscopy is the most reliable way to diagnose impingement, rotator cuff tears, glenoid labrum tear, capsule damage, and arthritis. In arthroscopy, the physician essentially inserts a tiny camera inside your shoulder to view any abnormalities directly. The procedure is minimally invasive and has a short recovery time if no repairs are made. If arthroscopically manageable repairs are seen to be needed, they can be done immediately.

Nonetheless, even with all their technological muscle, neither arthroscopy nor any of the imaging studies will reveal an abnormality if trigger points are the cause of your shoulder problem. They're useless for diagnosing myofascial pain, and this is what makes some shoulder problems "enigmatic" to the medical profession. The thesis of this book is that if trigger points were diagnosed and treated first, there would be much less need for imaging studies and their exorbitant cost, and medical treatment itself could become much less expensive.

Medical Treatment of the Shoulder

Traditional medicine sees shoulder pain and dysfunction primarily as a problem of joint injury or degeneration. Because physicians rarely consider myofascial trigger points in making a diagnosis, trigger points are seldom addressed by medical treatment or included in prescriptions for physical therapy. The reason for this is that few medical schools offer courses in the diagnosis and treatment of myofascial pain, and there's very little continuing education on the subject available for practicing physicians (Simons, Travell, and Simons 1999, 544-546, 604-606).

Medical books about pain and the shoulder are only beginning to take notice of trigger points and myofascial pain. The few short paragraphs that you find are apt to be mere short summaries of the work of Travell and Simons and of no practical value. An increasing number of articles reporting research on myofascial pain are beginning to appear in medical journals, but they tend to focus on scientific minutiae. Researchers show little interest in exploring innovations in manual treatment.

The relatively small number of doctors who treat trigger points are mainly self-educated through study and application of Travell and Simons's *Trigger Point Manual*. But because they're such a slim minority of medical practitioners, typical treatments of the shoulder still tend to be limited to surgery, injection of steroids, prescription drugs, and physical therapy. There have been medical advances, of course, but they're mostly just more of the same—new drugs for pain and new surgical techniques. New painkillers too often present new dangers to your health without helping with the underlying problems. Shoulder surgery, on the other hand, has evolved into a highly developed set of procedures that are successful more often than not.

The central issue with surgery is whether it's truly needed and whether the surgeon's skills rise to the level of competence, or even mediocrity. Great surgery is being done, but so is bad surgery, and some people end up in considerably worse shape after surgery than before. Before agreeing to undergo any surgery, it's worth your while to examine the various medical diagnoses of the shoulder, their specific treatments, and the significant hazards involved.

A doctor's first step in addressing your shoulder problem will be to assign it a diagnosis. On the basis of that diagnosis, your doctor will then recommend medication, surgery, or other medical procedures. The rest of this chapter will cover the most common diagnoses and the treatments usually recommended.

Inflammation

It's probably not the stiffness in your shoulder or the inconvenience of your lost range of motion that gets you to the doctor's office; it's the pain. The trouble is that, although pain is bringing you an important message, it seldom tells you exactly what that message means. It doesn't necessarily tell the doctor, either.

A routine medical examination for your shoulder pain by your primary health care provider, family practice physician, or general practitioner usually results in an on-the-spot, generic diagnosis of *arthritis*, *tendinitis*, or *bursitis*. These are names for inflammation of a joint, tendon, or bursa, respectively. In reality, the notion that your shoulder is suffering from inflammation is a canned explanation, based on no evidence beyond your statement that you have pain in your shoulder. Attributing your pain to inflammation, as though inflammation and pain were the same thing, is the mark of a superficial diagnosis. Inflammation can cause pain, but it's common to have pain without inflammation. Myofascial trigger points, which are the foremost cause of shoulder pain and stiffness, are very rarely associated with inflammation.

By definition, inflammation is characterized by four symptoms: pain, warmth, reddening, and swelling. Pain alone is not diagnostic of inflammation. You must have the other three symptoms too. Taken together, the four defining symptoms of inflammation embody a healing response to injury or disease. If you don't feel increased warmth in your shoulder and you don't see some degree of reddening and swelling, inflammation isn't the problem. Even when inflammation affects some part of your shoulder, your doctor needs to seek the cause, not simply treat the inflammatory symptoms.

Now that you know about myofascial pain, you'd probably guess that the trouble with your shoulder is more likely in the muscles than in the joints, tendons, or bursas. It may not be unreasonable to conclude that a doctor who makes the inflammation diagnosis simply doesn't know about trigger points and thus may not be able to solve your problem. The best you may get is a standard set of routine treatments and medications for a decidedly questionable diagnosis.

Anti-inflammatory Drugs

There's no question that good drugs have good uses, saving innumerable lives and making life bearable for millions of people. Even so, it's widely recognized by health care professionals and the public alike that huge numbers of people are unnecessarily and dangerously overmedicated. And in the constant, unremitting promotion of drugs in the media, pain medications are preeminent.

When you go to a conventional doctor for a shoulder problem, you'll almost always receive a prescription for a nonsteroidal anti-inflammatory drug (NSAID), along with the instruction to give it a try and come back if it doesn't help. But with a frozen shoulder, NSAIDs are simply not going to solve the problem. They may help with true physical injuries and disease, but they have minimal effects on myofascial pain. Worse, when taken for too long or in excessive quantities, anti-inflammatory drugs, even over-the-counter varieties, can cause irreversible damage to your heart, stomach, kidneys, and liver (Wirth, Orfaly, and Rockwood 2001, 120). Some people have even been killed by them, and yet they're handed out as though they were no more harmful than candy or vitamins.

New and supposedly improved anti-inflammatory drugs, such as the infamous COX-2 inhibitors, are no better solution for your shoulder problem, and they actually present greater life-threatening risks to your vital organs than the older anti-inflammatories (Wolfe et al. 2005, 281-286). If any of these substances cut your pain at all, remember that they're only masking it, giving you the illusion that the problem is solved. For a frozen shoulder, you need a real solution, not a sop. It's a tragedy that so many people desperately depend on pain medications, not knowing that simple treatments for myofascial trigger points could actually cure their problem, rather than just covering it up.

Muscle Relaxant Drugs

If the doctor believes your pain is from muscle spasm, you may get a prescription for a muscle relaxant. But myofascial trigger points aren't the same thing as muscle spasms and muscle relaxant drugs have negligible effects on referred myofascial pain. The prescribed dosages of muscle relaxant drugs aren't effective for pain, and they aren't even high enough to directly relax tense muscles. Instead, they have a merely sedative effect, which may or may not indirectly relax your muscles. Dosages are kept low because of the risk of adverse effects, which can include blurred vision, drowsiness, dizziness, heartburn, nausea, vomiting, constipation, and diarrhea. In the long term, muscle relaxants can worsen preexisting conditions such as glaucoma, an enlarged prostate, liver disease, and heart problems. A popular handbook on the misuse of prescription drugs, *Worst Pills, Best Pills*, puts a "Do Not Use" warning on all muscle relaxant drugs because of their side effects and lack of effectiveness (Wolfe et al. 2005, 483-487).

Narcotic Drugs for Pain

Combining anti-inflammatory drugs with narcotics, such as morphine, hydrocodone, oxycodone, and other codeine derivatives, boosts their painkilling effects and reduces their deleterious side effects. Familiar brand names are Demerol, Dilaudid, Lortab, Percocet, and Vicodin. The added narcotics are genuine painkillers, and they actually do help subdue most kinds of pain, including myofascial pain, but they're also highly addictive. In *Worst Pills, Best Pills*, Demerol and sixteen other brands of narcotic-containing painkillers also bear the "Do Not Use" warning (Wolfe et al. 2005, 260).

While people generally know that these combinations don't cure underlying conditions that cause pain, many fall into the trap of using them for pain relief. They are probably indispensable in the short term for treatment of serious shoulder injuries or diseases, but for obvious reasons it's best to be cautious. If used for myofascial pain, narcotic combinations should be seen only as emergency aid in the short term, while you're waiting for trigger point therapy to take effect.

Cortisone Injections

Cortisone injections are frequently given for persistent shoulder pain. They may grant you a longer period of local pain relief than drugs in pill form, but their dangers greatly outweigh any transitory benefit you may derive. Cortisone is a corticosteroid that weakens muscle fibers and tendon tissue and greatly increases the risk of tears, especially when you've had two injections or more. Fortunately, the word is out on the dangers of cortisone and most doctors use it very sparingly (Wirth, Orfaly, and Rockwood 2001, 138). You may sometimes read or hear that corticosteroids are injected into trigger points, but this is misinformation. Trigger point injections use relatively harmless local anesthetics, such as procaine.

Adhesive Capsulitis

As discussed earlier, a diagnosis of *adhesive capsulitis*, based on the presumption that the problem can only be in the joint, is now almost universally applied to frozen shoulder. This line of thought often leads to recommendations for invasive and sometimes expensive treatments, including forced manipulation under anesthesia (MUA), distension arthrography, arthroscopic capsular release, open capsular release, and trigger point injections.

Physicians generally agree that most cases of so-called adhesive capsulitis eventually heal on their own. This suggests that there are no actual adhesions in the joint, or if there are, that they're capable of being reabsorbed by the body in the normal course of spontaneous recovery. There's considerable doubt whether adhesions are present at all until your shoulder has been frozen for a year or more. The fact that trigger point therapy can dramatically shorten recovery time makes the presence of adhesions very doubtful. Still, the treatment of "adhesions" goes on (Simons, Travell, and Simons 1999, 604-606).

Manipulation Under Anesthesia

Doctors are becoming leery of *manipulation under anesthesia,* although many still resort to it. The tearing sounds heard during this process are assumed to be the tearing of adhesions and a sign of success, but postsurgical complications have shown that other events may be occurring. Forcible manipulation of your shoulder can tear the rotator cuff, the subscapularis muscle, or the glenoid labrum. It can also overstretch the nerves that supply the shoulder, arm, and hand. It's sometimes responsible for dislocations and recurrent instability of the shoulder. It has even been known to fracture the humerus. You should never agree to manipulation under anesthesia if you have any condition that weakens your bones, such as osteoporosis (Beyers and Bonutti 2004, 332; Wirth, Orfaly, and Rockwood 2001, 126; Cuomo 1999, 411-415).

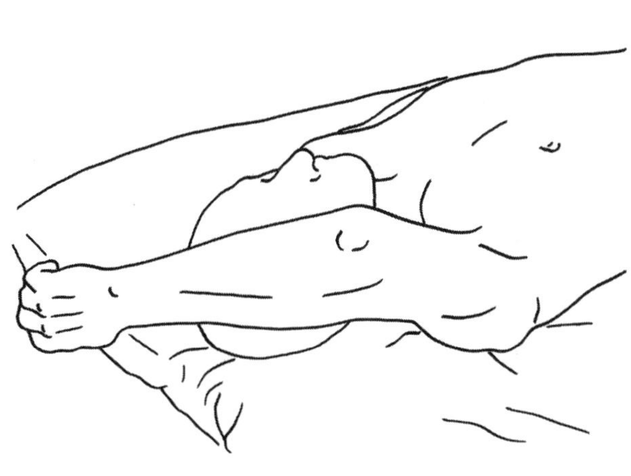

Figure 10.30 Manipulation under anesthesia. Maximum abduction of the arm risks tearing the subscapularis muscle or tendon.

For manipulation under anesthesia, you're put under general anesthesia and your arm is moved through what would be its normal range of motion. The goal is to reach three maximum positions: full abduction with your arm all the way over your head (Figure 10.30), full cross-body adduction (Figure 10.31), and full outward rotation (Figure 10.32). But, because anesthesia has no direct effect on myofascial trigger points, the muscles may resist these movements. If the forced stretching doesn't incidentally deactivate the trigger points, the procedure risks tearing the muscles

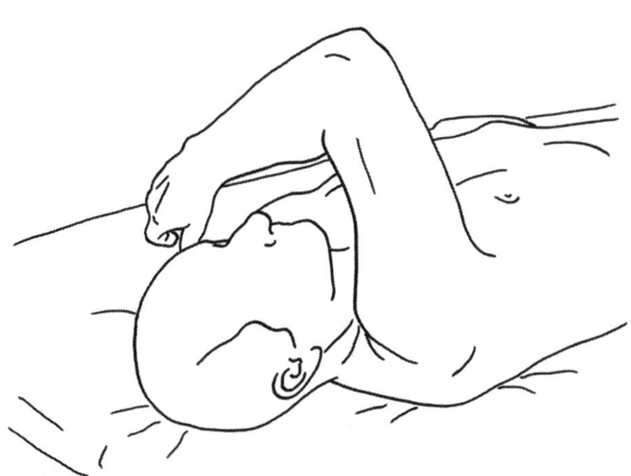

Figure 10.31 Manipulation under anesthesia. Maximum cross-body adduction risks tearing the infraspinatus, supraspinatus, and teres minor.

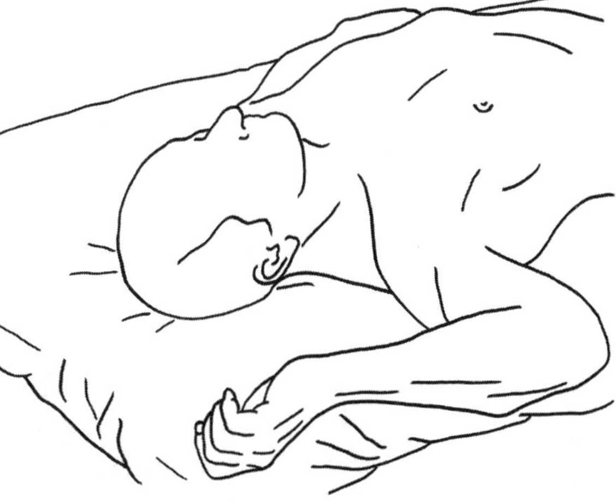

Figure 10.32 Manipulation under anesthesia. Maximum outward rotation risks dislocation and tearing of the subscapularis muscle and tendon.

and tendons of the rotator cuff. Manipulation under anesthesia does, however, sometimes succeed without injuring muscles or tendons. In these cases, it may be that the trigger points release during manipulation, just as they would with the spray and stretch technique.

Aftercare for manipulation under anesthesia includes a five-day interscalene nerve block to kill your pain while you begin an immediate program of physical therapy to keep your arm moving. Surgeons who do this procedure claim to produce pain-free outcomes, but a significant number of people continue to suffer for months afterward, sometimes with more pain than they originally had. You may also end up with a degree of permanent stiffness from scarring of tissue torn during manipulation (Cuomo 1999, 412-415).

Distension Arthrography

To avoid the risks of manipulation under anesthesia, your doctor may recommend *distension arthrography*. Also called *distension brisement* or *subacromial decompression*, this is a procedure in which adhesions are broken by injecting the shoulder joint with a saline solution containing an anesthetic, a radiocontrast substance, and a steroid. The pressure of the fluid forces the joint apart and tears any tissue binding it, and the joint is gently manipulated during the operation and afterward. Using a specialized X-ray technique, images of the joint taken before and after the procedure (*arthrograms*) tell the doctor whether the joint space has been increased (Cuomo 1999, 407; Cailliet 1991, 122).

Although orthopedic surgeons claim extraordinary success with distension arthrography, difficulties can compromise the results. It can be difficult to inject the joint space accurately and the fluid can be forced into surrounding tissues, in which case the procedure must be abandoned. And more to the point, if myofascial trigger points are the cause of the trouble, you probably won't experience any pain reduction.

Arthroscopic Capsular Release

Arthroscopic capsular release, or *arthroscopic capsulolysis*, is often combined with distension arthrography for more controlled loosening of the shoulder joint. In this method, the first step is distension, which increases the space available for insertion of arthroscopic implements. Then the space is cleared by removal of all adhesions and other redundant connective tissue. Often, your arm is moved through its entire range after capsular release.

Advantages of an arthroscopic approach are the opportunity for immediate treatment of conditions like rotator cuff tears, glenoid labrum tears, and arthritic or bony impingements. Disadvantages are that arthroscopy is more technically challenging and more costly, and it entails surgical risks, such as infection and inadvertent nerve damage (Nicholson 2003, 40-49).

Open Capsular Release

Open capsular release, or *open arthrolysis*, is done when you have osteoporosis or if you've had previous fractures. It's the procedure surgeons resort to after failed manipulation under anesthesia or an unsatisfactory arthroscopic operation. The surgery begins with a long incision in the front of your shoulder, allowing the surgeon a relatively unimpeded view of important parts of your shoulder and freer access for surgical tools. Open release may require cutting and reattaching the deltoid muscle, which can result in some degree of weakening, even with good physical therapy. Because of the extensive cutting required, you'll have more pain and will need a longer recovery period than the other procedures entail.

Other possible downsides are risk of infections, inadvertent nerve damage, and postsurgical stiffness due to scarring of skin, muscle, and other tissues (Cuomo 1999, 415).

Physicians who specialize in treating shoulders seem to agree that you should expect a full year to pass before you regain a pain-free full range of motion in your shoulder—with surgery or without. Given that there's evidence that most postsurgical complications are caused by the surgeon (Cuomo 1999, 415), it seems that there isn't a convincing argument for surgery or any other medical procedures unless you've tried absolutely everything else. In the future, the timely use of trigger point therapy may reduce the prevalence of shoulder surgery, relegating it to its rightful role in repair of physical injuries and damage due to degenerative diseases.

Trigger Point Injection

In *trigger point injection*, a local anesthetic that wears off quickly (procaine hydrochloride, or Novocain), is injected directly into trigger points to deactivate them. But trigger points can be difficult to locate precisely enough to inject. They can't always be felt clearly with the fingers, especially if they're buried deep in a thick muscle. The insertion of the needle can be unpleasantly painful, and it may leave some postinjection soreness, which can take several days to subside. Another downside is that your body also has to get rid of the anesthetic, and this limits the number of trigger points that can be injected at any one time.

In contrast, trigger points are usually quite easy to find on yourself because of the intimate feedback provided by their sensitivity to pressure. Experienced and well-trained massage therapists also usually have no difficulty finding and successfully treating even the most elusive trigger points. In a single session, a massage therapist can give attention to every trigger point you may have, with no risk beyond low-grade soreness for a day or two.

All other considerations aside, injection may be the quickest treatment for myofascial pain if the trigger points haven't been in place too long. Even so, chronic pain from long-standing trigger points may require dozens of injections. This means repeated visits to the doctor, along with the accompanying inconvenience, injection pain, and expense. If you depend on injection therapy, you'll be seeing a lot of your doctor and your insurer may not be willing to pay for it all (Simons, Travell, and Simons 1999, 150-166). Although Janet Travell pioneered research into the effectiveness of trigger point injections and found them to work well, Travell and Simons still advocate trying more conservative treatments first. Specifically, they recommend giving spray and stretch and trigger point massage a chance to work before resorting to trigger point injection (Simons, Travell, and Simons 1999, 605-609).

Subacromial Syndromes

Subacromial syndromes are abnormal conditions in the various tissues lying between the underside of the acromion and the top of the humeral head. These conditions are all interrelated, and the diagnostic terms are often used interchangeably when the differences are poorly understood. The various specific diagnoses are impingement syndrome, supraspinatus tendinitis, subacromial bursitis, bicipital tendinitis, and rotator cuff tears (Furia and Brown 2004, 103-106). Arthritis can be included in this group when degeneration of bone and cartilage causes increased compression in the subacromial space.

Impingement Syndrome

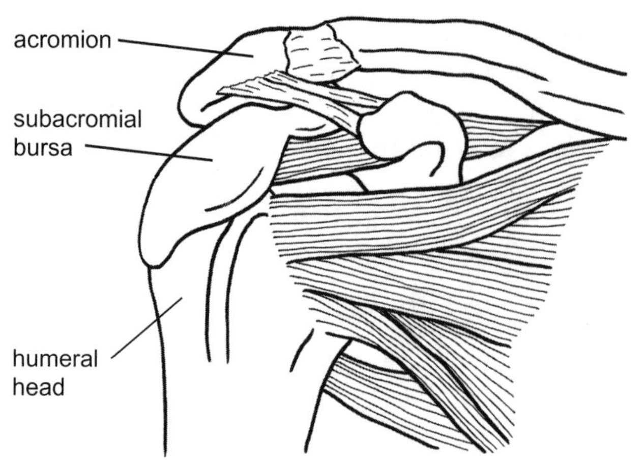

Figure 10.33 The subacromial bursa may be removed to increase the space between the acromion and the humeral head.

Various tests are used in the diagnosis of *impingement syndrome*, in which raising your arm causes sharp pain in your shoulder (see Figures 10.7, 10.8, and 10.9). Impingement is defined as excessive compression of the rotator cuff and subacromial bursa between the acromion and the head of the humerus. The greatest pain occurs as the arm actively rises through the "painful arc" from 60 to 120 degrees. If an injection of anesthetic under the acromion completely deadens the pain during this movement, it confirms the diagnosis of impingement syndrome. Physicians usually want to try conservative treatment for this condition before considering surgery (Wirth, Orfaly, and Rockwood 2001, 137).

Surgical treatment of impingement syndrome attempts to increase the subacromial space by means of *arthroscopic debridement* (removal of damaged tissue) and *acromioplasty* to reduce the size or shape of the acromion. During the arthroscopic operation, the subacromial bursa may be removed (Figure 10.33), especially if it's found to be grossly swollen and full of calcium deposits. Sometimes the acromioclavicular ligament and the outer end of the collarbone are also removed, in addition to any calcium deposits in the supraspinatus tendon (Figure 10.34).

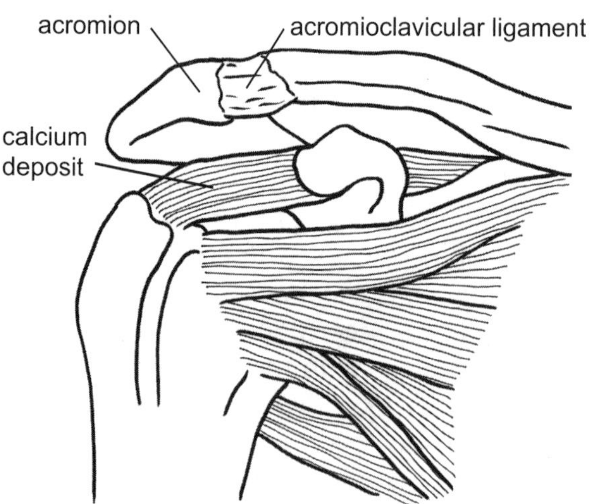

Figure 10.34 The site where calcium deposits may form in the supraspinatus tendon

Some surgeons believe that a hooked or abnormally shaped acromion (Figure 10.35) is a significant cause of impingement and also a major factor in rotator cuff tears (Sher 1999, 11-15). A mechanized burr is typically used to remove this "excess" bone from the undersurface of the acromion. *Acromionectomy*, or the removal of a significant portion of the acromion (Figure 10.36), is controversial, but some surgeons may choose to do it (Williams 1999, 93-98). In the past, some have advocated dispensing with the entire acromion, viewing it as a useless structure. More recently, the acromion has come to be seen as providing solid protection for the glenohumeral joint and helping to stabilize the shoulder during movements of the arm (Arroyo and Flatow 1999, 42).

Travell and Simons believe that impingement is usually caused by trigger points in the rotator muscles. Any disturbance in the balance of strength and functioning of these muscles allows the head of the humerus to ride up on the glenoid fossa, causing chronic compression of the bursa and supraspinatus tendon. This could result in the various kinds of

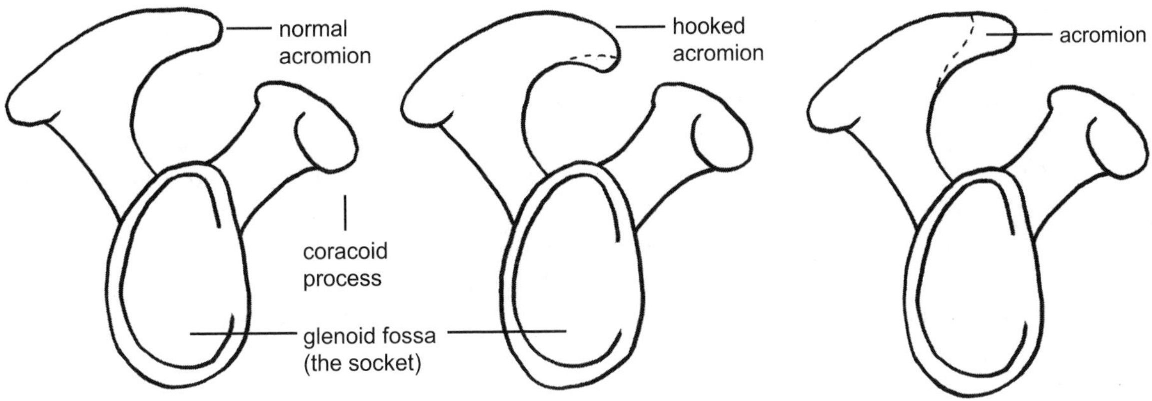

Figure 10.35 Side views of the shoulder socket. The hooked acromion on the right would be reshaped to resemble the normal one on the left.

Figure 10.36 Side view of the right shoulder socket showing removal of a large part of the acromion

deterioration that occur in the subacromial space. Release of the trigger points causing impingement could allow damaged tissue to heal on its own without resorting to surgery (Simons, Travell, and Simons 1999, 545-546).

Supraspinatus Tendinitis

Because of its importance in raising the arm, the supraspinatus tendon is at increased risk of damage from subacromial impingement. This topmost part of the rotator cuff is the place where most of the tears occur. Most people over sixty-five are believed to have degeneration and some degree of tearing in this tendon. *Supraspinatus tendinitis* is the pain, swelling, and fraying of the tendon preliminary to an actual tear (Cailliet 1991, 54).

With enough physical abuse from impingement, calcium deposits can form in the supraspinatus tendon and subacromial bursa, causing calcific tendinitis and subdeltoid bursitis. These "calcium boils" in a tendon or bursa can be aspirated or removed surgically (Cailliet 1991, 63-68). Trigger point therapy, however, could take away the abnormal compression and allow the area to heal naturally.

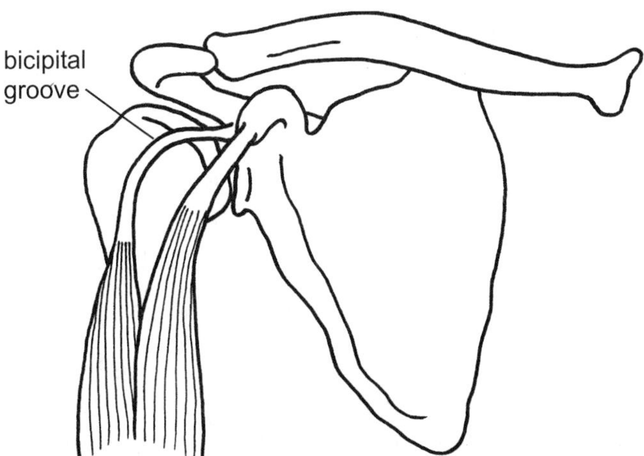

Figure 10.37 Front view of the right shoulder showing both biceps tendons. The tendon of the long head lies in the bicipital groove.

Bicipital Tendinitis

The tendon of the long head of the biceps lies in the bicipital groove in the front and top of the humeral head (Figure 10.37). The tendon needs to be free to slide up and down in this groove as the arm moves. Ligaments help keep the tendon in its groove, and synovial fluid keeps it lubricated. Strain, overuse, impingement, or damage to tissues surrounding the biceps tendon can restrict its movement, resulting in chronic pain and a diagnosis of *bicipital tendinitis*. However, deltoid and infraspinatus trigger points are actually the most common cause of pain and tenderness in this area. Of course, genuine injuries are possible.

Damage to the ligaments can allow the tendon to slip out of its groove. Also, age and overuse can erode the top of the humerus, effectively making the bicipital groove more shallow and allowing the bicipital tendon to pop out more easily (Cailliet 1991, 57). To explore this possibility, the examiner presses on the tendon while inwardly and outwardly rotating the arm. A positive test is an audible or palpable snap, along with pain (Cappel et al. 2001, 95-96). Under extreme strain or overuse, the biceps and its tendons are vulnerable to tearing, which requires skilled surgical repairs.

Rotator Cuff Injuries

Rotator cuff tears rarely occur in people younger than thirty, but 50 percent of people over forty with shoulder pain are believed to have some degree of tearing (Wirth, Orfaly, and Rockwood 2001, 107-108). But a tear in your rotator cuff may not be as disastrous as it sounds. An ultrasound study revealed that a torn rotator cuff can be present without pain or noticeable decrease in function. Among people over seventy with no symptoms, half had tears, and about 80 percent of the people over eighty had painless tears (Milgrom et al. 1995, 296-298). Since other muscles can compensate for any loss of function from a rotator cuff tear, surgery may not be an absolute requirement. The clear implication is that treatment should be based on symptoms, not on what an MRI shows.

Contributing causes of rotator cuff tears are aging, trauma, falls, dislocations, and fractures. Tendon tears generally occur more often in women and athletes, and genetics may play a role (Cailliet 1991, 95-96). As noted earlier, Travell and Simons believe that myofascial trigger points are the primary cause of impingement and the ultimate tearing of the rotator cuff.

The supraspinatus tendon is the part of the rotator cuff most often damaged by impingement by the head of the humerus. Compression of this tendon tends to cut off its circulation and undermine its ability to repair itself. Some physicians blame 95 percent of rotator cuff tears on subacromial compression and the ensuing loss of circulation in the area (Cailliet 1991, 59-60, 102). Excessive subacromial compression also keeps the tendon from moving freely under the acromion when you move your arm. This puts added strain on the tendon when the supraspinatus muscle contracts.

Degeneration of the supraspinatus tendon begins with tiny tears of individual superficial fibers, then progresses to a detectible partial tear, most often on the tendon's upper surface (Figure 10.38). Any remaining ability to raise or rotate your arm indicates only a partial tear, but ultimately an MRI or ultrasound must be used to determine whether a tear is partial or complete, or whether a tear actually exists. Since imaging is so costly, some physicians prefer to wait to see whether conservative treatment allows the tear to heal naturally. Studies show that nonoperative treatment is successful more than half the time, and one study showed a 92 percent success rate (Arroyo and Flatow 1999, 32-37).

Travell and Simons agree that partial tears in the rotator cuff can heal on their own, especially when aided by trigger point therapy to reduce stress on the subacromial area (Simons, Travell, and Simons 1999, 545). Surgical repair may be needed for complete tears in

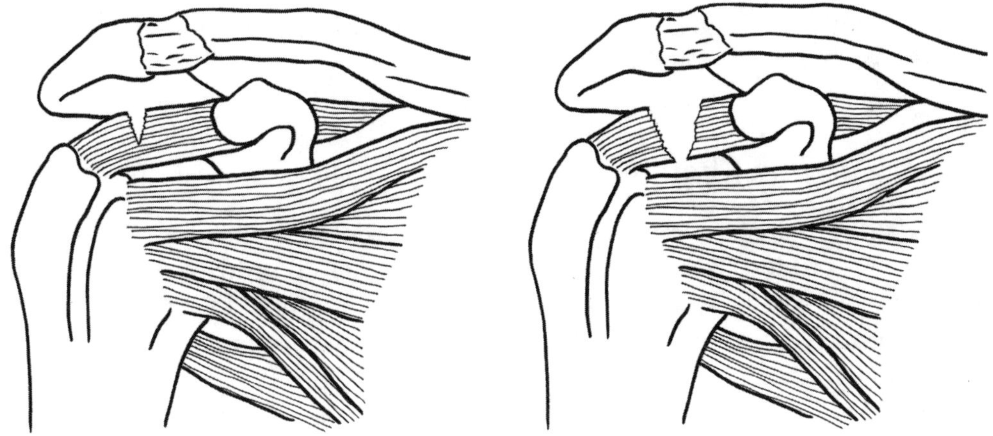

Figure 10.38 Partial and complete rotator cuff tears under the acromion in the supraspinatus tendon

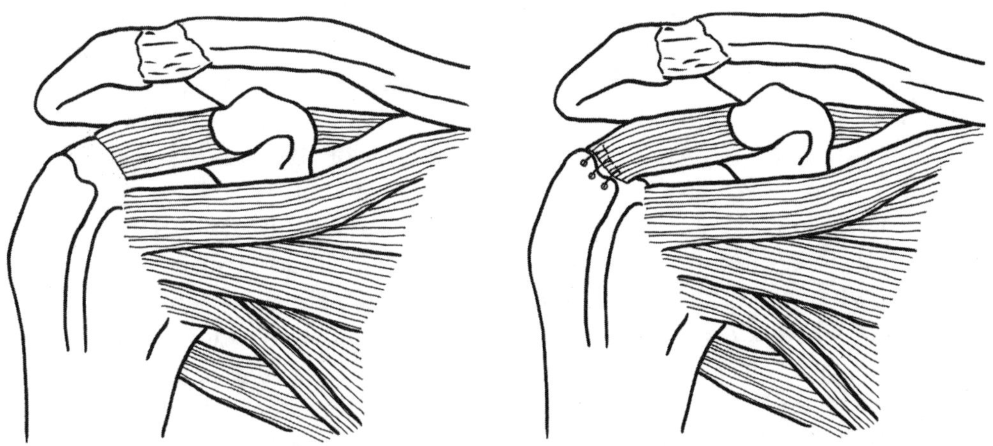

Figure 10.39 Repair of a complete tear in the supraspinatus tendon. The remnant is removed from the head of the humerus, then the tendon is trimmed and sutured to anchors embedded in the bone.

any of the rotator cuff tendons because normal muscle contraction retracts the torn tendon too far for self-healing (Figure 10.39).

There are two basic approaches to rotator cuff repair, arthroscopic surgery and open surgery. The arthroscopic method is used mainly for the supraspinatus tendon. Open surgery is usually reserved for the subscapularis and infraspinatus tendons. Since the deltoid covers all parts of the shoulder and must be cut and moved aside for open surgery, the advantage to arthroscopy is that detachment of the deltoid muscle can be avoided (Arroyo and Flatow 1999, 37-49).

The outcome of surgery depends almost exclusively on the ability of the surgeon. Surgical techniques are highly developed and well disseminated throughout the medical world, and if the surgeon is well-trained and experienced, the results are usually good. Things can go wrong, of course, with both arthroscopic and open surgery. The sutures can stretch or pull out, loose anchors in the humeral head can damage the joint, the deltoid muscle reattachment can tear loose, and nerves may be accidentally cut. Despite the risks, 80 percent of patients report relief of pain and improvement in function (Arroyo and Flatow 1999, 46-53). A partially torn tendon is usually strong six weeks after surgery, and a full tear requires three months. In both cases, a careful regimen of physical therapy is advisable to minimize the risk of frozen shoulder.

Arthritis of the Shoulder

Pain and stiffness in the ball-and-socket joint caused by arthritis can be the initiating factor in a frozen shoulder. Both osteoarthritis and rheumatoid arthritis normally take many months or years to develop, so pain from these causes comes on slowly and intermittently. You would expect to have signs of arthritis in other parts of your body long before you become afflicted with a frozen shoulder (Fehringer 2004, 119-121).

Glenohumeral arthritis of the shoulder causes destruction of joint cartilage, loss of joint space, decreased range of motion, tenderness to touch in the front and back of the joint, and bone-on-bone crepitus (grinding noises and sensations). There's usually no swelling in the joint and the pain is worst in the back of your shoulder. Initially, the cartilage that covers the humeral head first becomes degraded and rough (Figure 10.40), and eventually the cartilage is worn away and the bony surface of the humeral head is exposed. Thick growths called *osteophytes* (spurs) may develop around the bare surface. On an X-ray, this gives the humeral head the appearance of a balding head with a ring of hair, known as the *Friar Tuck sign*. A "goat beard" of spurs often forms on the undersurface of the humeral head. The glenoid socket may also wear down from abrasion (Fehringer 2004, 119-121).

Medication and surgery are the only options for the treatment of glenohumeral arthritis. Three surgical procedures are common. One option is to surgically remove some of the arthritic overgrowth and spurs with *arthroscopic synovectomy* and debridement. A second procedure, which is heavily promoted and possibly the most common, is joint replacement by *hemiarthroplasty* or *complete arthroplasty*. The third method is *glenohumeral arthrodesis*, or surgical fusion of the ball and socket. This extreme procedure is sometimes necessary if joint replacement fails due to loosening of prosthetic components and bone loss limits further reconstruction and implantation. Although full movement is no longer possible, fusion does allow limited use of the arm (Fehringer 2004, 121-124; Wirth, Orfaly, and Rockwood 2001, 118-120).

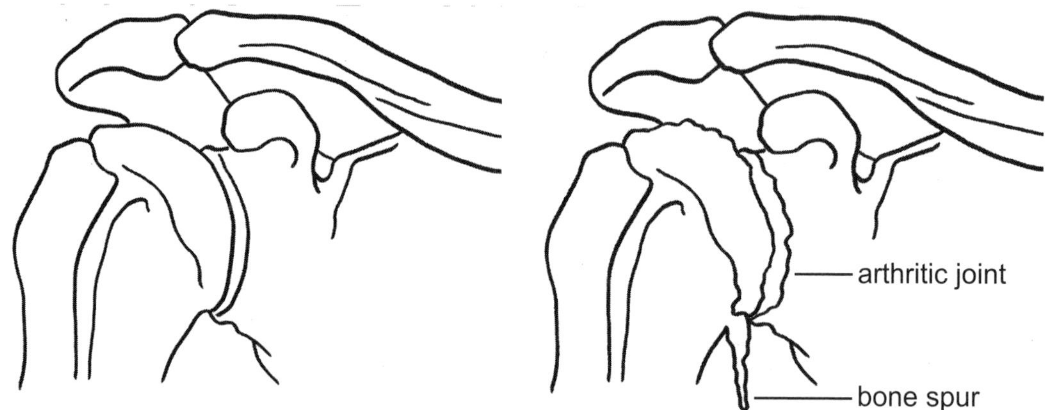

Figure 10.40 Front views of the right shoulder comparing a normal glenohumeral joint with a joint afflicted with arthritic degeneration

Shoulder Joint Replacement Surgery

Joint replacement surgery has undergone phenomenal development in recent years. The two primary methods in current use for the shoulder are *hemiarthroplasty*, replacement of just the humeral head (the ball), and *total arthroplasty*, replacement of both the ball and the socket. The prosthesis for the ball is long enough to extend down into the center of the humerus (Figure 10.41). When surgeons replace the ball, they must save the *tuberosities*, the bony outer part of the humeral head where the rotator cuff tendons attach (Figure 10.42). It's not possible to satisfactorily attach the muscles to the prosthetic ball, which is made of an alloy of steel. The implanted humeral prosthesis is secured with an adhesive cement (Figure 10.43). Reconstruction of the glenoid fossa or socket involves implanting a small plastic liner. Unfortunately, the prosthetic socket is subject to loosening because of the thinness of the glenoid bone it's attached to.

Even the best surgical outcome and the latest improvements in the hardware don't promise infinite durability and freedom from difficulties. The longevity of joint replacement is generally limited to about fifteen years if all goes well. Durability depends on the surgeon's experience and skills and on the quality and design of the prosthetic devices. The parts must be exactly the right size, the fit must be perfect, the muscles must be strong enough to keep the joint correctly articulated, and everything must be firmly anchored into solid bone.

After initially successful surgery, things can still go wrong. The prosthesis cement can loosen, and implanted parts can be damaged by overuse and excessive loads. Stiffness and pain can become worse than ever. When you read about the 80 or 90 percent success rate for these surgeries, you have to wonder about the other 10 or 20 percent that weren't successful. Occasionally, at the end of a long struggle with shoulder pain and multiple surgeries, the final solution has been fusion of the shoulder. Sometimes complete removal of the head of the humerus is necessary, leaving only the muscles and Dacron tape to hold the arm on and allow minimum function (Fehringer 2004, 122-123; Griggs et al. 1999, 358).

Despite the risks of a bad outcome, shoulder replacement surgery is a well-established medical procedure that seems to have helped many people escape debilitating pain and loss of function. A really good surgeon can accomplish everyday miracles. The question is, how do you find that really good surgeon? Remember what Ann Landers said about doctors, that half of them were in the bottom half of their class.

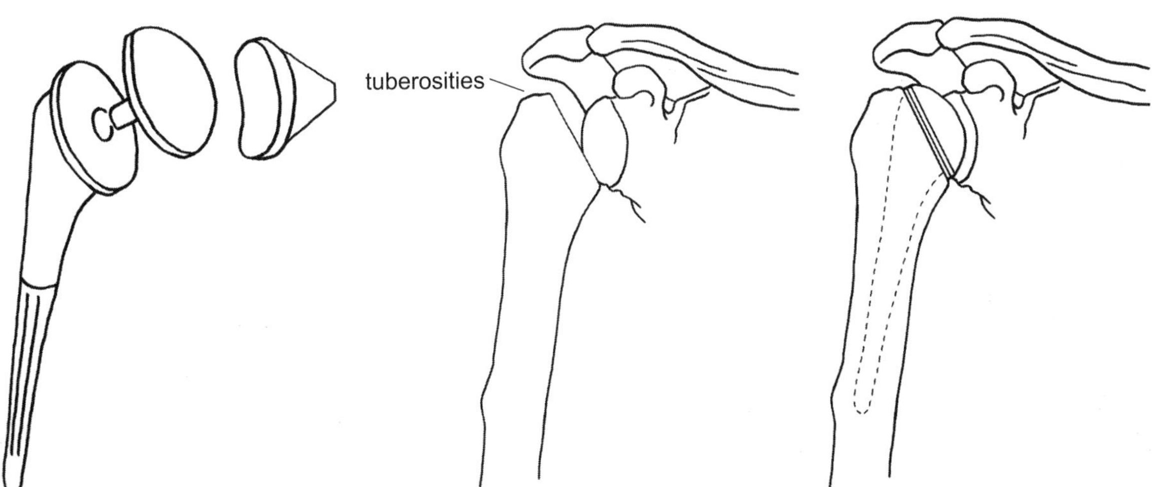

Figure 10.41 Prostheses for replacing the ball and socket

Figure 10.42 The defective head of the humerus is removed.

Figure 10.43 The humeral head prosthesis is cemented in place.

Trigger Points and Mainstream Medicine

Trigger points are a genuine medical phenomenon, and in most cases they're the fundamental cause of frozen shoulder. Doctors are on the front line in the war against pain, and yet most of them remain uninformed about this most important medical cause of myofascial pain and disability.

It's a disgrace to the medical profession that, all across this county, people who haven't been to medical school are successfully self-treating medical problems, including frozen shoulder, that baffle their doctors. Thousands of ordinary people have learned how to effectively treat their own myofascial pain with self-applied trigger point massage. Among health care professionals, who should be in the lead in developing and disseminating this therapy, it's mostly massage therapists and a few physical therapists who have mastered trigger point therapy, rarely the physicians.

Physicians in every specialty sorely need to become informed about trigger points and myofascial pain. Patients with problems ranging from knee pain and plantar fasciitis to headaches and frozen shoulder continue to suffer needlessly because their doctors are unable to cure them. And all the while, the cure is right at hand. Travell and Simons have worked out the solution to these problems and many others. Nevertheless, mainstream medicine goes on ignoring this wonderful opportunity to do better by their patients. With the investment of only a little bit of time, physicians could dramatically improve the practice of medicine and finally learn how to cure many of the kinds of pain that they still refer to as "enigmatic" or "idiopathic."

If you have any success in treating your own shoulder, by all means tell your doctor about it, particularly if your doctor's treatment failed to help you. You may get a cold reception, but it's worth a shot because some of them are ready for this information. Doctors have pain just like you do, and they can be just as exasperated and mystified by it as you have been. There may be doctors in your community who have shoulder pain, maybe even frozen shoulder, who might be delighted to know about this book. Be the bearer of good news. You may never hear about it, but you might make a real difference. A single physician who knows about trigger points can bring relief to hundreds, if not thousands, of people every year. That's something worth aiming at.

References

Acland, R. 1995. *Video Atlas of Human Anatomy.* Baltimore: Lippincott, Williams, and Wilkins.

American Physical Therapy Association. 2003. *Guide to Physical Therapist Practice.* 2nd edition, revised. Alexandria, VA: American Physical Therapy Association.

Apley, A. G., and L. Solomon. 1997. *Physical Examination in Orthopaedics.* London: Arnold Publishers.

Arroyo, J. S., and E. L. Flatow. 1999. Management of rotator cuff disease: Intact and repairable cuff. Chapter 2 in J. P. Iannotti and G. R. Williams (Eds.), *Disorders of the Shoulder: Diagnosis and Management*. Baltimore: Lippincott, Williams, and Wilkins.

Beyers, M., and P. Bonutti. 2004. Frozen shoulder. Chapter 11 in R. A. Donatelli (Ed.), *Physical Therapy of the Shoulder*. 4th edition. St. Louis: Churchill Livingstone.

Bochetta, A., F. Bernardi, M. Pedditzi, A. Loveselli, F. Velluzzi, E. Martino, et al. 1991. Thyroid abnormalities during lithium treatment. *Acta Psychiatrica Scandinavica* 83(3): 193-198.

Bonica, J. J., and A. E. Sola. 1990. Other painful disorders of the upper limb. Chapter 52 in J. J. Bonica, J. D. Loeser, C. R. Chapman, et al. (Eds.), *The Management of Pain*. 2nd edition. Philadelphia: Lea and Febiger.

Bork, B. E., T. M. Cook, J. C. Rosecrance, K. A. Engelhardt, M. E. Thomason, I. J. Wauford, et al. 1996. Work-related musculoskeletal disorders among physical therapists. *Physical Therapy* 76(8):827-835.

Bridgman, J. F. 1972. Periarthritis of the shoulder and diabetes mellitus. *Annals of the Rheumatic Diseases* 31(1):31-69.

Cailliet, R. 1991. *Shoulder Pain.* 3rd edition. Philadelphia: F. A. Davis Company.

Cantu, R. I., and A. J. Grodin. 1992. *Myofascial Manipulation: Theory and Clinical Application.* Gaithersburg, MD: Aspen Publishers.

Cappel, K., M. A. Clark, G. J. Davies, and T. S. Ellenbecker. 2001. Clinical examination of the shoulder. Chapter 5 in B. J. Tovin and B. H. Greenfield (Eds.), *Evaluation and Treatment of the Shoulder: An Integration of the Guide to Physical Therapist Practice.* Philadelphia: F. A. Davis Company.

Chaitow, L., and J. W. DeLany. 2000. *The Upper Body.* Vol. 1 of *Clinical Application of Neuromuscular Techniques.* London: Churchill Livingstone.

Codman, E. A. 1934. *The Shoulder.* Malabar, FL: Krieger Publishing Company.

Condon, S. M., and R. S. Hutton. 1987. Soleus muscle electromyographic activity and ankle dorsiflexion range of motion during four stretching procedures. *Physical Therapy* 67(1):24-30.

Cromie, J. E., V. J. Robertson, and M. O. Best. 2000. Work-related musculoskeletal disorders in physical therapists: Prevalence, severity, risks, and responses. *Physical Therapy* 80(4):336-351.

Cuomo, F. 1999. Management of rotator cuff disease: Intact and repairable cuff. Chapter 15 in J. P. Iannotti and G. R. Williams (Eds.), *Disorders of the Shoulder: Diagnosis and Management.* Baltimore: Lippincott, Williams, and Wilkins.

Danneskiold-Samoe, B., E. Christiansen, B. Lund, and R. B. Andersen. 1983. Regional muscle tension and pain ("fibrositis"): Effect of massage on myoglobin in plasma. *Scandinavian Journal of Rehabilitation Medicine* 15(1):17-20.

Davies, C. 2001. *The Trigger Point Therapy Workbook.* 1st edition. Oakland, CA: New Harbinger Publications.

———. 2004. *The Trigger Point Therapy Workbook.* 2nd edition. Oakland, CA: New Harbinger Publications.

Diercks, R. L., and M. Stevens. 2004. Gentle thawing of the frozen shoulder: A prospective study of supervised neglect versus intensive physical therapy in seventy-seven patients with frozen shoulder syndrome followed up for two years. *Journal of Shoulder and Elbow Surgery* 13(5):499-502.

Donatelli, R. A. 2004. Functional anatomy and mechanics. Chapter 2 in R. A. Donatelli (Ed.), *Physical Therapy of the Shoulder.* 4th edition. St. Louis: Churchill Livingstone.

Donatelli, R. A., J. P. Irwin, M. A. Johanson, and B. Z. Gonzalez-King. 2004. Differential soft tissue diagnosis. Chapter 4 in R. A. Donatelli (Ed.), *Physical Therapy of the Shoulder.* 4th edition. St. Louis: Churchill Livingstone.

Edeiken, J., and C. C. Wolferth. 1936. Persistent pain in the shoulder region following myocardial infarction. *American Journal of Medical Sciences* 191:201-210.

Edgelow, P. I. 2004. Neurovascular consequences of cumulative trauma disorders affecting the thoracic outlet: A patient-centered treatment approach. Chapter 7 in R. A. Donatelli (Ed.), *Physical Therapy of the Shoulder.* 4th edition. St. Louis: Churchill Livingstone.

Fassbender, H. G., and K. Wegner. 1973. Morphologie und Pathogenese des Weichteilrheumatismus. *Zeitung Rheumaforsch* 33:355-374.

Fehringer, E. V. 2004. Arthritis, arthroplasty, and arthrodesis of the shoulder. Chapter 26 in D. E. Brown and R. D. Neumann (Eds.), *Orthopedic Secrets.* 3rd edition. Philadelphia: Hanley and Belfus.

Fishbain, D. S., M. Goldberg, B. R. Meagher, R. Steele, and H. Rosomoff. 1986. Male and female chronic pain patients categorized by DSM-III psychiatric diagnostic criteria. *Pain* 26(2):181-197.

Fishman, S., and L. Berger. 2000. *The War on Pain.* New York: HarperCollins.

Foster, D. W., and A. H. Rubenstein. 1980. Hypoglycemia, insulinoma, and other hormone-secreting tumors of the pancreas. Chapter 340 in K. J. Isselbacher, R. D. Adams, E. Braunwald, R. G. Petersdorf, and J. B. Martin (Eds.), *Harrison's Principles of Internal Medicine.* 9th edition. New York: McGraw-Hill.

Fouri, L. J. 1991. The scapulocostal syndrome. *South African Medical Journal* 79(12):721-724.

Freiwald, J., M. Engelhardt, M. Jager, and A. Gnewuch. 1998a. Stretching—possibilities and limits. *Therapeutische Umschau* 55(4):267-272.

Freiwald, J., M. Engelhardt, M. Jager, A. Gnewuch, I. Reuter, K. Wiemann, et al. 1998b. Stretching—do current explanatory models suffice? *Sportverletz Sportschaden* 12(2):54-59.

Froriep, R. 1843. *Ein beitrag zur pathologie und therapie des rheumatismus.* Weimar.

Fulton, J. F. 1947. *Howell's Textbook of Physiology.* 15th edition. Philadelphia: W. B. Saunders Company.

Furia, J. P., and D. E. Brown. 2004. Subacromial syndromes. Chapter 22 in D. E. Brown and R. D. Neumann (Eds.), *Orthopedic Secrets.* 3rd edition. Philadelphia: Hanley and Belfus.

Gerber, C. 1999. Massive rotator cuff tears. Chapter 3 in J. P. Iannotti and G. R. Williams (Eds.), *Disorders of the Shoulder: Diagnosis and Management.* Baltimore: Lippincott, Williams, and Wilkins.

Gerwin, R. D. 1995. A study of 96 subjects examined both for fibromyalgia and myofascial pain. *Journal of Musculoskeletal Pain* 3(Suppl. 1):121.

Gray, J. C. 2004. Visceral referred pain to the shoulder. Chapter 13 in R. A. Donatelli (Ed.), *Physical Therapy of the Shoulder.* 4th edition. St. Louis: Churchill Livingstone.

Griggs, S. M., G. B. Holloway, G. R. Williams Jr., and J. P. Iannotti. 1999. Treatment of locked anterior and posterior dislocations of the shoulder. Chapter 13 in J. P. Iannotti and G. R. Williams (Eds.), *Disorders of the Shoulder: Diagnosis and Management.* Baltimore: Lippincott, Williams, and Wilkins.

Hackett, R. M. 2000. Personal communication.

Hagberg, M. 1981. Electromyographic signs of shoulder muscular fatigue in two elevated arm positions. *American Journal of Physical Medicine* 60(3):111-121.

Hawley, R. J., Jr. 1996. Thoracic outlet syndrome (a reply) [Letter]. *Muscle and Nerve* 19(2):254-256.

Holder, N. L., H. A. Clark, J. M. DiBlasio, C. L. Hughes, J. W. Scherpf, L. Harding, et al. 1999. Cause, prevalence, and response to occupational musculoskeletal injuries reported by physical therapists and physical therapist assistants. *Physical Therapy* 79(7):642-652.

Hsieh, L. L., C. H. Kuo, M. F. Yen, and T. H. Chen. 2004. A randomized controlled clinical trial for low back pain treated by acupressure and physical therapy. *Preventive Medicine* 39(1):168-176.

Irwin, S. 2004. The guide to practice. Chapter 1 in R. A. Donatelli (Ed.), *Physical Therapy of the Shoulder*. 4th edition. St. Louis: Churchill Livingstone.

Jacob, S. W., C. A. Francone, and W. J. Lossow. 1978. *Structure and Function in Man.* Philadelphia: W. B. Saunders.

Jamison, J. R. 1994. Chiropractic holism: Accessing the placebo effect. *Journal of Manipulative and Physiological Therapeutics* 17(5):339-345.

Jensen, K. S., and C. A. Rockwood. 1997. Delayed primary repair of a kyrogenic spinal accessory nerve injury: A case report. *Clinical Orthopaedics and Related Research* 336:116-121.

Jonsson, B., and M. Hagberg. 1974. The effect of different working heights on the deltoid muscle: A preliminary methodological study. *Scandinavian Journal of Rehabilitation Medicine. Supplement* 3:26-32.

Kelley, W. N. 1980. Gout and other disorders of purine metabolism. Chapter 92 in K. J. Isselbacher, R. D. Adams, E. Braunwald, R. G. Petersdorf, and J. B. Martin (Eds.), *Harrison's Principles of Internal Medicine.* 9th edition. New York: McGraw-Hill.

Kendal, F. P., E. K. McCreary, and P. G. Provance. 1993. *Muscles: Testing and Function.* 4th edition. Baltimore: Lippincott, Williams, and Wilkins.

Kordella, T. 2002. Frozen shoulder and diabetes. *Diabetes Forecast* 55(8):60-64.

Kozin, S. H. 1999. Injuries of the brachial plexus. Chapter 30 in J. P. Iannotti and G. R. Williams (Eds.), *Disorders of the Shoulder: Diagnosis and Management.* Baltimore: Lippincott, Williams, and Wilkins.

Lange, M. 1931. *Die Muskelhaerten (Myogelosen); Ihre Entstehung und Heilung.* Munich: J. G. Lehmanns.

Lehtinen, J. T., J. C. Macy, E. Cassinelli, and J. J. Warner. 2004. The painful scapulothoracic articulation: Surgical management. *Clinical Orthopaedics and Related Research* 423:99-105.

Lewit, K. 1979. The needle effect in the relief of myofascial pain. *Pain* 6(1):83-90.

———. 1991. *Manipulative Therapy in Rehabilitation of the Locomotor System.* 2nd edition. Oxford: Butterworth Heinemann.

Long, C. 1956. Myofascial pain syndromes, part III: Some syndromes of the trunk and thigh. *Henry Ford Hospital Medical Bulletin* 4:22-28, 102-106.

McAtee, R. E. 1993. *Facilitated Stretching.* Champaign, IL: Human Kinetics Publishing.

McMahon, T. J., and R. A. Donatelli. 2004. Manual therapy techniques. Chapter 14 in R. A. Donatelli (Ed.), *Physical Therapy of the Shoulder.* 4th edition. St. Louis: Churchill Livingstone.

Melzack, R., E. J. Fox, and D. M. Stillwell. 1977. Trigger points and acupuncture points for pain: Correlations and implications. *Pain* 3(1):3-23.

Mense, S., and D. G. Simons. 2001. *Muscle Pain: Understanding Its Nature, Diagnosis, and Treatment.* Baltimore: Lippincott, Williams, and Wilkins.

Milgrom, C., M. Schaffler, S. Gilbert, and M. van Holsbeeck. 1995. Rotator-cuff changes in asymptomatic adults: The effect of age, hand dominance, and gender. *Journal of Bone and Joint Surgery. British Volume* 77(2):296-298.

Moore, M. A., and R. S. Hutton. 1980. Electromyographic investigation of muscle stretching techniques. *Medicine and Science in Sports and Exercise* 12(5):322-329.

Netter, F. 1989. *Atlas of Human Anatomy.* East Hanover, NJ: Novartis.

Nicholson, G. P. 2003. Arthroscopic capsular release for stiff shoulders: Effect of etiology on outcomes. *Arthroscopy* 19(1):40-49.

Ormandy, L. 1994. Scapulocostal syndrome. 1994. *Virginia Medical Quarterly* 121(2):105-108.

Pinci, J. 2005. Personal communication.

Prudden, B. 1980. *Pain Erasure: The Bonnie Prudden Way.* New York: M. Evans and Co.

Reynolds, M. D. 1981. Myofascial trigger point syndromes in the practice of rheumatology. *Archives of Physical Medicine and Rehabilitation* 62(3):111-114.

Rubin, D. 1981. Myofascial trigger point syndromes: An approach to management. *Archives of Physical Medicine Rehabilitation* 62(3):107-110.

Shah, J. P., T. M. Phillips, J. V. Danoff, and L. H. Gerber. 2005. An in vivo microanalytical technique for measuring the local biochemical milieu of human skeletal muscle. *Journal of Applied Physiology* 99(5):1977-84. Epub 2005 Jul 21.

Sher, J. S. 1999. Anatomy, biomechanics, and pathophysiology of rotator cuff disease. Chapter 1 in J. P. Iannotti and G. R. Williams (Eds.), *Disorders of the Shoulder: Diagnosis and Management.* Baltimore: Lippincott, Williams, and Wilkins.

Sherman, R. A. 1980. Published treatments of phantom limb pain. *American Journal of Physical Medicine and Rehabilitation* 59(5):232-244.

Simons, D. G. 1960. *Man High.* Garden City, NY: Doubleday and Company.

———. 2001. Personal communication.

———. 2005. Personal communication.

———. 2006. Personal communication.

Simons, D. G., J. G. Travell, and L. S. Simons. 1992. *Myofascial Pain and Dysfunction: The Trigger Point Manual.* Vol. 1, 2nd edition. Baltimore: Lippincott, Williams, and Wilkins.

———. 1999. *Myofascial Pain and Dysfunction: The Trigger Point Manual.* 2nd edition. Baltimore: Lippincott, Williams, and Wilkins.

Smith, L. K., E. L. Weiss, and L. D. Lehmkuhl. 1983. *Brunnstrom's Clinical Kinesiology.* 4th edition. Philadelphia: F. A. Davis Company.

———. 1996. *Brunnstrom's Clinical Kinesiology.* 5th edition. Philadelphia: F. A. Davis Company.

Snider, R. K., D. S. Brodke, J. S. Fischgrund, H. N. Herkowitz, A. M. Levine, J. T. Lovitt, et al. 2001. Spine. Section 8 in W. B. Green (Ed.), *Essentials of Musculoskeletal Care.* 2nd edition. Rosemont, IL: American Academy of Orthopaedic Surgeons.

Sola, A. E., and R. L. Williams. 1956. Myofascial pain syndromes. *Journal of Neurology* 6(2):91-95.

Sonkin, L. S. 1994. Myofascial pain due to metabolic disorders: Diagnosis and treatment. Chapter 3 in E. S. Rachlin (Ed.), *Myofascial Pain and Fibromyalgia.* St Louis: Mosby-Yearbook.

Spring, H., W. Schneider, and T. Tritschler. 1997. Stretching. *Orthopade* 26(11):981-986.

Sullivan, M. S., J. M. Kues, and T. P. Mayhew. 1996. Treatment categories for low back pain: A methodological approach. *Journal of Orthopaedic and Sports Physical Therapy* 24(6):359-364.

Thomas, C. L. (Ed.). 1997. *Taber's Cyclopedic Medical Dictionary.* Philadelphia: F. A. Davis Company.

Travell, J. G. 1968. *Office Hours: Day and Night.* New York: World Publishing Company.

Travell, J., S. Rinzler, and M. Herman. 1942. Pain and disability in the shoulder and arm: Treatment by intramuscular infiltration with procaine hydrochloride. *Journal of the American Medical Association* 120:417-422.

Travell, J., and D. Simons. 1983. *Myofascial Pain and Dysfunction: The Trigger Point Manual.* Vol. 1. Baltimore: Williams and Wilkins.

Upledger, J. E. 1997. *Your Inner Physician and You: CranioSacral Therapy and SomatoEmotional Release.* Berkeley: North Atlantic Books.

Williams, G. R., Jr. 1999. Complications of rotator cuff surgery. Chapter 4 in J. P. Iannotti and G. R. Williams (Eds.), *Disorders of the Shoulder: Diagnosis and Management.* Baltimore: Lippincott, Williams, and Wilkins.

Wirth, M. A., R. M. Orfaly, and C. A. Rockwood Jr. 2001. Shoulder. Section 2 in W. B. Greene (Ed.), *Essentials of Musculoskeletal Care.* 2nd edition. Rosemont, IL: American Academy of Orthopaedic Surgeons.

Wolfe, S. M., L. D. Sasich, R. E. Hope, and Public Citizen's Health Research Group. 2005. *Worst Pills, Best Pills: A Consumer's Guide to Avoiding Drug-Induced Death or Illness.* New York: Pocket Books.

Index

A

B

E

F

G

H

I

J

K

L

M

N

S

T

U

V

W

X

Y

Z

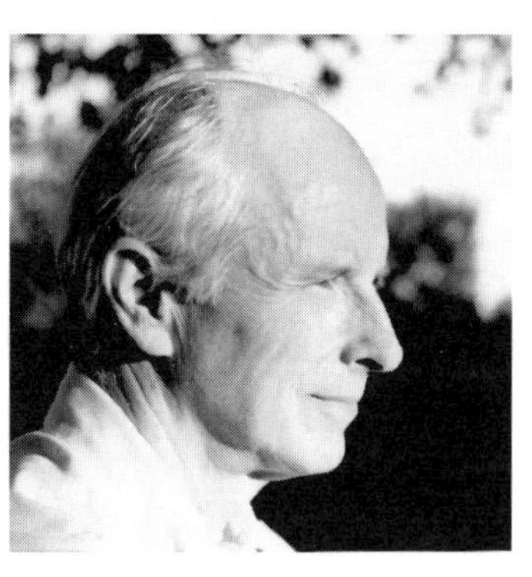

Clair Davies, NCTMB (Nationally Certified in Therapeutic Massage and Bodywork), is a member of the American Massage Therapy Association, and a graduate of the Utah College of Massage Therapy. He specializes in trigger point massage for the treatment of pain.

Mr. Davies's interest in massage began when he successfully self-treated a frozen shoulder with trigger point massage. Inspired by the experience, he began an intensive private study of trigger points and referred pain. He subsequently retired from a thriving piano service business to become a professional massage therapist. After tuning pianos for nearly forty years, he now "tunes" people.

From his home base in Lexington, Kentucky, Mr. Davies travels extensively with his daughter Amber, leading workshops and seminars on the self-treatment and clinical treatment of pain using trigger point massage. For information about dates, locations, and workshop format, go to www.TriggerPointBook.com.

break free from pain with the power of

TRIGGER POINT THERAPY

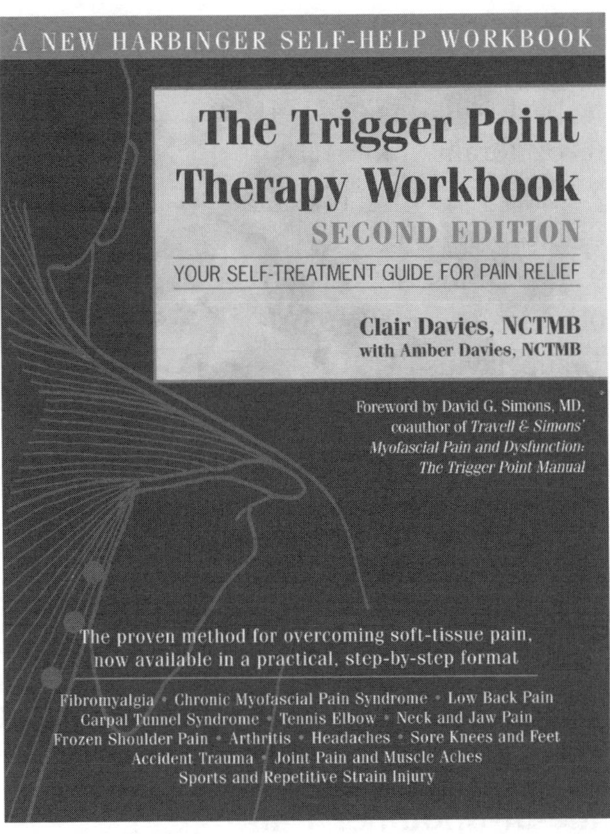

US $19.95 • ISBN-10:1572243759
ISBN-13: 9781572243750 • New Harbinger Item 3759

Millions have found relief from pain through the application of trigger point therapy. This gentle massage technique alleviates blockages in soft tissue that can cause pain and even refer it to other parts of the body.

This workbook teaches you exactly what to look for when assessing trigger points. Its clear illustrations show you where on the body trigger points form and the corresponding areas to which they refer pain. Then, in step-by-step detail, it explains how you can treat these sources of chronic pain with effective massage techniques you can do by yourself at any time.

If you've struggled with chronic pain without finding relief, you owe it to yourself to learn and practice the techniques in this workbook—easy, reliable skills that offer real, lasting relief without drugs, doctor visits, and costly medical bills.

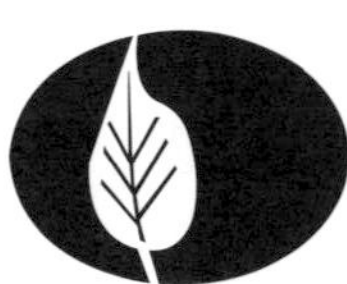

available from **newharbinger**publications
and fine booksellers everywhere

To order, call toll free **1-800-748-6273**
or visit our online bookstore at **www.newharbinger.com**

(V, MC, AMEX • prices subject to change without notice)

Trigger Point Guide: Shoulder Pain

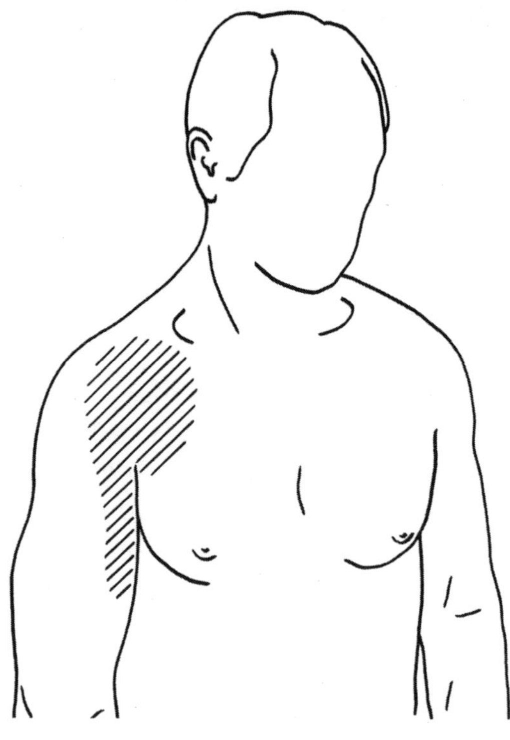

Front-of-Shoulder Pain

1. infraspinatus (135)
2. anterior deltoid (149)
3. scalenes (116)
4. supraspinatus (131)
5. pectoralis major (174)
6. pectoralis minor (180)
7. subscapularis (124)
8. biceps (189)
9. latissimus dorsi (143)
10. coracobrachiallis (197)
11. subclavius (179)
12. brachialis (191)

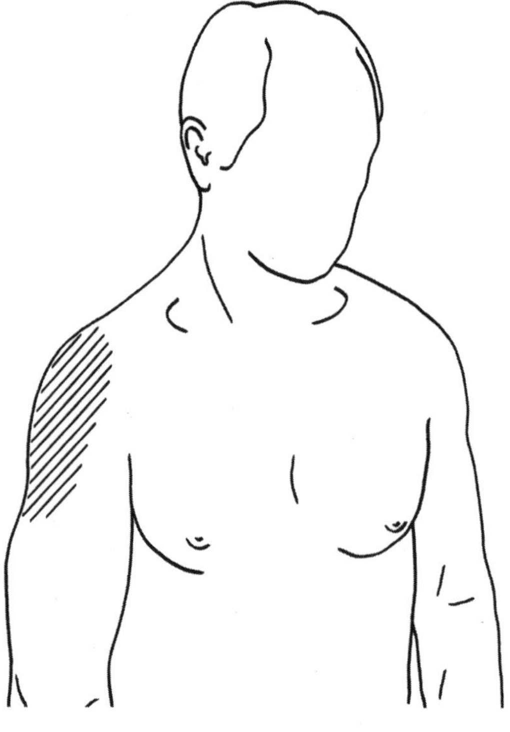

Side-of-Shoulder Pain

1. infraspinatus (135)
2. scalenes (116)
3. middle deltoid (149)
4. supraspinatus (131)